LIVER METASTASIS

DEVELOPMENTS IN ONCOLOGY

LIVER METASTASIS
Basic aspects, detection and management

edited by

Cornelis J.H. VAN DE VELDE, MD, PhD
Department of Surgery, University Hospital
Leiden, The Netherlands

Paul H. SUGARBAKER, MD
Colorectal Cancer Section, National Institutes of Health
Bethesda, Maryland, USA

1984 **MARTINUS NIJHOFF PUBLISHERS**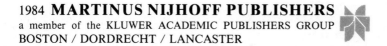
a member of the KLUWER ACADEMIC PUBLISHERS GROUP
BOSTON / DORDRECHT / LANCASTER

Distributors

for the United States and Canada: Kluwer Academic Publishers, 190 Old Derby Street, Hingham, MA 02043, USA
for the UK and Ireland: Kluwer Academic Publishers, MTP Press Limited, Falcon House, Queen Square, Lancaster LA1 1RN, England
for all other countries: Kluwer Academic Publishers Group, Distribution Center, P.O. Box 322, 3300 AH Dordrecht, The Netherlands

Library of Congress Cataloging in Publication Data

```
Liver metastasis.

    (Developments in oncology)
    Proceedings of the International Congress on Hepatic
Metastasis, sponsored by the University Hospital of
Leiden and the National Cancer Institute, USA; and
held in Leiden, May 24-26, 1984.
    Includes bibliographies and index.
    1. Liver--Cancer--Congresses.  2. Metastasis--
Congresses.  3. Cancer invasiveness--Congresses.
I. Velde, Cornelis J. H. van de.  II. Sugarbaker,
Paul H.  III. International Congress on Hepatic
Metastasis.  (1984 : Leiden, Netherlands)
IV. Academisch Ziekenhuis (Leiden, Netherlands)
V. National Cancer Institute (U.S.)  VI. Series.
RC280.L5L585  1984     616.99'436       84-16621
ISBN 0-89838-684-5
```

ISBN 0-89838-684-5 (this volume)

Book Information

This publication is based upon a Boerhaave course organized by the Faculty of Medicine, University of Leiden, The Netherlands in co-operation with the National Cancer Institute, Bethesda, Maryland, USA

PREFACE

B. CADY

   Hepatic metastases present one of the major therapeutic challenges
of cancer patient management, for it is the destruction of vital organ
function that makes cancer fatal, not local tumor growth. The process
of tumor cell dislodgement from the primary cancer, their spread through
the lymphatic and hematogenous channels, their lodgement in distant
sites, and their subsequent progressive growth tax our comprehension
and frustrate our therapies. The proceedings of this International
Congress on Hepatic Metastasis address these aspects of metastases to
the liver, and predominatly focus on metastatic colon cancer because
of its frequency, its prominent hepatic only pattern of spread, and
enticing preliminary data about prevention and control of small subsets of the afflicted population. Predictably, the "false technologies"
of Dr. Lewis Thomas that involve surgical, radiotherapeutic and chemotherapeutic attack on these metastases after elaborate diagnostic
studies take precedence because of the clinical imperatives of sick
patients. This is displayed in the preponderance of papers and interest in various diagnostic scanning techniques by means of radioisotopes, radiographically useful dyes, biochemical markers, interest
in developing accurate staging systems to categorize patients for
therapeutic comparisons, and interest in elaborate, and expensive,
technology to increase the effectiveness of chemotherapeutic agents
that are of limited benefit with simple intravenous administration.
   Behind this clinical enthusiasm, however, lies the research to
develop the "true technology," in Thomas' words, that will prevent
such clinical catastrophies as hepatic metastases. The first inkling
of such a "true technology" in liver cancer is the recent development
of hepatitis immunization to prevent subsequent hepatoma in endemic
areas of the world. In hepatic metastases from colon cancer, several

recent articles correlate worse prognosis and by inference liver metastases, with perioperative transfusions which induce a state of
relative immunosuppression. Such immunological modulation is beneficial in renal transplantation where immunosuppression is necessary,
but is harmful in colon cancer treatment where presumably immune com-
petence needs to be intact to prevent implantation and growth of disseminated cancer cells. The immunological aspects will clearly be
difficult to unravel as judged by the failure of non-specific immuno-
stimulation trials with BCG or MER to improve survival. However, with
such clues as seed may come harvests of research data. The work of
Fidler in defining the hepatic "homing" and lodgement of hematogenously
disseminated cells in animal models and of Folkman in defining angio-
neogenesis as a requirement for progressive growth after metastatic
cell lodgement have opened up whole new fields of investigation.

International conferences, as presented in this book, are enormous
stimuli for further work. New directions have been suggested in the
spirited discussion of the workshop sessions of the Congress. Besides
the necessity for laboratory research work, agreements need to be
achieved for a staging system, diagnostic criteria for response,
conditions for conducting and evaluating clinical trials in chemotherapy, both systemic and regional, and proper criteria for surgical
resection of metastases and even for hepatic transplantation. International meetings to review progress in hepatic metastases on a regular
basis and to set out new goals in biological understanding and therapeutic achievement are needed. Hopefully this book will be the first
in a series that measure progress in one of the most devastating complications of cancer.

CONTENTS

Treatment of Liver Metastases

New Treatment Modalities

Surgical Techniques in the Management of Hepatic Metastases

LIST OF MAJOR CONTRIBUTORS

K.R. Aigner, M.D., Department of Surgery, Justus-Liebig-University, Klinikstrasse 29, 63 Giessen, West Germany.

B. Cady, M.D., Professor of Surgery at the New England Deaconess Hospital, Harvard Medical School, Boston, MA 02115, U.S.A.

F.J. Cleton, M.D., Ph.D., Professor of Medicine, Chairman Dept. of Clinical Oncology, University Hospital, 2333 AA Leiden, The Netherlands.

F.C.A. den Hartog Jager, M.D., Dept. of Medicine, The Netherlands Cancer Institute, Plesmanlaan 121, 1066 CX Amsterdam, The Netherlands.

J. Jeekel, M.D., Ph.D. Professor of Surgery, Chairman Dept. of Surgery, University Hospital Dijkzigt, Dr. Molewaterplein 40, 3015 GD Rotterdam, The Netherlands.

M.M. Kemeny, M.D., Senior Surgeon, City of Hope National Medical Center, 1500 East Duarte Road, Duarte 91010, California, U.S.A.

T.J.A. Kuijpers, M.D., Dept. of Diagnostic Radiology, University Hospital, 2333 AA Leiden, The Netherlands.

J.P. Mach, M.D., Professor at the Ludwig Institute for Cancer Research, Ch. des Boveresses, CH-1066 Epalinges, Lausanne, Switzerland.

V.R. McCready, M.D., Consultant Nuclear Medicine, The Royal Marsden Hospital, Downs Road, Stutton, Surrey SM2 5PT, Great Britain.

J.G. McVie, M.D., Dept. of Medicine, The Netherlands Cancer Institute, Plesmanlaan 121, 1066 CX Amsterdam, The Netherlands.

D.L. Miller, M.D., Senior Radiologist, Dept. of Diagnostic Radiology, National Institutes of Health , Bethesda, Maryland 20205, U.S.A.

G.L. Nicolson, Professor of Cancer Research, Head of the Dept. of Tumor Biology, M.D. Anderson Hospital, 6723 Bertner Avenue, Houston, Texas 77030, U.S.A.

A.T. van Oosterom, M.D., Ph.D., Dept. of Clinical Oncology, University Hospital, Rijnsburgerweg 10, 2333 AA Leiden, The Netherlands.

E.K.J. Pauwels, Ph.D., Dept. of Diagnostic Radiology, Div. of Nuclear Medicine, University Hospital, Rijnsburgerweg 10, 2333 AA Leiden, The Netherlands.

J. Pettavel, M.D., Professor at the Dept. of Surgery, 10, Avenue de la Gare, Lausanne University Hospitals, 1003 Lausanne, Switzerland.

E. Roos, Ph.D., Division of Cell Biology, The Netherlands Cancer Institute, Plesmanlaan 121, 1066 CX Amsterdam, The Netherlands.

D.J. Ruiter, M.D., Ph.D., Dept. of Pathology, Faculty of Medicine, University of Leiden, 2333 AA Leiden, The Netherlands.

Ph.S. Schein,M.D., F.R.C.P., Research and Development, Smith Kline and French Laboratories, 1500 Spring Garden Street, P.O. Box 7929, Philadelphia 19101, U.S.A.

P.D. Schneider, M.D., F.A.C.S., Senior Surgeon, National Institutes of Health, Bethesda, Maryland 20205, U.S.A.

T.H. Shawker, Chief Ultrasound Dept., Diagnostic Radiology, National Institutes of Health, Bethesda, Maryland 20205, U.S.A.

J.L. Speyer, M.D. Dept. of Medicine, New York University Medical Center, 550 First Avenue, New.York, N.Y. 10016, U.S.A.

P.H. Sugarbaker, M.D., Head of the Colorectal Cancer Section, Surgery Branch, National Institutes of Healt, Bethesda, Maryland 20205, U.S.A.

G.J. van Steenis, M.D., Dept. of Clinical Cytology, University Hospital, Rijnsburgerweg 10, 2333 AA Leiden, The Netherlands.

I. Taylor, M.D., Ch.M., F.R.C.S., Professor of Surgery, University Surgical Unit of the Southampton General Hospital, 'F'-level, Tremona Road, Southampton SO1 6HU, Great Britain.

P. Thomas, M.D., Ph.D., Professor of Radiotherapy, Dept. of Clinical Oncology, University Hospital, Rijnsburgerweg 10, 2333 AA Leiden, The Netherlands.

C.H.N. Veenhof, M.D., Ph.D., Division of Medical Oncology, Dept. of Medicine, Medical Center of the University of Amsterdam, Meibergdreef 9, 1105 AZ Amsterdam, The Netherlands.

C.J.H. van de Velde, M.D., Ph.D. Dept. of Surgery, University Hospital, Rijnsburgerweg 10, 2333 AA Leiden, The Netherlands

M. Vermess, M.D., Associate Chief Radiologist, Dept. of Diagnostic Radiology, National Institutes of Health, Bethesda, Maryland 20205, U.S.A.

S. Wallace, M.D., Professor of Radiology, Dept. of Diagnostic Radiology, M.D. Anderson Hospital and Tumor Institute, 6723 Bertner Avenue, Houston, Texas 77030, U.S.A.

A.W. Wolkoff, M.D., Associate Professor of Medicine, Liver Research Center, Albert Einstein College of Medicine, 1300 Morris Park, Bronx, New York, N.Y. 10461, U.S.A.

C.B. Wood, F.R.C.S., Senior Lecturer in Surgery, Royal Postgraduate Medical School, Hammersmith Hospital, Ducane Road, London W12 OHS, Great Britain.

A. Zwaveling, M.D., Ph.D., Professor of Surgery, Chairman Dept. of Surgery, University Hospital, Rijnsburgerweg 10, 2333 AA Leiden, The Netherlands.

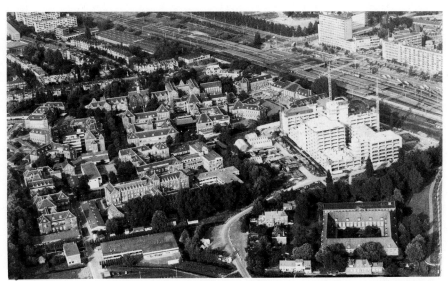

FIGURE 1
Aireal view of the University Hospital Leiden, The Netherlands

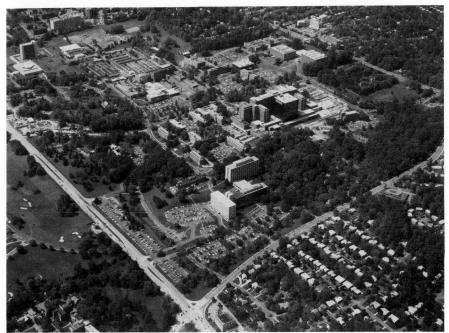

FIGURE 2
Aireal view of the National Institutes of Health, Bethesda, Maryland,
U.S.A.

INTRODUCTION

Paul H. Sugarbaker and Cornelis J.H. van de Velde
June, 1984, Leiden, The Netherlands

This book was derived from information shared by international authorities on hepatic metastases. Thirty formal presentations and 55 abstracts presentations were made at a meeting sponsored by the University Hospital of Leiden and the National Cancer Institute, USA on May 24-26, 1984. At Leiden in a warm and beautiful few days of Holland springtime, 270 participants and guest faculty organized their thoughts about this timely clinical problem. The speakers were gathered nearly equally from the United States, Great Britain and the Continent. The participants were also an international group; more than half the participants were from outside of Holland and over 40 were from the United States, Not only was this an international group, but all the relevant disciplines within the practice of medicine were represented. In a roll call of the audience, we noted that about half of the participants were surgeons, a large number were medical oncologists; but, radiation therapists, radiologists, full-time researchers, pathologists and biomedical engineers were present. Our aim in bringing this international and multidisciplinary group together was to share the best basic science and medical science ideas. With the co-ordinating activities of the Boerhaave Committee a pleasant, educational and stimulating experience was reported by all.

Speakers and program participants alike agreed that now was an appropriate time to review and then look ahead into the topic of hepatic metastases. For the first time, useful and reproducible animal models are available for studying tumor spread to the liver. New and more refined means by which to deliver chemotherapy to the liver have been introduced. Hepatic artery infusion, portal venous infusion and intraperitoneal chemotherapy make possible higher and more sustained levels of drug than have ever been possible in the past.

Also, totally implanted intravascular access devices allow improved quality of life for patients despite intensive treatments. Innovative techniques, such as regional liver perfusion, need exploration and assessment as a treatment tool. Ways of looking at the liver and accurately assessing tumor growth are also becoming available. Monoclonal antibodies, liver contrast agents, nuclear magnetic resonance and single photon emission tomography may allow tumor within the liver be be accurately localized, serially assessed and targeted for effective treatments.

Some problems areas needing further development to speed progess in managing hepatic metastases were identiefied. More effective drugs to treat gastrointestinal malignancies would greatly improve our ability to treat hepatic metastases. A more reliable small animal model for the study of hepatic metastases would allow the evaluation of potential treatment plans prior to their institution in human controlled trials. With the successful use of an animal model the optimal route of drug administration, the optimal combination of surgical, medical and radiation therapy treatments could be addressed. Questions about prevention of hepatic metastases could be answered within several years in an active laboratory. If these problems must be solved in the human experiment, controlled trials will consume several decades before the required information is gathered. Hypotheses regarding the tumor biology of hepatic metastases need to be formulated, tested, reformulated and used to enlarge our knowledge of this problem.

During the first two days of the Symposium, a large amount of basic science and clinical data was presented and discussed. In this book, as at the Symposium, the first session was devoted to the basic aspects of liver metastases. The outstanding work of Nicolson (Houston, U.S.A.) and Roos (Amsterdam) captured the interest of the entire group. In the second session clinical tests by which liver metastases can be detected and serially evaluated were presented. Exciting new liver imaging methods using EOE-13 were reported by Miller (Bethesda, U.S.A.). The thoughtful presentation by Pettavel (Lausanne, Switzerland) regarding the necessity of a standardized staging system for hepatic tumors seemed to be universally accepted by the group. In the session devoted to the treatment of liver metastases, presentations reviewed the surgical, chemotherapeutic and radiation therapy treatments that have

been employed in the near and distant past. As presented by Wallace
(Houston, U.S.A.), Taylor (Southampton, England, Van Oosterom (Leiden),
Speyer (New York) and Schneider (Bethesda, U.S.A.) new and innovative
means of delivering the few effective chemotherapeutic agents are
emerging. The continued evaluation of intraportal, intrahepatic artery
and intraperitoneal chemotherapy will be an exciting new chapter in
the medical history that will be written over the next few years.
In the session on new treatment modalities the speakers reviewed current
clinical research protocols that point to a significant interaction of
basic sciences and clinical medicine.

In order to round out the conference, a video session was held in
the evening. Technical Aspects of the Surgical Management of Hepatic
Metastases were presented and make-up this section of the book. A review of new commercially available devices was presented and evaluated
by Symposium participants. It was emphasized throughout this meeting
that progress in patient care can only be made if the techniques utilized can be completed with an acceptable morbidity and mortality.

On the third and final day of the Symposium, many of the participants gathered together for a Workshop. This Workshop was designed to
take the great volume of information presented at the Symposium and
synthesize it into a working body of knowledge and techniques. The
proceedings of this Workshop make-up the final chapter of this book.
The staging of hepatic metastases and response criteria in clinical
trials were openly discussed by both speakers and participants. The
group tried to reach a consensus that would make international collaboration possible in the future. Also, a consensus regarding surgical
attempts to potentially curatively resect hepatic metastases was formulated. Finally the group tried to agree upon a matrix for a protocol
in which promising new treatments modalities could be reliably tested.
Although the specific treatments to be employed were not discussed,
the eligibility requirements, exclusions, monitoring, endpoints, and
statistical analysis of hepatic metastases in controlled clinical
trials were presented. The collected thoughts and ideas of this general
discussion constitute the final chapter of this book. The worth of this
book may be found, the authors hope, in its use in planning future
research, managing patients and conducting clinical trials.

BASIC ASPECTS OF LIVER METASTASIS

INVASION OF THE LIVER BY TUMOR CELLS

E. ROOS

1. INTRODUCTION

The liver is one of the most frequently affected target sites for disseminating cancer. It is seeded by tumors draining into the portal circulation and in addition often by blood cell neoplasms. Particularly certain lymphomas have a striking propensity to infiltrate extensively and spread diffusely through liver tissue. To investigate the mechanisms underlying these processes, we examined interactions of tumor cells with cells in the intact liver using electron microscopy and reproduced the observed phenomena in cultures of isolated liver cells. The in vitro models were then employed to study the molecular details. In this paper I will present an overview of our observations in vivo and in vitro, and results of our studies aimed at the identification of cell surface molecules, both on liver cells and tumor cells, involved in their interaction. Furthermore, recent findings concerning the invasive and metastatic behaviour of T-cell hybridomas will be described. This study was based on our observation that activated normal T-lymphocytes infiltrate hepatocyte monolayers similarly as metastatic lymphoma cells. We established that this property of activated T-cells could be conferred upon non-invasive T-lymphoma cells by cell fusion. The resulting T-cell hybridomas were not only highly invasive, but also highly metastatic.

Since these observations have been or will be extensively described elsewhere (1-13), the results will be summarized only briefly.

2. METHODS

2.1. The intact liver

Details of the methods have been described elsewhere, as indicated. Briefly, murine tumor cells that had been grown in ascites or in suspension culture were injected into a small mesenteric vein of syngeneic mice (1,2) or were added to the medium that perfused an isolated mouse liver (3,4). In case of lymphoma cells, liver metastases could also be obtained after injection into the tail vein (1). Livers were fixed at various intervals, and sections were examined in the electron microscope.

2.2. Liver cell cultures

Liver cells were dispersed by collagenase perfusion and hepatocytes were isolated by low speed centrifugation (5). From the supernatant endothelial cells were purified using density gradient centrifugation and unit gravity sedimentation (6). We used mainly cells isolated from rat livers, but observations were similar with syngeneic murine liver cells. The cells were seeded in serum-free medium in serum-coated wells. Tumor cells were added to endothelial cell cultures 1 h later, and the cultures were fixed after an additional 1-4 hours. Hepatocytes were washed after 2 h and cultured overnight in serum-containing medium. The supernatant was removed, tumor cells were added in serum-free medium and the cultures fixed at intervals up to 24 h. During processing for EM, cells were detached while in propylene oxide and embedded as a pellet of culture fragments (5). Interactions were quantified by counting cells in sections through these pellets using the light or electron microscope (7).

2.3. Antibodies

Polyclonal antibodies were raised in rabbits against rat liver plasma membrane subfractions or against intact tumor cells, and monovalent Fab fragments were prepared as described (8). Monoclonal antibodies were prepared using spleen cells of mice injected several times with rat liver plasma membranes.

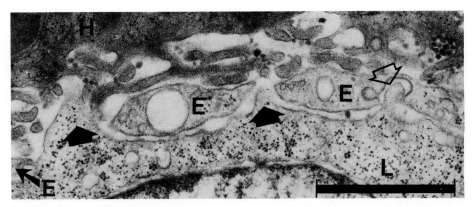

Fig.1. A metastatic lymphoma cell (L) in a liver sinusoid extends protrusions into (open arrow) and through (black arrows) an endothelial cell (E); H: hepatocyte; bar: 1 µm.

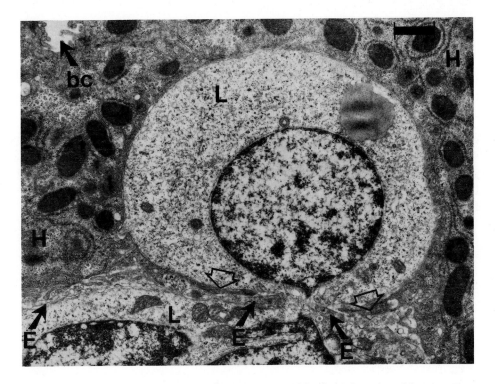

Fig.2. Extravasation of a lymphoma cell (L) in the liver. Note passage through a narrow gap in the endothelium (E), close association between membranes of lymphoma cell and hepatocytes (H), particularly the encirclement by thin rims of hepatocytic cytoplasm (open arrows); bc: bile canaliculus; bar: 1 µm.

Hybridomas were prepared as soon as Fab fragments prepared from their sera inhibited interactions. Hybridoma supernatants were screened for effect on adhesion of ^{51}Cr-labeled tumor cells to hepatocyte cultures in microtiter wells. Rats were immunized with tumor cells and as soon as inhibitory antibodies were present in serum, (rat x mouse) hybridomas were prepared. In case of lymphoma cells, the ^{51}Cr-adhesion test could not be used because of high and variable background levels. Supernatants were therefore prescreened by ELISA for reaction with invasive lymphoma cell lines but not with lymphoma cells that did not adhere to hepatocytes and did not absorb inhibitory antibodies from the rabbit antisera. Hybridomas were then grown to larger numbers and inhibition by antibodies tested using microscopy as described above.

2.4. T-cell hybridomas

Murine spleen T-cells were activated with ConA or in a mixed lymphocyte culture with irradiated allogeneic spleen cells. T-cell hybridomas were prepared by fusion of non-invasive BW5147 T-lymphoma cells with either activated or non-stimulated T-cells. BW cells are sensitive to HAT and normal T-cells do not survive in culture, so T-cell hybridomas were selected in HAT-medium.

3. RESULTS
3.1. The intact liver

3.1.1. Lymphoma cells. Within a few hours after arrest in the liver, many cells of highly metastatic lymphomas infil-trated the blood vessel wall and the underlying hepatocyte layer. Many protrusions were extended that induced gaps within, and not between, endothelial cells (Fig. 1). Some of these swelled and invaginated hepatocytes (Fig. 2). Thus, the cell was gradually displaced to an extravascular location (Fig. 3). The association between hepatocyte and tumor cell surface was strikingly close, the hepatocyte often seemingly engulfing the tumor cell (Fig. 2). Lymphoma cells injected into the tail vein were first arrested in the lungs, and arrived in the liver with a delay of 2 days.

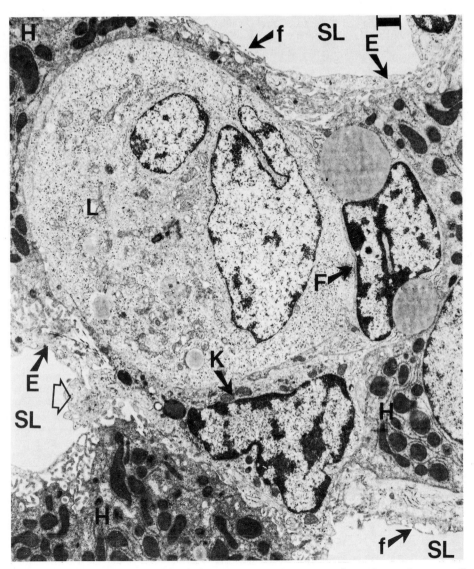

Fig.3. A lymphoma cell (L), in an extravascular location, a few hours after intraportal injection. The lymphoma cell is easily recognized because of its highly irregular nucleus and in addition intracisternal virus particles (not visible at this magnification). Note surrounding blood vessels (SL: sinusoidal lumen), sinusoidal endothelial cells with typical fenestrations (f; compare with figs. 5&6), a liver macrophage or Kupffer cell (K), partly protruding into the sinusoid (open arrow), and hepatic fat cell (F); H: hepatocyte; bar: 1 μm.

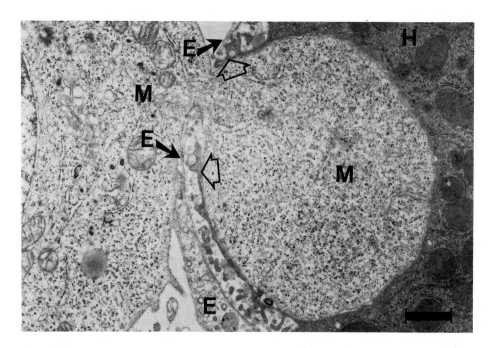

Fig.4. Extravasation of a mammary carcinoma cell (M) in the liver a few hours after intraportal injection. Note small gap in the endothelium (E), close association with hepatocyte (H), particularly encirclement by thin rims of hepatocytic cytoplasm (open arrows). Bar: 1 μm.

There they rapidly infiltrated, in striking difference with the absence of infiltration in the lungs (1). The highly invasive lymphoma cells gave rapidly rise to considerably enlarged, diffusely infiltrated livers.

3.1.2. Mammary carcinoma cells. The morphology of infiltration by TA3 mammary tumor cells was similar to that of lymphoma cells (Fig. 4). However, only a small percentage, less than 0.1%, were observed in an advanced stage of infiltration, in accordance with the relatively small number of isolated metastatic nodules obtained in vivo (4).

3.2. Liver cell cultures

3.2.1. Endothelial cells. Metastatic lymphoma cells adhered to hepatic endothelial cells (Fig. 5). In the presence of rat serum, the latter cells even tended to engulf the lymphoma cells

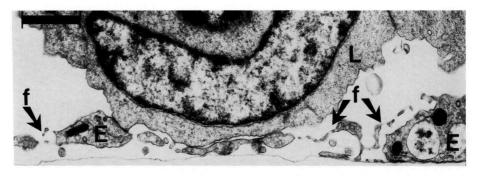

Fig.5. A lymphoma cell (L) adhering to a freshly isolated liver endothelial cell (E) in vitro. Note fenestrations (f). Bar: 1 μm.

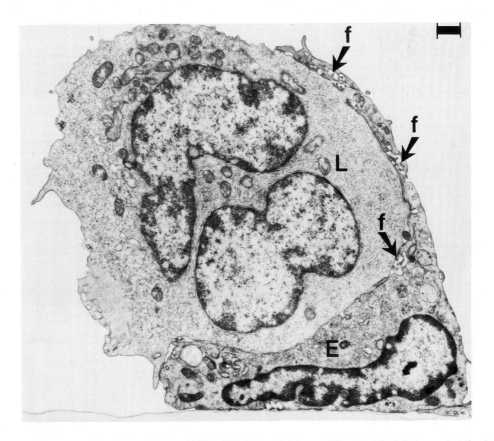

Fig.6. A lymphoma cell (L) adhering to, and partially encircled by a sinusoidal liver endothelial cell in vitro, in the presence of 5% rat serum. Note fenestrations (f). Bar: 1 μm.

(Fig. 6), an indication for strong interaction. The reason for this effect of rat serum is not known. In contrast, non-metastatic leukemia cells, and also TA3 mammary tumor cells did not adhere to endothelial cells. These results are described more extensively in (6).

3.2.2. Hepatocytes. Both metastatic lymphoma and mammary carcinoma cells adhered to hepatocyte monolayers. The lymphoma cells rapidly infiltrated between, and accumulated under the hepatocytes (Fig. 7). After a few hours the monolayer was diffusely infiltrated (Fig. 8), comparable to what can be observed in vivo. Non-metastatic lymphoma cells did not interact with hepatocytes. Mammary carcinoma cells also intruded, but in a different manner: The cells invaginated hepatocytes, not necessarily at a hepatocyte boundary, and thus "sunk" into the monolayer. A minority of cells exhibited this behaviour and it was relatively slow (5). The morphological differences indicated different mechanisms for mammary tumor as compared to lymphoma cells. This was affirmed by the observation that invagination by mammary, but not lymphoid tumor cells was greatly enhanced by microtubule-disrupting drugs (7). Also adhesion per sé was differently affected: inhibition in case of lymphoid cells but no effect with mammary tumor cells (7). The same was true for certain other drugs (9). Thus, adhesion mechanisms were apparently different. Indeed, we found that adhesion was mediated by distinct surface molecules, as described below.

3.3. Effect of antibodies

3.3.1. Polyclonal antibodies. Monovalent Fab-fragments of polyclonal antibodies raised against liver plasma membranes affected adhesion and infiltration of both lymphoid and mammary tumor cell types. Antibodies against preparations enriched in membranes facing the blood vessel inhibited adhesion, but distinct antisera had different effects on the two cell types, indicating that different hepatocyte surface molecules were involved (9). Antibodies against contiguous face plasma membranes inhibited infiltration of lymphoid cells, in addition to adhesion per sé. Apparently a distinct hepatocyte surface molecule is involved

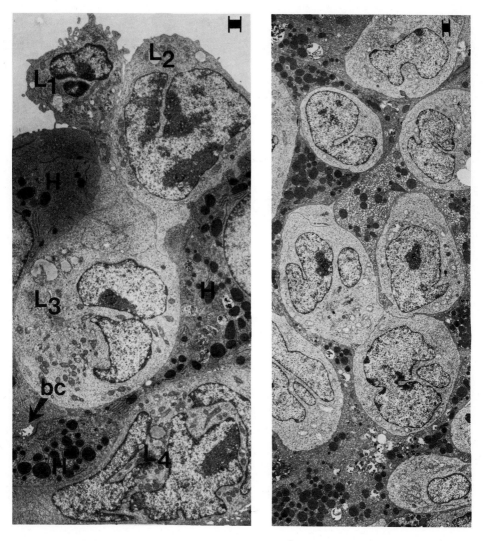

Fig.7.(Left). A hepatocyte (H) culture _in vitro_, infiltrated by lymphoma cells. Two lymphoma cells ($\overline{L_1 \& L_2}$) are moving between hepatocytes, another (L_3) is located within the culture. Finally, many lymphoma cells accumulate between hepatocytes and substrate (L_4). Note reconstituted bile canaliculus (bc). Bar: 1 µm.

Fig.8.(Right). A hepatocyte culture, infiltrated by lymphoma cells. The section was cut parallel to the substrate. This pattern of diffusely spread cells is quite comparable to what can be seen _in vivo_. Bar: 1 µm.

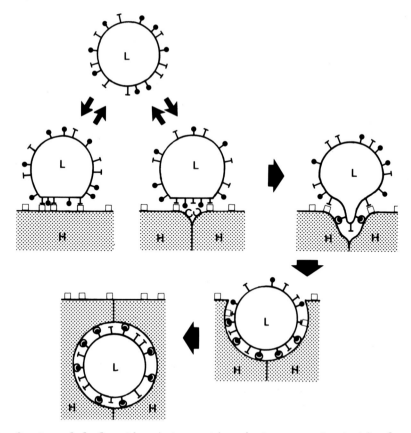

Fig.9. A model for the interaction between metastatic lymphoma cells (L) and hepatocytes (H), based on the effects of antisera raised against liver plasma mambrane subfractions and against lymphoma cells. The cells reversibly adhere to an adhesion molecule (□) located at the exposed surface of hepatocytes, but infiltrate at a boundary between two hepatocytes after adhesion to a second adhesion molecule (U), located at the contiguous surface. The latter interaction induces invagination of hepatocytes.

in the infiltration step (8). A model based on these findings is depicted in Fig. 9. Antibodies raised against the tumor cells inhibited adhesion of the appropriate cell type, but not of the other, again indicative for distinct surface molecules. Finally, also anti-endothelial cell antibodies were inhibitory. Although not yet clearly established, our results suggest that one molecule, which is present on both endothelial cells and hepatocytes,mediates adhesion of lymphoid cells. The model

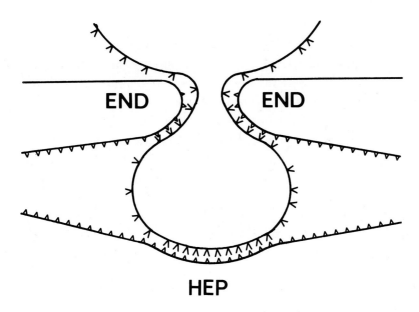

Fig.10. A model for extravasation of lymphoma cells. They adhere to an adhesion molecule on endothelial cells, that is supposed to be located predominantly on the extravascular surface. Thus, the lymphoma cell is provided with anchorage sites which facilitate extravasation. Next, the lymphoma cell adheres to hepatocytes. We have indications, but no definite evidence that the involved hepatocyte molecule may be the same as the one on the endothelial cell.

Table 1. Distinct cellular adhesion molecules (CAM) involved in interaction between tumor cells and liver cells

CAM	Expressed on	Mediating adhesion to
Lh-CAM	Lymphoma cells	Hepatocytes
Mh-CAM	Mammary tumor cells	Hepatocytes
Hl-CAM	Hepatocytes	Lymphoma cells
Hm-CAM	Hepatocytes	Mammary tumor cells
El-CAM	Endothelial cells	Lymphoma cells

Note: Hl-CAM may be identical to El-CAM (see fig. 10)

depicted in Fig. 10 illustrates how this molecule might stimulate extravasation of lymphoid cells.

The different adhesion molecules for the existence of which evidence was obtained using polyclonal antibodies, are summarized in Table 1.

3.3.2. <u>Monoclonal antibodies</u>. Presently we are preparing monoclonal antibodies against the involved adhesion molecules. So far, antibodies directed against Hm-CAM and Lh-CAM (see Table 1) were obtained. The latter have not yet been characterized. The former are two IgM antibodies, designated OPAR-1 and -2, that inhibited adhesion of mammary tumor cells, and also of prostate carcinoma and hepatoma cells, to hepatocytes. Adhesion of lymphoma and melanoma cells was not affected. An immunoblot of SDS-PAGE-separated liver plasma membrane proteins showed bands at molecular weights of approx. 140 and 110 kDa (10).

Immuno-EM on frozen liver sections revealed that the antigen was abundantly present at the sinusoidal surface of hepatocytes. It was also localized between hepatocytes and on Kupffer cells, but not on hepatic fat cells and, interestingly, not on hepatic sinusoidal endothelial cells, to which mammary tumor cells do not to adhere (see 3.2.1.). Immunohistochemistry on a section through a whole neonatal rat indicated that the antigen was not localized in other major metastatic target sites. Surprisingly, it was found in a fibrillar form in the skin (10). This tissue distribution and the molecular weight are reminiscent of procollagen. The possibility that Hm-CAM is identical to procollagen is being investigated.

3.4. T-cell hybridomas

3.4.1. <u>Activated T-lymphocytes</u>. We discovered that activated non-neoplastic T-lymphocytes heavily infiltrated hepatocyte cultures, in contrast to unstimulated spleen T-cells (11). T-cells activated by allogeneic cells <u>in vitro</u> and <u>in vivo</u>, or by concanavalin A, exhibited this property. Also spleen T-cells from mice that had been injected intraperitoneally with allogeneic cells were invasive. The same was true for human cytotoxic T-cell lines (unpublished).

3.4.2. <u>Fusion in vivo</u>. De Baetselier et al. (12) recently established that BW5147 lymphoma cells could give rise to highly metastatic variants <u>in vivo</u>, apparently by spontaneous fusion with normal host T-lymphocytes. We established that these variants were invasive in hepatocyte cultures, whereas the parental cell line was not. This led us to the assumption that the metastatic variants had acquired their invasive potential from the host fusion partner, which presumably had been an activated T-cell.

3.4.3. Fusion in vitro. If the above notion is correct, it should be possible to generate highly metastatic T-cell lymphomas by fusion between BW5147 cells and activated T-cells; and possibly non-invasive hybridomas by fusion with non-stimulated T-cells. For such fusions we used T-cells activated in 5-day mixed lymphocyte cultures (MLC), in which the irradiated stimulator cells were derived from Balb/c ($H2^d$) mice, and the respon-

Table 2. Invasiveness of T-cell hybridomas

Fusion	Mouse	Source[1]	Cell lines	Invasive
2	AKR	MLC	2	2/2
3	CBA	MLC	4	4/4
4	AKR	MLC	4	4/4
5	AKR	Spl	3	1/3
6	CBA	MLC	12	12/12
7	CBA	Spl	13	13/13

[1]Source of lymphocytes: MLC: mixed lymphocyte culture; Spl: (unstimulated) spleen

der cells either from AKR (syngeneic to BW5147) or CBA mice. Alternatively we used T-cell-enriched unstimulated spleen cells also either from AKR or CBA. These mice are H2-compatible ($H2^k$) but on a different genetic background, including the Thy.1 T-cell marker (Thy.1.1 in AKR and Thy.1.2 in CBA). Thus, the cell lines obtained after fusion with CBA cells could unequivocally be shown to be derived from fusion because of their expression of both Thy.1.1 and Thy.1.2. Being syngeneic to AKR mice was the advantage of AKR x BW hybridomas. Indeed, CBA x BW hybridomas were rejected in both CBA and AKR mice, so that in vivo studies in either strain were impossible.

As shown in Table 2, all MLC-derived T-cells gave rise to invasive hybridomas. Indeed, many cell lines were even more

invasive than several of the highly metastatic T-cell lymphomas
we used in our previous studies (13). One of the hybridomas lost
invasiveness within a few weeks in culture, and from others we
obtained non-invasive variants by cloning, including an interesting variant, which readily adhered to but hardly infiltrated
the hepatocyte monolayer.

In one fusion experiment with non-stimulated spleen cells
three cell lines arose, of which two were non-invasive (TAS5,
see Table 2). In another case, however, all the obtained cell
lines were invasive (TCS7, Table 2). This result might be explained by assuming that in the latter experiment the spleen
contained activated T-cells which are generally known to be
better fusers and thus were probably selected by the fusion
process.

After tail vein injection into AKR mice, three invasive cell
lines tested so far gave rise to wide-spread metastasis, whereas three non-invasive cell lines, the one that had lost invasiveness in culture and two lines derived from unstimulated spleen
cells, did not form metastases. Affected organs were liver,
kidneys, ovaria, spleen and sometimes mesentery or thymus. The
liver was always enlarged, often more than three-fold, and
diffusely infiltrated throughout (13).

4. DISCUSSION
4.1. In vitro models.

To investigate the mechanisms underlying invasive processes
in the liver, our approach has been to start with the study of
phenomena in the intact liver, and subsequently to reproduce
observations in vitro using the same tumor cells and freshly
isolated liver cells. This approach ensures that processes
relevant for the in vivo situation are studied, yet provides
for the convenience of in vitro experimentation that should
enable an analysis at the molecular level.

4.2. Surface molecules

Using antibodies against tumor and liver cells that inhibited
their mutual interaction, several cell surface components were

shown to be involved. Lymphoid and epithelial tumor cells employed different adhesion molecules that interact with distinct hepatocyte components. The one component identified so far, Hm-CAM (see Table 1), was distinct from hepatocyte adhesion molecules described by others (14-18). Furthermore, its tissue distribution as established by immunohistochemistry, is such that it can only play a role in metastasis to the liver, but not to other organs. These results point to considerable specificity in interactions between tumor cells and normal cells, and are compatible with the notion that organ-preferent metastasis may sometimes be due to lack or presence of adhesion molecules necessary to invade particular organs. On the other hand, specificity may be limited in certain cases, e.g. in the lungs, since it was recently found that a tumor component mediating adhesion during formation of lung metastases (19), is expressed by several distinct tumor cell types (20).

4.3. Steps in invasion

Invasion of tumor cells into a target tissue is a complex multi-step process. The cells interact with the endothelium, and adhere to and pass through basement membrane. Next, the cells adhere to parenchymal cells and finally they invade between them. Particularly, the interaction with basement membrane is considered important in other tissues (21-23). However, a basement membrane is virtually absent in liver, so this step can be ignored.

In contrast to metastatic lymphoma cells, mammary tumor cells did not adhere to liver endothelial cells, yet they were 100% efficiently arrested in the liver (4), indicating that arrest is due to sieving rather than to endothelial adhesiveness. Whereas metastatic lymphoma cells adhered to liver endothelial cells, non-metastatic lymphoma cells did not, suggesting that this type of interaction contributes to invasiveness. If so, it is not likely that the involved adhesion molecule is predominantly localized at the luminal side of the endothelium, because that would tend to lock the cells inside the vessel. Localization at the extravascular side, as depicted in Fig. 10, is perhaps more likely because in that case the molecule would provide for extravascular anchorage and thus promote extravasation. In this context it is striking that mammary tumor cells readily extend small protrusions through the endothelium in vivo (4), comparable to the lymphoma cells (3), but that they very rarely proceed beyond this stage. Thus, the absence of an appropriate adhesion molecule for these cells at the endothelium may be an important factor determining their relatively low colonization potential.

In case of lymphoma cells, our results indicate that two different hepatocyte surface molecules mediate two subsequent steps, the interaction with the sinusoidal hepatocyte surface and the intrusion between contiguous surfaces (see Fig. 9). This again adds to the complexity of the process. Hopefully, the recent isolation of a T-cell hybridoma variant which adheres to but does not infiltrate between hepatocytes will help us to dissect the mechanisms involved.

4.4. Normal versus neoplastic lymphoid cells

Invasiveness is a normal property of several haematopoietic cell types at certain stages of maturation. The fact that certain lymphoid tumors are hardly invasive in contrast to the extraordinary invasiveness of others, suggested to us that the latter lymphomas might be arrested at maturation stages in which invasiveness is normally constitutively expressed. This notion was supported by our observation that activation of T-lymphocytes rendered them invasive in hepatocyte cultures. Our results with T-cell hybridomas show that this normal property can be conferred onto relatively benign lymphoma cells, resulting in very highly malignant tumors. Thus, activated T-cells should perhaps be regarded as "semi-malignant", because they express a property of malignant cells, invasiveness, but lack infinite growth. However, when infinite growth is introduced by fusion with a lymphoma cell, the normal T-cell's invasiveness leads to highly malignant behaviour.

4.5. T-cell hybridomas as research tool

T-cell hybridomas might become an important tool for metastasis research, because they can easily be generated, are very highly invasive, and metastasize widely after tail vein injection. In addition, within cloned cell lines variants arise which lack one or more important properties, probably due to chromosome loss. This, and the availability of closely related, but non-invasive T-cell hybridomas, should facilitate comparative studies and should enable the dissection of the multiple factors involved in this complex phenomenon. Finally, the close correlation between invasiveness and metastatic capacity observed with these cells lends credit to the notion that invasiveness is a property of major importance for metastasis formation.

ACKNOWLEDGEMENTS

Part of the results described were obtained by Drs O.P. Middelkoop and J. Calafat. Contributions were made by Drs K.P. Dingemans (University of Amsterdam), P. de Baetselier (Free University, Brussels, Belgium), A. Tulp and M.J. Sukart. Expert technical assistance was provided by I.V. Van de Pavert, P. Van Bavel, A. Korving-Peters, H. Janssen, M.G. Barnhoorn and M.A.A. Van der Kraan, and secretaial assistence by G.G.H. Meyerink. The critical support of Drs C.A. Feltkamp and D.A.M. Mesland is gratefully acknowledged. Part of the work was made possible by grant NKI 80-6 from the KWF-Netherlands Cancer Foundation.

REFERENCES

1. Dingemans KP. 1973. Behaviour of intravenously injected lymlymphoma cells. A morphologic study. J Natl Cancer Inst 51, 1883-1895.
2. Dingemans KP. 1974. Invasion of liver tissue by blood-borne mammary carcinoma cells. J Natl Cancer Inst 53, 1813-1824.
3. Roos E, Dingemans KP, Van de Pavert IV, Van den Bergh Weerman M. 1977. Invasion of lymphosarcoma cells into the perfused mouse liver. J Natl Cancer Inst 58, 399-407.
4. Roos E, Dingemans KP, Van de Pavert IV, Van den Bergh Weerman M. 1978. Mammary carcinoma cells in mouse liver: Infiltration of liver tissue and interaction with Kupffer cells. Br J Cancer 38, 88-99.
5. Roos E, Van de Pavert IV, Middelkoop OP. 1981. Infiltration of tumour cells into cultures of isolated hepatocytes. J Cell Science 47, 385-397.
6. Roos E, Tulp A, Middelkoop OP, Van de Pavert IV. 1984. Interactions between lymphoid tumor cells and isolated liver endothelial cells. JNCI 72(5) in press.

18

7. Roos E, Van de Pavert IV. 1982. Effect of tubulin-binding agents on the infiltration of tumour cells into primary hepatocyte cultures. J Cell Sci 55, 233-245.
8. Middelkoop OP, Roos E, Van de Pavert IV. 1982. Infiltration of lymphosarcoma cells into hepatocyte cultures: inhibition by univalent antibodies against liver plasma membranes and lymphosarcoma cells. J Cell Sci 56, 461-470.
9. Roos E, Middelkoop OP, Van de Pavert IV. 1984. Adhesion of tumor cells to hepatocytes: Different mechanisms for mammary carcinoma compared with lymphosarcoma cells (submitted).
10. Middelkoop OP, Van Bavel P, Calafat J, Roos E. 1984. Identification of a hepatocyte cell surface molecule involved in the adhesion of metastatic murine mammary carcinoma cells to hepatocytes (submitted).
11. Roos E, Van de Pavert, IV. 1983. Antigen-activated T-lymphocytes infiltrate hepatocyte cultures in a manner comparable to liver-colonizing lymphosarcoma cells. Clin Exp Metastasis 1, 173-180.
12. De Baetselier P, Roos E, Brys L, Remels L & Feldman M. 1984. Generation of an invasive and metastatic variant of a non-metastatic T-cell lymphoma by in vivo fusion with a normal host cell (submitted).
13. Roos E, De Baetselier P, Stukart MJ. 1984. Invasive and metastatic potential of T-cell hybridomas (submitted).
14. Ocklind C, Öbrink B. 1982. Intercellular adhesion of rat hepatocytes. Identification of a cell surface glycoprotein involved in the initial adhesion process. J Biol Chem 257, 6788-6795.
15. Gallin WJ, Edelman GM, Cunningham BA. 1983. Characterization of L-CAM, a major cell adhesion molecule from embryonic liver cells. Proc Natl Acad Sci USA 80, 1038-1042.
16. Imhof BA, Vollmers HP, Goodman SL, Birchmeier W. 1983. Cell-cell interaction and polarity of epithelial cells: specific perturbation using a monoclonal antibody. Cell 35, 667-675.
17. Ogou SI, Yoshida-Noro C, Takeichi M. 1983. Calcium-dependent cell-cell adhesion molecules common to hepatocytes and teratocarcinoma stem cells. J Cell Biol 97, 944-948.
18. Ocklind C, Odin P, Öbrink B. 1984. Two different cell adhesion molecules-cell CAM 105 and a calcium-dependent protein-occur on the surface of rat hepatocytes. Exp Cell Res 151, 29-45.
19. Vollmers HP, Birchmeier W. 1983. Monoclonal antibodies inhibit the adhesion of murine B16 melanoma cells in vitro and block lung metastasis in vivo. Proc Natl Acad Sci USA 80, 3729-3733.
20. Vollmers HP, Birchmeier W. 1983. Monoclonal antibodies that prevent adhesion of B16 melanoma cells and reduce metastases in mice: cross-reaction with human tumor cells. Proc Natl Acad Sci USA 80, 6863-6867.
21. Terranova VP, Liotta LA, Russo RG, Martin GR. 1982. Role of laminin in the attachment and metastasis of murine tumor cells. Cancer Res 42, 2265-2269.

22. Salo T, Liotta LA, Keski-Oja J, Turpeenniemi-Hujanen T, Tryggvason K. 1982. Secretion of basement membrane collagen degrading enzyme and plasminogen activator by transformed cells-role in metastasis. Int J Cancer 30, 669-673.
23. Kramer RH, Vogel KG, Nicolson GL. 1982. Solubilization and degradation of subendothelial matrix glycoproteins and proteoglycans by metastatic tumor cells. J Biol Chem 257, 2678-2686.

THE ROLE OF CELL SURFACE DETERMINANTS IN LARGE CELL
LYMPHOMA METASTASIS TO LIVER

GARTH L. NICOLSON

1. INTRODUCTION

Malignant tumor cells circumvent the normal controls which maintain
proper cellular interactions with other normal cells and maintain their unique
position and distribution within tissues. This can result in aberrant behavior
and escape from the primary tumor mass, transport to near and distant sites,
and eventually colonization of these sites to form metastases (1,2,3,4).
Although the spread of metastatic cells may, in some cases, appear to be due to
fetal-like characteristics (5), the ultimate success of metastasis formation is
also dependent upon unique host as well as tumor-cell properties (4,6,7,8).

To study tumor cell properties important in the metastatic process,
animal tumor models have been established by sequential selection in vivo or in
vitro to obtain variant cells with enhanced metastatic and organ colonization
behaviors (2,3,4,6). Using such techniques, metastatic systems have been
developed that show preferential colonization of liver (9,10,11,12). One such
system, based on the large cell lymphoma line RAW117, has been used in our
laboratory to examine tumor and host characteristics important in blood-borne
colonization of liver (9,12,13,14). This tumor system was derived from parental
RAW117-P large cell lymphoma or lymphosarcoma, which is a tumor line of
recent origin that colonizes lungs, liver, spleen, and lymph nodes at low
frequency in BALB/c mice (15). Metastatic variant sublines have been
sequentially selected from RAW117-P for their abilities to colonize liver, and
after ten such in vivo selections subline RAW117-H10 was established (9). The
highly metastatic RAWll7-H10 variant subline rapidly kills its host and forms
more than 200 times as many gross surface liver tumor nodules after
intravenous or subcutaneous injection than does the parental RAW117-P line
(9,13,16).

Examination of cell surface properties of RAW117 parental and variant
sublines indicate that there are specific changes in the more metastatic cells.

These differences include: exposure of cell-surface proteins (16) and glycoproteins (13,14), amounts of viral antigens (13) and lectin binding sites (13,14), growth characteristics (17), partitioning behavior in aqueous two-phase systems (18), and sensitivities to host immune response mechanisms (17,19). In addition, we have found that liver-colonizing RAW117 cells express another cell surface antigen(s) (12) and is related to and crossreacts with a murine fetal antigen(s) involved in liver cell adhesion (20). Immunologic reagents against the fetal antigen(s) inhibit in vitro RAW117-H10 adhesion to liver cells in vitro (21) and inhibit in vivo liver colonization by RAW117-H10 cells (12,21).

2.   PROCEDURE

2.1. Material and methods

    2.1.1. Cells. RAW117 parental (RAW117-P) cells and sublines selected 5 times (RAW117-H5) or 10 times (RAW117-H10), for liver colonization, respectively, were established and grown in culture in Dulbecco-modified Eagle's medium (DME) containing 10% fetal bovine serum (FBS) as described previously (9,13,16). The procedures for in vitro selection of lectin-binding variant sublines based on their nonadherence to immobilized lectins are reported elsewhere (14). Clones were established from RAW117-P, from in vivo selected subline RAW117-H10 and from the in vitro selected sublines RAW117-P Con-A^{a10} (selected sequentially 10 times for lack of binding to immobilized concanavalin-A) and in RAW117-H10 WGA^{a10} (selected sequentially 10 times for lack of binding to immobilized wheat germ agglutinin as described by Reading et al. (14). Cell cultures were used within 10 passages from frozen stocks of low passage cells to eliminate possible drift in metastatic properties (12). Cultures were tested for the presence of Mycoplasmas using Hoechst 33258 staining (22) and were found to be negative. Embryonic mouse liver (EML) cells and embryonic mouse brain (EMB) cells were isolated from the organs of embryos 17-20 days gestation and prepared as described previously (20,23).

    2.1.2. RAW117 experimental metastasis assays. RAW117 sublines were assayed for organ colonization by intravenous injection of 5-10 x 10^3 viable tumor cells in 0.1 ml phosphate-buffered saline (PBS) (9). Experiments continued until the mice died or were sacrificed at specific times after injection. Visible surface tumor nodules were counted in all major organs and were confirmed by histologic examination (13,14).

2.1.3. Quantitative antigen analysis. Quantitative analysis of viral antigens was performed by competition radioimmunoassay as described (13). Antigen content was determined by comparison of sample curves with those obtained with purified antigens.

2.1.4. Quantitative adhesion assays. Individual cells were obtained from radiolabeled minced tissue as described (23). Tissue from approximately 45 mouse livers or brains from 17-19 day-old embryos was labeled in 3 ml HEPES-buffered media (25% HEPES-buffered Hank's balanced salt solution, 60% HEPES-buffered medium 199, 15% heat-inactivated chicken serum, 2 mg per ml DNAse, 100 µg/ml penicillin, 0.25 µg/ml fungizone, 100 µg/ml streptomycin) with 100 µCi ^{3}H-leucine at 37^0 C for 3-4 hrs. Labeled tissue was rinsed and the cells prepared, resulting in cells with a specific activity of 0.1-0.02 cpm/cell (20,21,23). RAW117 lymphoma cells were labeled in suspension at a concentration of 1×10^7 cells in 1 ml of HEPES-buffered media containing 40 µCi [^{14}C]-labeled, mixed amino acids (Schwartz/Mann, reconstituted protein hydrolysate) by incubation for 1-3 hrs at 37^0 C. Cells were washed twice in the HEPES buffer before use, resulting in cells with a specific activity of 0.1-0.5 cpm/cell (21).

2.1.5. Antibody inhibition of cell adhesion and experimental metastasis. Antisera against EML cells was prepared according to McGuire et al. (21). This antisera inhibited EML cell aggregation but had no effect on EMB cell or other organ cell aggregations. Rabbit anti-H-2K^k sera was made against affinity-purified H-2K^k glycoproteins as described previously (21). This antisera reacted with public specificities of the H-2 α and β $_2$-microglobulin chains and was not haplotype specific. All antisera were heated to 56^0C for 40 minutes to destroy complement before use.

Divalent F(ab')$_2$ and monovalent Fab' antibody fragments were prepared by the procedures of Nisonoff et al. (24,25). Residual F$_c$-containing components were removed by absorption with formalin-fixed Staphlococcus aureus (Calbiochem-Behring). Fab' antibody fragments were prepared by reductive alkylation using 2-mercaptoethanol and iodoacetimide (26).

RAW117 cells were treated with whole antibody, F(ab')$_2$ or Fab' antibody fragments as described (21). Cells (1×10^6) were suspended with various concentrations of anti-EML, anti-EML F(ab')$_2$, or anti-EML Fab' antibody fragments. Control cells were incubated in PBS. After incubation for 2 hrs at

Table I
Biologic properties of in vivo- and in vitro-selected RAW117 large cell lymphoma/lymphosarcoma variants sublines*

Subline	Selection	Average No. (range) of visible tumor colonies[‡]		
		Liver	Lung	Other sites
RAW117-P	None	0.5 (0-3)	0.4 (0-1)	2/10 spleen
RAW117-P Con A[a10]	10X immobilized con-canavalin A	112 (9-250)	1 (0-4)	6/10 spleen
RAW117-H5	5X liver colonization	25 (9-42)	0.6 (0-2)	3/10 spleen
RAW117-H10	10X liver colonization	230 (92-250)	1 (1-5)	9/10 spleen
RAW117-H10 WGA[a10]	10X liver colonization and 10X immobilized wheat-germ agglutinin	1 (0-5)	0.5 (0-2)	none

*Data of Nicolson et al. (12).

[‡]5×10^3 viable lymphosarcoma cells were injected intravenously into groups of 10 BALB/c mice and number of visible tumor nodules determined after 10 days.

4°C on a tube rotor, the cells were washed 3 times by centrifugation and resuspension in PBS, and viabilities were determined by dye exclusion. The washed cells were injected intravenously ($5{-}10 \times 10^{3}$) into BALB/c mice as described (12,21). All animals died of experimental metastases or were killed at 31-63 days post injection, and major organs were examined for the presence of tumor nodules.

2.1.6. Cytolysis and cytostasis of RAW117 cells. Peritoneal exudate cells solicited with thioglycolate pretreatment of BALB/c mice were obtained as described (19). Cells were seeded onto tissue culture plates and were washed once with media plus 10% FBS to remove nonadherent cells. Nonspecific esterase staining indicated 95-98% of the cells were esterase-positive. These adherent macrophage monolayers were treated with poly I:C (40 µg/ml; P-L Biochemicals) in DME containing 0.1% lactalbumin hydrolysate for 1 hr to activate macrophages. Half of the cultures received media without poly I:C. RAW117 target cells were added as single-cell suspensions to the macrophage monolayers at a density of 2×10^{4} cells/ml for cytostasis assays and 5×10^{4} cells/ml for cytolysis assays (effector:target ratios of 5:1, 10:1, and 25:1). After 72 hrs, target cells were suspended and counted in triplicate according to Miner and Nicolson (19). Statistical analysis for significance was determined by one-way analysis of variance and Mann-Whitney U test.

2.2. Results

2.2.1. Metastatic and cell surface properties of RAW117 cells. The biological properties of RAW117-P and sublines selected in vivo for liver colonization or in vitro for loss of adherence to immobilized lectins are shown in Table 1. Selection using immobilized lectins resulted in either an increase (RAW117-P selected using immobilized Con-A) or decrease (RAW117-H10 selected using immobilized WGA) in metastatic liver colonization. Cell surface properties correlating with metastatic potential in the RAW117 system are loss of Con-A binding sites (13,14), increased partitioning behavior in poly(ethylene glycol):dextran aqueous phase using counter-current distribution (18), and loss of cell surface RNA tumor virus antigen gp70 (12,13). The relationship of this last parameter to liver metastasis showed a very high correlation (r=0.93) between the quantity of gp70 determined by competion radioimmune analysis of several clones derived from RAW117 sublines and metastatic potential determined in liver colonization assays (Fig. 1).

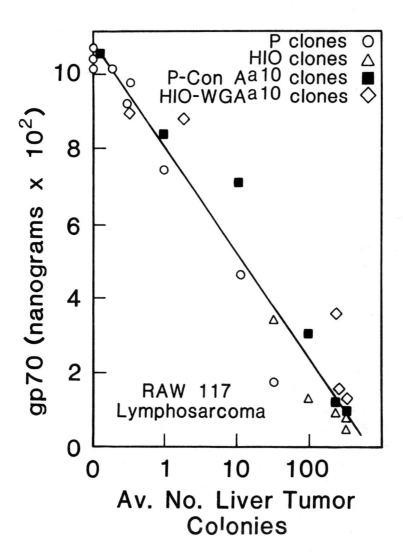

FIGURE 1. Relationship of the content of RNA-tumor virus envelope glyco-protein gp70 to liver tumor colonization in various RAW117 lymphosarcoma cell clones. Antigen content is expressed as ng/10⁶ cells, and liver tumor colonization is expressed as the average number (*n*=10) of gross liver tumor colonies formed in 12 days after injection intravenously of 1 x 10³ cells. See text for details. Data of Nicolson et al. (12).

2.2.2. Relationship of RAW117 clls to embryonic murine liver cells. We have found that RAW117 cells show adhesive specificites toward embryonic liver cells. This was determined in a double label coaggregation assay, and using this assay RAW117-H10 cells had an approximately 4 times greater rate of adherence to embryonic murine liver (EML) than to embryonic murine brain (EMB) cells. In contrast, RAW117-P cells displayed no selectivity in binding to EMB or EML cells (Table 2).

We examined RAW117 cells for the presence of liver cross-reactive antigens using polyclonal xenoantibody preparations directed against EML cells. These antibody preparations block organ-specific homotypic adhesion of EML cells in vitro (20). The amount of the fetal liver antigen(s) expressed on RAW117 sublines correlated with liver colonization potentials (H10>H5>P) in quantitative absorption assays (21).

To examine the effect of the anti-EML reagents on liver colonization, we pretreated RAW117 cells in vitro and injected them into syngeneic mice. Treatment of RAW117-H10 cells with anti-EML $F(ab')_2$ or Fab' antibody fragments essentially blocked experimental liver metastasis (Table 3). In contrast, treatment of RAW117-H10 cells with anti-H-2 $F(ab')_2$ or Fab' had no effect on the number of liver tumor nodules that formed, and all animals died at the expected times post injection (Table 3). Treatment of RAW117-H10 cells with low concentrations of the anti-EML $F(ab')_2$ resulted in the binding of lower amounts of immunoglobulin fragments that did not prevent host death from multiple experimental liver metastases, while higher concentrations of anti-EML $F(ab')_2$ that essentially saturated the anti-EML-binding sites reduced mortality (21).

Quantitative binding of anti-EML and anti-H-2 immunoglobulins or their $F(ab')_2$ antibody fragments was measured using excess anti-immunoglobulin followed by Staphlococcus aureus ^{125}I protein A binding (21). The amounts of cell-bound anti-H-2 immunoglobulin or their $F(ab')_2$ fragments ranged from approximately 40-70% of the maximum levels of cell bound anti-EML $F(ab')_2$. While the binding of anti-H-2 immunoglobulin or $F(ab')_2$ was somewhat lower than anti-EML, anti-EML $F(ab')_2$ was still effective in reducing metastasis at binding levels comparable to anti-H-2 (Table 4). Examination of the organs of animals injected with anti-EML $F(ab')_2$ or anti-EML Fab'-treated RAW117-H10 cells did not reveal micrometastases in liver or spleen; however, approximately

Table 2
Coaggregation of RAW117 variant cells with embryonic mouse cells*

Aggregate type[+]	No. aggregates counted	Mean of normalized ratios of individual aggregates[‡]	Selectivity ratio	
P/EMB	20	1.04	$\frac{P/EML}{P/EMB}$	= 0.66
H10/EMB	20	0.73		
P/EML	10	0.69	$\frac{H10/EML}{H10/EMB}$	= 3.63
H10/EML	10	2.65		

*Data of McGuire et al. (21); EMB=embryonic mouse brain; EML=embryonic mouse liver

[+][3]H-labeled embryo cells (2.5-10x10[6]) were incubated under shear with RAW117 cells (1-2x10[6]) in a total volume of 1.5 ml medium for 1 hour at 37°C. Individual cell aggregates were removed, washed, and counted.

[‡]Data normalized to initial 1:1 RAW117/embryo cells.

Table 3
Biologic properties of RAW117-H10 cells after treatment with anti-embryonic mouse liver (EMB) or anti-H-2 antibody F(ab')$_2$ or Fab' fragments*

No. of experiments	Antibody F(ab')$_2$ or Fab' (amount/10^6 cells)	No. animals with >200 liver tumors/ No. animals at 21-63 days post injection	No. animals with spleen tumors/total No. animals at 31-63 days post injection	No. animals with lung tumors/total No. animals at 31-63 days post injection
8	None	36/37 †‡	36/37 †‡	†
8	Anti-H-2 F(ab')$_2$ (1-10 mg)	30/33 †‡	30/33 †‡	†
8	Anti-EML F(ab')$_2$ (0.8-1 mg)	3/30 ‡	3/30 ‡	19/30
1	Anti-H-2 Fab' (10 mg)	5/5	5/5	†
1	Anti-EML Fab' (10 mg)	0/4	0/4	4/4

*Data of McGuire et al. (21).

‡By the chi square test, data from the first 3 groups does not fit random occurence of tumors for the total population of 100 animals (χ^2_2 = 21.3, p <0.0005). By analyzing the groups, the anti-H-2-treated group does not differ significantly from the control groups (χ^2_2 = 0.125, p=0.70), and the anti-EML group is significantly different from the control groups (χ^2_2 = 26.3, p <0.0005).

†Mice died prior to appearance of gross lung lesions.

Table 4
Concentration dependence of anti-embryonic mouse liver (EMB) $F(ab')_2$ on inhibition of RAW117-H10 liver colonization*

Antibody $F(ab')_2$ (mg/1X10^6 cells)[†]	Percent $F(ab')_2$ bound[‡]	No. animals with >200 liver tumors/total No. animals at 25 days post injection
0	0	5/5[§]
0.005	25	4/5[§]
0.25	37	3/5
0.5	63	2/5
1.5	100	0/5

*Data of McGuire et al. (21).

†For conditions see Table 3.

‡Determined by indirect antibody, <u>Staphylococcus aureus</u> ^{125}I-protein A binding.

§Mice died prior to the end of the assay.

Table 5
In vitro cytolysis and cytostasis of RAW117 cells mediated by poly I:C-activated peritoneal macrophages*

Cell line RAW117	Effector: Target[†]	Ave. No. Target cells[‡] ($\times 10^{-2}$)	% Cytolysis[§]	Ave. No. Target cells[II] ($\times 10^{-2}$)	% Cytostasis**
P	none	2146 ± 104	-	115296 ± 611	-
	5:1	1352 ± 72	36[¶]	101025 ± 282	13[††]
	10:1	1201 ± 108	44[¶]	92071 ± 771	20[††]
	25:1	865 ± 67	60[¶]	314 ± 87	74[††]
H10	none	2075 ± 34	-	12631 ± 318	-
	5:1	1708 ± 108	18[¶]	12510 ± 293	1[††]
	10:1	1510 ± 137	27[¶]	12422 ± 205	2[††]
	25:1	1370 ± 84	33[¶]	12365 ± 201	3[††]

*Data of Miner and Nicolson (19).

[†]Effectors were thioglycolate elicited peritoneal macrophages from BALB/c mice which were activated in vitro with poly I:C. Targets were metastatic RAW117 lymphosarcoma cells. For details see Materials and Methods.

[‡]2×10^5 target cells were treated with mitomycin-C and plated in the presence or absence of macrophages.

[§]Percent cytolysis was calculated as equal to $[(C-E)/T] \times 100$ where E and C are remaining number of target cells in wells with or without macrophages, respectively.

[¶]The difference among control and both experimental populations for P and H10 assays was significant at the 0.001 level by one-way analysis of variance.

[II]2×10^4 dividing target cells were plated in the presence or absence of macrophages.

**Percent cytostasis was calculated as $[(1-(E-T)/(C-T)] \times 100$ where E and C are the remaining number of target cells in wells with or without macrophages, respectively.

[††]The difference between P and H10 experimental populations was significant at the 0.005 level by one-way analysis of variance. However there was no significant difference among the H10 populations.

two months after injection, a few small tumor nodules were found in the lungs. These lung tumor nodules grew, invaded slowly, and required over 60 days to kill the mice (21).

2.2.3. <u>Sensitivities of RAW117 cells to host response</u>. We have conducted both <u>in vitro</u> (19) and <u>in vivo</u> (17) experiments to determine whether mice can respond to RAW117 cells. Impairment of anti-tumor responses by using 400R irradiated or variously aged BALB/c nude (nu/nu) mice was not effective in modifying the metastatic properties of any of the RAW117 cell lines or clones (17). In contrast, inhibiting macrophage function by placing chlorine in the drinking water or giving animals injections of Trypan blue, silica particles, carageenan, cyclophosphamid, or pristane dramatically enhanced the malignant properties of RAW117-P cells but had little or no effect on the highly metastatic RAW117 cells <u>in vivo</u> (17). These results suggested that macrophages may suppress RAW117 cells of low metastatic potential. Therefore, we examined RAW117-P and selected sublines and clones for their sensitivities <u>in vitro</u> to poly I:C activated syngeneic macrophages in cytolysis and cytostasis assays. Activated but not unactivated macrophages had differing effects on RAW117 sublines and clones (19). The least metastatic cell line (RAW117-P) was the most sensitive to activated macrophage-mediated cytolysis and cytostasis, while the most metastatic subline (RAW117-H10) was the least sensitive in such assays (Table 5). Differences in cytolysis and cytostasis between RAW117-P cells and highly malignant RAW117-H10 cells were significant at the 0.002 and 0.001 levels, respectively, by the Mann-Whitney U test using data from 6 independent experiments (Table 5). RAW117 sublines and clones of intermediate metastatic potential between RAW117-P and RAW117-H10 yielded differing results in cytolysis or cytostasis assays (19). In other experiments, we determined that macrophages rather than NC or NK cells were mediating the cytolysis and cytostasis activities (19).

2.3. <u>Discussion</u>

Cell surface biochemical data indicates that the loss of gp70 in the highly malignant RAW117 cells correlates with metastatic potential suggesting that immune responses might be involved in suppressing cells of high gp70 content. We found no evidence for T, NK, or NC cell-mediated host response against RAW117 cells (17). However, we did note differences in macrophage-mediated cytolysis and cytostasis between RAW117 cells of low and high malignant potential (Table 5 and reference 19). That macrophage-mediated host responses were important in suppressing RAW117 cells of low metastatic potential was confirmed in vivo by impairing macrophage function, resulting in increased malignancy of parental but not RAW117-H10 cells (17). Although the number of experimental metastases appear to be affected by host macrophage-mediated responses, the organ specificity of RAW117 cells could not be explained by this mechanism (12).

In examining the adhesive specificities of RAW117 cells, we found that these cells adhere selectively to isolated liver cells in relation to their liver colonization properties (21). This selectivity was not seen with other organ cells, such as those isolated from brain or lung. Kieran and Longenecker (27), have also found that RAW117 cells bind more effectively to mouse liver than other organs in frozen section cell-binding assays. They also noted that RAW117-H10 cells bound approximately 7 times better to liver compared to RAW117-P cells. Thus, the specificity of organ colonization may be determined by cell-cell recognition (4,6,28).

Antibodies made against cell surface antigens have been used to block blood-borne colonization of metastatic cells (10,20,29). In our studies we have used polyclonal antibodies to cell adhesion components on the target organ cells rather than to the tumor cell itself. Antibodies made against fetal liver cells, which block fetal liver cell-cell aggregation, inhibited liver colonization of RAW117 cells (21). In quantitative absorption studies, cell surface antigens cross reacting with liver adhesion molecules were found on RAW117 cells, as well as on adult mouse liver and spleen cells (21). The binding of this polyclonal reagent to RAW117 sublines occurred in relation to their liver colonizing potentials (H10>H5>P). Anti-EML Fab' antibody fragments significantly decreased RAW117-H10 cell adhesion to EML cells in vitro and inhibited experimental blood-borne metastasis and prolonged the life expectancy of animals injected with RAW117-H10 cells (21). We used antibody fragments lacking the F_c portions of their structure in order to preclude a role for complement, ADDC or monocyte cell attack of the antibody-coated cells in vivo. We found that anti-H-2 antibody fragments had no effect on RAW117 cell adhesive or malignant properties, and that anti-EML Fab'-treated RAW117-H10 cells produced small numbers of lung lesions. Thus the antibody-coated RAW117-H10 cells were not simply trapped in the lungs. This was confirmed using radiolabeled anti-EML-treated RAW117 cells. Injection of these cells in vivo indicated that the antibody coated cells arrive at and depart the lungs at rates similar to untreated cells (21).

Our studies suggest that one of the initial steps of organ colonization by RAW117 cells is mediated by an organ adhesion system which may exist on endothelial as well as parenchymal cells (6). However, the ultimate growth and metastsis of a tumor also involves many other host and tumor factors such as escape from host responses. These are discussed in more detail elsewhere (4,6,31,32,33).

ACKNOWLEDGMENTS

We gratefully acknowledge the assistance of Adele Brodginski, Eleanor Felonia and Pat Bramlett. These studies were supported by U. S. National Cancer Institute Grant RO1-CA29571.

REFERENCES

1. Fidler IJ. 1978. In vitro tumoricidal activity of macrophages against virus-transformed lines with temperature-dependent transformed phenotypic characteristics. Cell Immunol. 38:131-146.
2. Nicolson GL, Poste G. 1982. Tumor cell diversity and host responses in cancer metastasis. I. Properties of metastatic cells. Curr. Prob. Cancer 7(6):1-83.
3. Nicolson GL, and Poste G. 1983a. Tumor cell diversity and host responses in cancer metastasis. II. Host immune responses and therapy of metastases. Curr. Prob. Cancer 7(7):1-43.
4. Nicolson GL, Poste G. 1983b. Tumor implantation and invasion at metastatic sites. Int. Rev. Exp. Pathol. 25:77-181.
5. Franks LM. 1978. Structure and biological malignancy of tumors. In Chemotherapy of Cancer Dissemination and Metastasis (S. Garattini and G. Franchi, eds.), Raven Press, New York.
6. Nicolson GL. 1982. Cancer Metastasis: Organ colonization and the cell surface properties of malignant cells. Biochim. Biophys. Acta 695:113.176.
7. Sugarbaker EV. 1981. Patterns of metastasis in human malignancies. Cancer Biol. Res. 2:235-278.
8. Poste G. 1982. Experimental systems for analysis of the malignant phenotype. Cancer Metastasis Rev. 1:141-199.
9. Brunson KW, Nicolson GL. 1978. Selection and biologic properties of malignant variants of a murine lymphosarcoma. J. Natl. Cancer Inst. 61:1499-1503.
10. Shearman PJ, Longenecker BM. 1980. Selection for virulence and organ-specific metastasis of herpes virus-transformed lymphoma cells. Int. J. Cancer 25:363-369.

34

11. Schirrmacher V, Shantz G, Clauer K, Komitowski D, Zimmermann H-P, Loahmann-Matthes M-L. 1979. Tumor metastases and cell-mediated immunity in a model system in DBA/2 mice. I. Tumor invasiveness in vitro and metastasis formation in vivo. Int. J. Cancer 23:233-244.

12. Nicolson GL, Mascali JJ, McGuire EJ. 1982. Metastatic RAW117 lymphosarcoma as a model for malignant-normal cell interactions. Possible roles for cell surface antigens in determining the quantity and location of secondary tumors. Oncodevelop. Biol. Med. 4:149-159.

13. Reading CL, Belloni PN, Nicolson GL. 1980a. Selection and in vivo properties of lectin-attachment variants of malignant murine lymphosarcoma cell lines. J. Natl. Cancer Inst. 64:1241-1249.

14. Reading CL, Brunson KW, Torriani M, Nicolson GL. 1980b. Malignancies of metastatic murine lymphosarcoma cell lines and clones correlate with decreased cell surface display of RNA tumor virus envelope glycoprotein gp70. Proc. Natl. Acad. Sci. U.S.A. 77:5943-5947.

15. Raschke WC, Ralph P, Watson J, Sklar M, Coon H. 1975. Oncogenic transformation of murine lymphoid cells by in vitro infection with Abelson leukemia virus. J. Natl. Cancer Inst. 54:1249-1253.

16. Nicolson GL, Reading CL, Brunson KW. 1980. Blood-brone tumor metastasis: Some properties of selected tumor cell variants of differing malignancies. In Tumor Progression (R.G. Crispen, ed.), Elsevier North Holland, Inc., Amsterdam.

17. Reading CL, Kraemer PM, Miner KM, Nicolson, GL. 1983. In vivo and in vitro properties of malignant variants of RAW117 metastatic murine lymphoma/lymphosarcoma. Clin. Expl. Metastasis 1:135-151.

18. Miner KM, Walter H, Nicolson GL. 1981. Subfractionation of malignant variants of metastatic murine lymphosarcoma cells by countercurrent distribution in two-polymer aqueous phases. Biochemistry 20:6244-6250.

19. Miner KM, Nicolson GL. 1983. Differences in the sensitivities of murine metastatic lymphoma/lymphosarcoma cells to macrophage-mediated cytolysis and/or cytostasis. Cancer Res. 43:2063-2071.

20. Grady SR, Nielsen LD, McGuire EJ. 1982. Organ and class specificity of cell adhesion blocking antisera. Exp. Cell Res. 142:169-180.

21. McGuire EJ, Mascali JJ, Grady SR, Nicolson GL. 1984. Involvement of cell-cell adhesion molecules in liver colonization by metastatic murine lymphoma/lymphosarcoma variants. Clin. Exp. Metastasis, in press.

22. Chen TR. 1977. In situ detection of mycoplasma contamination in cell cultures by fluorescent Hoechst 33258 stain. Exp. Cell Res. 140:255.262.

23. Grady SR, McGuire EJ. 1976. Intercellular adhesive selectivity. III. Species selectivity of embryonic liver intercellular adhesion. J. Cell Biol. 71:96-106.

24. Nisonoff A, Wissler FC, Lipman LN, Woernley BL. 1960. Properties of the major component of a peptic digest of rabbit antibody. Science 132:1770-1771.

25. Nisonoff A, Markus G, Wissler FC. 1961. Separation of univalent fragments of rabbit antibody by reduction of a single, labile disulfide bond. Nature 189:293-295.

26. Galfre G, Howe SC, Milstein C, Butcher GW, Howard JC. 1977. Antibodies to major histocompatibility antigens produced by hybrid cell lines. Nature (London) 266:550-552.

27. Kieran MW, Longenecker BM. 1983. Organ specific metastasis with special reference to avian system. Cancer Metastasis Rev. 2:165-182.

28. Schirrmacher V, Cheinsong-Popov R, Arnheiter H. 1980. Hepatocyte-tumor interaction in vitro. I. Conditions for rosette formtion and inhibtion by anti-H-2 antibody. J. Exp. Med. 151:984-989.

29. Shearman PJ and Longenecker BM. 1981. Clonal variation and functional correlation of organ specific metastasis and an organ-specific metastasis associated antigen. Int. J. Cancer 27:387-395.
30. Vollmers HP, Birchmeier W. 1983. Monoclonal antibodies inhibit the adhesion of mouse B16 melanoma cells in vitro and block lung metastasis in vivo (cancer/cell adhesion/syngeneic immunization). Proc. Natl. Acad. Sci. U.S.A. 80:3729-3733.
31. Nicolson GL. 1984a. Cell surface molecules and tumor metastatsis. Regulation of metastatic diversity. Exp. Cell Res. 150:3-22.
32. Nicolson GL. 1984b. Generation of phenotypic diversity and progression in metastatic tumors. Cancer Metastasis Rev. 3:25-42.
33. Nicolson GL. 1984c. Tumor progress, oncogenes and the evolution of metastatic phenotypic diversity. Clin. Exp. Metastasis 2: in press.

INTERRELATION OF ANIMAL TUMOR MODELS TO THE CLINICAL
PROBLEM OF THE TREATMENT OF HEPATIC METASTASES

A. Zwaveling

HISTORICAL SURVEY

After a 'dormant' phase of many years the problems presented by liver metastases are again of great interest to both
experimental researchers and clinicians. Purely mechanical
theories are being replaced by experimentally acquired in-
sights into the biological behaviour of tumor and host.
Halsted's concept was that the metastatic process consisted
of separate lymphogenous and haematogenous routes of spread
that with time should follow one another. This simple view
has been replaced by another; it is now obvious that we are
dealing with an expression of a disturbed tumor-host relationship. This does not mean that in daily practice the old
theories cannot contribute towards diagnosis and therapy.
Here also, Walter's Theory of metastases based upon the filtering properties of the various capillary beds has been
shown to be much too simplistic; yet, it still gives the clinician direction in his search for metastases. The theory
can only be considered a 'rule-of-thumb'; an exception to
it is well illustrated by the behaviour of metastasis from
breast carcinoma. Walter's Theory cannot predict why one so
seldom sees metastases in skeletal muscle, kidney or spleen,
Also why some tumors nearly always and others almost never
metastasize. Not explained is the fact that only a small
minority of cells entering blood or lymphatic vessels are
able to grow elsewhere. Why is it that the number of cells
in the circulation and the chance of successful implantation
does not increase in all cases as the size of the tumor increases. With a review of these questions it becomes ever
more obvious that Paget's ideas of the metastatic process

expressed in 1889 need review. He suggested that both 'seed and soil', 'grain and terrain', play a role. 'Seed' in this case being the properties of the metastasized tumor cell, and 'soil' the conditions in the microenvironment where the cell has landed.

I will not speak about the investigations done by Sugar-baker[2], Nicholson[3], Porte[4], Fidler[5] and others over the last few years. These studies have deepened our understanding of factors influencing the metastatic process. This is especially true of the immunological factors, and the process of selection and survival of specific cell populations. A primary tumor does not appear to be a collection of identical cells. As the tumor grows there is a rapid development of phenotypically heterogenous cell populations which have differing properties. This is expressed as differing potentials to metastasizes and differing sensitivities to chemotherapeutic agents. A metastasis that originates from a single clone may develop different abnormal cell populations. This may result in therapeutic problems with a single treatment modality.

ANIMAL MODELS

The metastatic process has been investigated in many experimental animal models. In these models one tries to approximate the human situations as closely as possible. Mouse and rat models are principally used because of the availability of genetically identical strains and matched tumors. Tumors used may arise 'spontaneously' or chemically or virally induced. The host-tumor relationship is much different from that in man; the experimental animals have short life-spans, the tumors grow rapidly and they are strongly immunogenic. The xenograft technique utilizing congenitally athymic nude mice has been successfully employed. In it the soil element and so immune reactions are to a large degree eliminated. Unfortunately metastasization proceeds with difficulty here. Tissue culture and Bogden assay are also little suited to the study of the metastatic process.

Waiting for spontaneous metastases in a model usually

yields disappointing results. This is due to the rapid growth
of the primary tumor. By timely removal of the primary after
micro-metastases have occurred, this model may be successfully
studied. The use of intravenous techniques is easier. The
study of lung metastases is in this case the principal object
of study.

Liver metastases can only be induced by intravenous infusion of malignant cells after a laparotomy. Usually the injection is made into a branch of the portal vein. This model does
not incorporate the problems that a metastasizing cell encoun-
ters by its detachment and migration. Local extravasation of
tumor, failure of implantation and intrahepatic growth do occur, just as in more physiological conditions. In both experimental and natural situations trans-organ-passage and recirculation with eventual metastasis elsewhere can occur.

Our first experiments in Leiden to obtain a good liver
metastasis model were not entirely successful. Cotino[6] did
not succeed in inducing liver metastases in rats using Walker
256 tumor injected into a caecal vein. Extensive retroperitoneal lymph node metastases did occur, and lung metastases were
seen. To investigate the effect of intra-arterial infusion
of 5-FU upon liver metastases Cotino had to be satisfied with
transhepatic inoculation of cells. Extensive lymphatic metastases were seen again after this; however, without interfe-
ring with a satisfactory assessment of the treatment under
investigation.

Verbeek[7] also performed a similar study, and only succeeded in inducing liver metastases with portal vein infusions
in a few instances. He used both a rhabdomyosarcoma and a
squamous cell carcinoma. By performing a re-laparotomy and
liver massage (as described by Fisher and Fisher[8]), four
weeks after inoculation, it was still possible to 'activate'
a number of dormant cancer cells. This was also true if cyclo-
phosphamide was administered two days before inoculation. This
has been attributed to blocking of the natural killer cells
(Riccardi et al[9]). The results are shown in Table 1.

At the moment our group in Leiden is investigating the

EθMθ	LL	EL	survival in days	average survival	EθMθ	LL	EL	survival in days	average survival
1	35	-	68		1	4	-	81	
2	3	+	91		2	2	-	109	
3	1	-	131		3	2	-	117	
4	1	-	132	195,2	4	1	-	128	111,6
5	4	+	86		5	3	-	101	
6	1	-	123		6	1	-	134	
7	-	-			7	-	-		
8	-	-			8	-	-		

EθEθ	LL	EL	survival in days	average survival	EθEθ	LL	EL	survival in days	average survival
1	2	-	105		1	2	-	112	
2	3	-	80		2	1	-	115	
3	1	-	122		3	-	-		
4	1	-	121	106,4	4	-	-		113,5
5	3	+	104		5	-	-		
6	-	-			6	-	-		
7	-	-			7	-	-		
8	-	-			8	-	-		

Table 1.

Survival, number of liver localizations and extrahepatic
localizations after inoculation of an average of 20 x 10[6]
squamous cell carcinoma cells in rats.
1. EθMθ: Endoxan pretreatment, no liver-massage
2. EθMθ: No endoxan pretreatment, with liver massage
3. EθMθ: Endoxan pretreatment and liver massage
4. EθMθ: No endoxan pretreatment, no liver massage
LL: Liver localisations
EL: Extrahepatic localisations

utilization of 5-FU and its metabolites in normal liver tissue
and in metastases. De Brauw (personal communication), induces
liver metastases simply by inoculation into a central branch
of the portal vein with a suspension of tumor cells originating from a chemical induced colonic carcinoma. Using 0.5×10^6
viable cells he achieved tumor growth in 80% of the animals.
But the growth of tumor was very slow. Probably the anatomic
origin of the tumor used plays a large role in the occurrence
of visible metastases in the liver after intraportal inoculation.

The colon tumor model developed in our laboratory by Zoetmulder[10] is an example of an orthotopic model with spontaneous
liver metastases. Lewis lung carcinoma cells are directly injected into the caecum wall of mice, after which tumor growth
was observed in the liver within 2 - 3 weeks in two thirds of
the animals. After 4 weeks there were liver metastases in 60%
of the mice; also 50% had lung, 40% peritoneal, and 20% regional lymph node metastases. Survival after removal of the primary one week after inoculation was 80%, after two weeks 20%
and after 3 weeks, none survived. If the primary was removed
after two weeks, there were still no obvious macroscopic metastases, but with time it was found that 60% had developed
liver metastases.

Murine experiments are unsuitable for developing techniques
which are applicable to humans, as is the case with isolated
regional liver perfusion(Van de Velde[11]). Large experimental
animals must be used, preferably those whose anatomy and physiology are close to human, so that pharmacokinetic studies
are also possible. Pigs are good experimental animals in which
to study the problems of isolated liver perfusion. Unfortunately, liver metastases are unable to be induced in these animals.
In order to study the effects on metastases of isolated liver
perfusion during which very high doses of cancer chemotherapeutic agents may be administered, we returned to the rodent.
We are now studying the pharmacodynamics of 5-FU and its metabolites on normal liver tissue and liver metastases by micro-
perfusions in the rat model described above.

As soon as we have models that reflect the human situation, we can investigate how the microenvironment of metastases can be manipulated; not only by chemotherapy, but also by surgery and immunotherapy.

So far, neither seed nor soil in the experimental models are comparable with those in man. For accurate knowledge we must go to man himself. Initial investigations are necessary to determine what the possibilities are, and to find the safety margins. After careful Phase I studies one must ask: does it help? Does the patient derive any real benefit in terms of better survival or a longer disease free interval? Is the cost/benefit ratio acceptable for both monetary and psychological considerations? Only a carefully designed clinical trial can answer these questions.

MAGNITUDE OF THE PROBLEM

Liver metastases are a clinical problem of great magnitude. This is true because tumors of the digestive tract, lung and breast frequently metastasize to the liver. Liver metastases are demonstrable in about 20% of patients with colon and rectal tumors at the time of the initial therapy. At the Academisch Ziekenhuis we observed a 14% incidence. By estimation, about half of the patients with colorectal carcinomas die of this form of metastasis. Once metastases are visible, the median survival is then only 5 months. The Roswell Park data on 9700 autopsies, analyzed by Pickren et al[12], showed that of 8055 patients with metastases, liver metastases were seen in 4444 of these. The tumors which most frequently metastasize to the liver are pancreas (75%), breast (60%), gallbladder and extrahepatic bile ducts (60.5%), colon and rectum (56.8%) and stomach (48.9%).

TREATMENT OF LIVER METASTASES

These figures show the magnitude of the problem of liver metastases, and make it clear why so much energy is expended in the research and treatment of them. The results of treatment depend upon many factors, especially upon the number and size of the metastases. In order to make comparison between series possible it is very desirable that a generally accepted clear staging system of liver growth is devised. How can liver metastases be treated? In Table 2   an overview is given. Some methods are not suitable for adjuvant therapy; others may be used as both adjuvant therapy and as treatment of macroscopic liver metastases. Combinations of the methods are possible in a number of cases.

Prevention of liver metastases by adjuvant chemotherapy has been repeatedly attempted. Why are the results of adjuvant chemotherapy so disappointing? One would expect that a small amount of remaining tumor tissue would be easily destroyed by a chemotherapeutic agent to which it is sensitive. De Vita[13] presented a summary of this problem in his James Ewing lecture in 1983. Justifiably, he emphasized the theories of Goldy and Caldman[14], concerning the development of resistance to chemotherapeutic agents. In genetically unstable, fast growing malignant cell lines permanent mutation to a phenotypic drug resistance can occur spontaneously. Unfortunately, occurrence of such resistance is not seen in normal regenerating tissues such as bone marrow. During chemotherapy small numbers of resistant cells may be spared. These multiply, and an initially successful treatment, possibly a total remission, may fail. These resistant cells may themselves metastasize, regardless of the fact that they too arose in metastases. The smaller tne tumor, the less the chance of resistant cell lines. This indicates that the therapy must begin as quickly as possible; in the case of adjuvant therapy, possibly at the time of operation of the primary tumor. Resistant clones must be prevented. Unfortunately, in a number of cases, the metastatic tumors will result from resistant clones from the primary tumor, and so early treatment will produce no benefit.

Surgery of metastases is the oldest method and is often applied with good results in man. The problem is that surgery of liver metastases can only be used in patients in whom the part of the liver to be spared appears to be free of tumor.

Table 2.

MODES OF TREATMENT OF LIVER METASTASES

SURGERY

CHEMOTHERAPY

    systemic (oral; i.v.)
    intra-arterial
    intra-portal
    isolated perfusion

DEVASCULARISATION

    operative
    percutaneous

} event.
  combinations

RADIOTHERAPY

IMMUNOTHERAPY

CRYOSURGERY

The best results are achieved with solitary metastases and results in more than 30% 5-year survival. About 10 percent synchronous metastases of colorectal tumors come into consideration for resection. The operative mortality is, depending upon the magnitude of the resection, 0 - 10%. If possible solitary metastases should be surgically removed. Unfortunately, such a situation appears only in a limited number of patients. Resection may be followed by chemotherapeutic treatment.

Radiotherapy has only recently been used in clinical research protocols. Early on isotopes were regionally introduced by means of infusion of radio-active microspheres, but later externally applied irradiation with 20-30 Gy over 2 - 5 weeks was used. Undesirable effects appear to be minimal, with shrinkage of tumor and relief of symptoms seen in 80% of patients. This is much higher than with chemotherapy. It is possible that sensitizers may better the results still further.

Chemotherapy was initially **systemically** administered, either orally or intravenously. Many variations have been used: short term administration, long term with or without intervals, very high dose, loading doses followed by continuous administration, combinations either simultaneously or successively. All have given poor results. Usually about 20% remission is reported, mostly of short duration.

Better results are to be expected of intra-arterial or intra-portal administration. A canula is either operatively or percutaneously introduced into the hepatic artery or portal vein, and a chemotherapeutic agent is chronically infused directly into the liver. The method has been made even more interesting by the development of subcutaneously implantable pumps that can be percutaneously re-charged. Here too, many dosages are applied with several kinds of chemotherapeutic agents and still no one knows what is the best. The results are neither consistant nor are they often comparable, and no breakthrough has yet been documented. Also these devices are very expensive. The combination of chemotherapy with hyperthermia appears to yield little extra success.

An investigation has been started into the value of intra-portal administration of 5-FU or an adjuvant therapy with operated colorectal tumors. Intraportal infusion after ligation of the hepatic artery may result in prolonged survival; the controlled trials are in progress.

Special delivery methods in chemotherapeutic agents via the hepatic artery may also be carried out by these means, e.g. by infusion of microspheres filled with cytostatics.

Isolated liver perfusion has been performed by Aigner in Giessen. Studies in Leiden will begin soon. Results of Phase I and II Trials are eagerly awaited.

Dearterialization procedures of the liver appear to have a short lasting effect. They may give improved results when applied in conjunction with intra-arterial or intraportal infusions. It is unable to be said whether the results are better than with perfusions alone. Further controlled studies are needed.

Immunotherapy has recently presented great new potential. Now very specific monoclonal antibodies against specific human antigens have become available. They can be used for antibody mediated tumor cell killing. Also antibody conjugated to toxic agents, a kind of armed monoclonal antibody, has been suggested.

Liposomes as carriers of immunomodulators to render macrophages cytotoxic against metastatic tumor cells is another approach with an immunological background. In some places research is progressing, but the results are as yet unclear.

Cryosurgery of liver metastases that lay near or on the liver surface is a simple, local effective method that is far to infrequently applied in cases where the metastases are found in both lobes. Research in our laboratory has shown that the tumor must be frozen and rapidly thawed several times, after which it can completely disappear (Zonnevylle[15]).

OVERVIEW

Looking over the whole, there is a battle on many fronts: from basic research via applied research, to clinical investigation, to arrive at a better understanding of the occur-

rence, diagnosis and treatment of liver metastases. We shall
not be able to standardize the treatment in the near future,
but it is important to exchange experiences. We are gaining
more insight into what are purposeful or purposeless diagnostic investigations. We must arrive at a generally acceptable
staging method so as to better compare our results. Last but
not least collaborative investigations have to be arranged.
There is still much work to be done.

REFERENCES

1. Paget S. 1889. The distribution of secondary growth in
   cancer of the breast. Lancet 1: 571.
2. Sugarbaker EV. 1979. Cancer metastasis: a product of tumor-
   host interactions. Curr Probl Cancer III/7.
3. Nicolson GL, Porte G. 1982. Tumor cell diversity and host
   responses in cancer metastasis - Part I. Curr Probl Cancer
   VII/6.
4. Porte G, Fidler IJ. 1980. The pathogenesis of cancer metastasis. Nature 283: 139.
5. Fidler IJ. 1976. Patterns of tumor cell arrest and development. In: Weiss L, (ed.). Fundamental aspects of metastasis. Amsterdam, North Holland Publ. Comp., pp. 275-289.
6. Cotino HH. 1974. Intra-arteriële infusie van de rattelever
   in vivo. Thesis Leiden.
7. Verbeek PCM. 1983. De waarde van locale toediening van
   kankerchemotherapeutica bij levermetastasen. Thesis Leiden.
8. Fisher B, Fisher ER. 1959. Experimental studies of factors
   influencing hepatic metastases. III Effect of surgical
   trauma with special reference to liver injury. Ann Surg
   150: 731.
9. Riccardi C, et al. 1980. In vivo natural reactivity of
   mice against tumor cells. Int J Cancer 25: 475.
10. Zoetmulder FAN. 1982. Modelstudies over het colorectale
    carcinoom. Thesis Leiden.
11. Velde CJH van de, Kothuis BJL, Barenbrug HWM, Tjaden UR.
    A successful technique of in vivo isolated chemotherapeu-
    tic liver perfusion in the pig with survival. J Surg Res
    (submitted for publication).
12. Pickren JW, et al. 1982. Liver metastases: Analysis of
    autopsy data. In: Weiss L, Gilbert HA, (eds.). Liver
    metastases. Boston, Hall Med. Publ., pp. 2-18.
13. DeVita Jr. V. 1983. The relationship between tumor mass
    and resistance to chemotherapy. Cancer 51: 1209.
14. Goldie JH Coldman AJ. 1979. A mathematical model for
    relating drug sensitivity of tumors to their spontaneous
    mutation rate. Cancer Treat Rep 63: 172
15. Zonnevylle JA. 1981. De invloed van cryochirurgie en
    electrocoagulatie op het metastaseringsproces. Thesis
    Leiden

NATURAL HISTORY OF LIVER METASTASES

CB WOOD

INTRODUCTION

The liver is a favourite site for metastatic spread from many cancers, particularly those of the gastrointestinal tract. Between 15 and 25 per cent of patients with primary tumours of the colon and rectum have liver metastases detected at the time of the initial presentation (1,2,3). In up to 30 per cent of patients, the presence of liver metastases remains undetected at the time of initial surgery and these become apparent during the postoperative period. In post-mortem studies, the incidence of liver metastases is even higher (4). The proportion of patients with liver metastases increases with progressive spread of the primary tumour (2).

There is no doubt that the presence of liver metastases carries a very dismal prognosis since few effective methods of treatment are available at the present time. The average survival time is approximately 6 months although there are occasional reports of long-term survivors. In general, most patients with untreated liver metastases are dead within two years from the time of diagnosis (5,6,3).

Although the overall picture is depressing, there are several factors which influence the overall prognosis. There is now considerable evidence to show that for patients with liver metastases, the survival pattern is related to the extent of secondary spread within the liver. The presence or absence of extrahepatic spread of tumour also influences prognosis. Furthermore, the management of the primary tumour has an important bearing on the outcome of the patients with hepatic metastases, and in recent years there have been some promising developments in the use of cytotoxic agents, admin-

istered in a variety of ways to the liver, and also the
increasing use of surgical techniques to treat liver metastases. It is worth while considering each of these factors in
more detail.

In a study of patients with primary tumours of the pancreas, biliary tract and stomach, as well as colon and rectum,
Jaffe et al (1968) found the median survival time of 136 days
for patients with solitary liver metastases, 93 days for
patients with tumour localised to one lobe of the liver, and
72 days for patients with widespread liver metastases (5).
Similarly, Nielsen, Balsley & Jensen (1971) reported a mean
survival rate of 18 months for patients with "few" liver
metastases compared with 9 months for those with "several"
metastases and only 5 months for patients with "multiple"
metastatic disease (7). In the retrospective study by the
author (3) of 110 patients with liver metastases at the time
of presentation with colorectal cancer, the one-year survival
rate was 5.7 per cent of patients with widespread liver metastases, but was 27 per cent for metastases localised to a
segment or lobe of the liver. As well as confirming that
survival related to the extent of metastatic spread within
the liver, this study also showed that the presence of extra-
hepatic metastases played a significant role in the influencing prognosis.

In patients with localised liver metastases, but with
evidence of tumour spread at other sites, the main survival
was 10.6 months with a 27 per cent one-year survival. However, in the same group of patients in whom the liver metastases were the sole evidence of metastatic spread, the
mean survival was 17 months and a 50 per cent one-year survival. The same pattern is seen in the group with solitary
liver metastases. Those patients with extrahepatic tumour
spread had a mean survival of 16.7 months and a 60 per cent
one-year survival. By comparison, those with solitary liver
metastases alone had a mean survival of 25 months and a 100
per cent one-year survival. Thus, the volume of tumour has
an important bearing on prognosis.

On the basis of this retrospective analysis, a detailed
prospective study was initiated in which 404 patients with
colorectal cancer seen in a 3-year period were assessed for
the extent of liver involvement of tumour. One hundred and
four patients had liver metastases at the time of initial
presentation. Of these, 15 (14%) had solitary metastases,
13 (13%) had metastases localised to a segment or lobe of
the liver, and 76 (73%) had widespread metastases. None of
these patients had specific treatment for their liver metastases. The 5-year survival figures show that all patients
with localised or widespread metastases were dead by 4 years,
most of them dying within the first 2-3 years. However, (16) ?
per cent of patients with solitary metastases were still
alive at 5 years. These results give confirmation that prognosis is related to the extent of liver involvement with
tumour and that the natural history of patients with solitary metastases is reasonably good in the short-term outlook.

The available evidence would suggest that removal of
the primary tumour will improve prognosis, as well as provide better palliation (6). In a prospective study of
patients with liver metastases from tumours in the colon and
rectum, 76 (75%) had metastases involving both lobes of the
liver. The one-year survival rate for patients who had
resection of the primary tumour was 32 per cent, but only 15
per cent of those in whom the primary lesion was not resected were alive at one year. Of course, other factors may
have influenced the decision to resect the primary tumour or
not. Nevertheless, the evidence is in favour of removal of
the primary tumour, performing a local excision or a sphinc-
ter-sparing procedure whenever possible, or possibly fulgura-
tion in more advanced cases (8).

Thus, there is ample evidence to show that several factors can influence the overall prognosis for patients with
liver metastases. The most encouraging results are obtained
in those patients with solitary metastatic disease of the
liver. Not only is the survival pattern much better in
these patients, compared to those with diffuse involvement

of the liver, but they are also potential candidates for hepatic resectional surgery provided there is no other evidence
of metastatic spread. In a collected review of the literature, Foster (1970) found a 5-year survival rate of 21 per
cent in patients undergoing liver resection for metastases
(9). For some years this 5 year survival rate remained the
standard reference point for the results of liver resection.
However, in 1976, Wolfson & Adson reported the results of the
Mayo Clinic experience (10); 60 patients who had resection
of hepatic metastases from colorectal cancer, with multiple
lesions being removed from 20 patients and solitary lesions
in the remaining 40. No patients who had resection of multiple secondary deposits were alive at 5 years. However, the
prospect for those with resection of apparently solitary
metastases was significantly better, with 5 and 10 year survival rates of 42 per cent and 28 per cent respectively.
Somewhat similar results were reported by Wanebo et al (1978)
who published their experience with 25 patients having resection of solitary liver metastases (8). In their group, 9
(36%) survived 4 years after resection compared with only 3
(17%) of 18 patients with unresected solitary metastases.
With these encouraging results, and a better understanding
of the detailed anatomy of the segments of the liver, hepatic
resection of secondary tumour is being performed with increasing frequency. It is not always necessary to excise
major segments or lobes of the liver since removal of a small
section of liver is sufficient if the metastases are located
peripherally. However, resection is only possible in between
5 and 10 per cent of all patients with liver metastases from
primary lesions in the large bowel. Thus, in routine surgical practice, one is unlikely to see a large number of
patients requiring such surgery. Nevertheless, in centres
with an understanding of the nuances in the surgical techniques and experience of the postoperative sequelae, liver
resection carries acceptable operative mortality (11,12) and
the long-term results are encouraging.

    Whereas liver resection has offered the possibility of

a long-term influence on prognosis, other methods of treatment, particularly for widespread liver metastases, have been singularly unimpressive. Cytotoxic agents have been administered in a variety of ways, either systemically or directly to liver via the hepatic artery or portal vein (13,14,15). Hepatic artery ligation, with or without chemotherapy has also been advocated (16,17). Many of these studies have claimed objective tumour regression and improved survival rates for the methods of treatment, although any improvement in survival has been shortlived.

It is absolutely essential, when considering these various forms of treatment, whether surgical resection or palliative therapy with cytotoxic agents, immunotherapy or radiotherapy, that the results be carefully compared with the natural history of the disease. Furthermore, the various factors mentioned above must also be taken into account before making any dramatic claim for the treatment modality. Thus, the results of the natural history of untreated liver metastases are vital to our better understanding of the disease process and for assessing and comparing with the various forms of treatment. It has been shown already that patients with solitary metastases have a much better outcome than patients with widespread metastases, so that a larger proportion with solitary lesions in any one treatment group would bias the results in favour of that group of patients. An attempt to relate the results of regional infusion chemotherapy to the extent of liver metastases was made by Cady & Oberfield in 1974 (14). Fifty-five patients with liver metastases had infusion with 5-Fluro-2-deoxyuridine (5-Fudr), via the hepatic artery. In the group with less than 25 per cent of the liver involved with secondary tumour, the median survival time was 16 months but the median survival time was only 8 months in those with 50 per cent or more of the liver involved with tumour. Thus, any comparative study of treatment regimens should randomise for the degree of liver involvement with tumour.

DETECTION

There is no doubt that the less the degree of liver involvement with tumour, the better is the prognosis and greater is the chance of improving palliation. Thus, the earliest possible detection of liver metastases is an admirable goal, although the techniques available for detection have, until recently, been rather disappointing. Liver function tests have the advantage of being easy to perform and can be done readily in all centres. However, liver function tests lack the sensitivity and specificity to be an accurate guide to the presence of secondary tumour in the liver.

Carcinoembryonic antigen (CEA) is a useful tumour marker for colorectal cancer and a recent concensus statement from the National Institute of Health (1982) concluded that CEA was the best currently available, non-invasive technique for postoperative surveillance of tumour recurrence after large bowel cancer surgery (18). Moertel et al (1978) have noted the deficiencies of the CEA assay, particularly in relation to detection of local tumour recurrence (19). However, the sensitivity of the CEA assay is much better in detection of liver metastases. In addition, there are two distinct patterns of CEA rise after apparently curative surgery: a fast rise associated with distant metastases and a slow rise, which was noted mainly in patients with local recurrence (20).

In addition to biochemical and immunological tests, there are also now available several means of scanning the liver. Of these, CT scanning appears to be the most reliable for detection of liver metastases. A recent study by Findlay et al (1982) compared the CEA assay and CT scanning and showed that CT imaging was far superior at detecting liver metastases than CEA and was able to detect disease at a much earlier stage (21). However, it is true to say that the two techniques are not strictly comparable since CEA is a non-specific screening agent whilst CT scanning gives a more direct view of the liver architecture.

With recent advances, such as NMR scanning and radiolabelled monoclonal antibodies, it is to be hoped that the early detection of liver metastases will become a standard part of tumour management and coupled with improvements in the therapeutic options, there should be an encouraging improvement in the prognosis of this condition.

REFERENCES

1. Bengmark S, Hafstrom L. 1969. The natural history of primary and secondary malignant tumours of the liver. Cancer 23: 198-202.
2. Morris MJ, Newland RC, Pheils MT, MacPherson JG. 1977. Hepatic metastases from colorectal carcinoma: An analysis of survival rates and histopathology. Australian and New Zealand Journal of Surgery 47: 365-368.
3. Wood CB, Gillis CR, Blumgart LH. 1976. A retrospective study of the natural history of patients with liver metastases from colorectal cancer. Clinical Oncology 2: 285-288.
4. Goligher JC. 1975. Surgery of the anus, rectum and colon, 3rd edn. Bailliere Tindall, London, p 505.
5. Jaffe BM, Donegan WL, Watson F, Spratt JS Jr. 1968. Factors influencing survival in patients with untreated hepatic metastases. Surgery, Gynecology and Obstetrics 127: 1-11.
6. Oxley EM, Ellis H. 1969. Prognosis of carcinoma of the large bowel in the presence of liver metastases. British Journal of Surgery 56: 149-152.
7. Nielsen J, Balsley I, Jensen HE. 1971. Carcinoma of the colon with liver metastases. Operative indications and prognosis. Acta Chirurgica Scandinavica 137: 463-465.
8. Wanebo HJ, Semoglou C, Attiyeh F, Stearns MJ Jr. 1978. Surgical management of patients with primary operable colorectal cancer and synchronous liver metastases. American Journal of Surgery 135: 81-85.
9. Foster JH. 1970. Survival after liver resection for cancer. Cancer 26: 493-502.
10. Wilson SM, Adson MA. 1976. Surgical treatment of hepatic metastases from colorectal cancers. Archives of Surgery 111: 330-334.
11. Adson MA, Sheedy PF. 1974. Resection of primary hepatic malignant lesions. Archives of Surgery 108: 599-603.
12. Blumgart LH, Drury JK, Wood CB. 1979. Hepatic resection for trauma, tumour and biliary obstruction. British Journal of Surgery 66: 762-769.
13. Watkins E Jr, Khazei AM, Nahra KS. 1970. Surgical basis for arterial infusion chemotherapy of disseminated carcinoma of the liver. Surgery, Gynecology and Obstetrics 130: 581-605.
14. Cady B, Oberfield RA. 1974. Regional infusion chemotherapy of hepatic metastases from carcinoma of the colon. American Journal of Surgery 127: 220-227.
15. Taylor I. 1978. Cytotoxic perfusion for colorectal liver metastases. British Journal of Surgery 65: 109-114.

Hughes Surgery Jan 1989 solitary mets (n=509) 37% 5yr survival

54

16. Murray-Lyon IM, Parsons VA, Blendis LM, Dawson JL, Rake MO, Laws JW, Williams R. 1970. Treatment of secondary hepatic tumours by ligation of hepatic artery and infusion of cytotoxic drugs. Lancet ii: 172-175.
17. Larmi TKI, Karkola P, Klintrup HE, Heikkinen E. 1974. Treatment of patients with hepatic tumours and jaundice by ligation of the hepatic artery. Archives of Surgery 108: 178-183.
18. National Health Concensus Statement 1982.
19. Moertell CG, Schutt AJ, Go VLW. 1978. Carcinoembryonic antigen test for recurrent colorectal carcinoma. Inadequacy for early detection. Journal of the American Medical Association 239: 1065-1066.
20. Findlay G. and McArdle CS. 1982. Incidence and detection of occult hepatic metastases in colorectal carcinoma. British Medical Journal 285: 211.
21. Wood CB, Blumgart LH, Gillis CR, Hole D and Malcolm AJ. 1981. Local tumour invasion as a prognostic factor in colorectal cancer. British Journal of Surgery 68: 326.

METHODS FOR PREVENTION OF METASTASES IN THE PERIOPERATIVE
PHASE

J. JEEKEL, TH. WIGGERS, R.L. MARQUET

In many patients with a malignant tumor dissemination of
cancer cells will already have taken place at the moment of
detection of the primary tumor. The primary tumor is usually
detected late in the disease, and it is questionable whether
the physician will be able to prevent further dissemination
just in the relatively short time from the moment of
detection until operation of the primary tumor. Methods for
prevention of metastases can only be applied successfully
when significant metastases develop in this short period.

The process of development of metastases is probably more
complex than the old concept of tumor spread from the primary
tumor, growing to a critical size, then orderly spreading
regionally and at last systemically. Much more it is a
process early in the development of the primary tumor, in
which dissemination is dependent upon characteristics of the
cancer cells and host tissue,according to the so-called seed
and soil theory (1). Seeding then is dependent upon the
number of cells in the lymphatic and venous pathways, the
structure of cancer cell membranes, the ability to produce
certain enzymes (2), and a number of factors in the host.
Especially immunological factors of the host may play an
important role.

Dissemination of cancer cells may not only be caused by
the primary tumor but also by metastasis itself. According
to the cascade theory, metastases in certain organs may themselves cause dissemination. In fact in a certain stage of
the disease tumor seedings may act functionally as primary

tumors and cause metastases.

The primary tumor itself may exert some influence on the growth of metastaes either by factors from the tumor which inhibit growth or suppress the immune system of the host (3, 4, 5, 6). Operation of the primary tumor certainly has a profound effect on the immune response of the patient as has been demonstrated with a variety of operations. Furthermore it is known that during operation considerable dissemination of tumor cells occurs which can be measured in peripheral veins and in the case of colo/rectal cancer in the portal vein (7). In as many as 50% of patients tumor cells can be demonstrated during operation versus 4% before operation. Before entering the circulation angio-invasive growth has to take place. Talbot (8) studied the angio-invasive growth in 703 colon cancers. He found a correlation between venous invasion of tumor cells and the percentage of liver metastases in the follow-up period. Thus it is possible that significant metastasis occurs during operation of the primary tumor. If this holds true, then special operation techniques might reduce the number of cancer cells dislodged during the operation. Furthermore immune stimulation of the host in the perioperative phase may improve the defense of the host against circulating tumor cells.

In this chapter we will describe a few methods in the perioperative phase that might reduce the incidence of metastases.

Perioperative procedures

As patients may experience marked immunosuppression during and shortly after operation, it may be important to stimulate the immune apparatus during this period. Routine perioperative treatment as for example with blood trans-fusions may also exert an influence on the immune response. It is well known from renal transplantation in man that blood transfusions have a profound positive influence on graft survival. The underlying mechanism is hitherto largely unknown. It can be expected that blood transfusions do have an effect on tumor growth and in fact this has been described by Tartter (11). We have investigated the effect of a single blood transfusion administered preoperatively on tumor growth in WAG rats. Two syngeneic tumors were used: a radiation-induced basal cell carcinoma of the skin (T1) and a chemically induced adenocarcinoma of the duodenum (T2).The T1 tumor exhibits strong immunogenic properties, the T2 is only weakly immunogenic. After subcutaneous implantation the doubling time of T1 appeared to be 2-5 days and of the adeno-carcinoma 14 days. Upon intravenous inoculation of isolated T1 cells lung nodules could be counted after 14 days. 7-14 days before tumor challenge 1 ml BN blood was injected intra-venously into WAG rats. Controls received syngeneic blood. The T1 tumor was administered either as a subcutaneous implantation of 2x 2 mm pieces or by intravenous injection of 10^5 tumor cells. The T2 tumor was implanted subcutaneous-ly only. Subcutaneous growth of tumor T1 was not significant-ly inhibited by the allogeneic blood transfusions in 8 animals, but a 50% reduction of lung nodules was observed 3 weeks after inoculation, which is significant ($p < 0.01$). Blood transfusion also evoked a strong inhibitory effect on the growth of subcutaneously implanted T2 tumor, tested with 8 animals in each experimental group. It thus appears that allogeneic blood transfusion can induce a significant reduction of tumor growth depending on tumor type and site of implantation.

Stimulation of the immune response may be undertaken before and after the operative procedure. We have embarked upon an experimental study towards the effect of interferon, and reported on the effect of partially purified rat interferon on the growth of a transplantable adenocarcinoma of the colon and liposarcoma in rats (10). Interferon treatment resulted in a significant reduction of tumor growth. Yet, more studies are needed to investigate prediction of responsiveness, timing and dosage and the effect of combination therapy of interferon with chemotherapy. The effectiveness of interferon in preventing metastases is still unknown.

Peroperative procedures

Accepting the concept that tumor spread occurs during operation by touching the tumor, which increases the number of cancer cells in lymphatic and venous pathways, R. Turnbull in 1967 devised a technique by which the tumor is not touched until the vascular pedicle of the colon segment with tumor has been ligated (9). He described in patients with Dukes C cancer a significant higher 5-year survival compared to historical controls. It is difficult though to conclude from this study that the no-touch isolation technique is valid, as the control group was historical and not comparable for various other reasons, one being the extent of resection. Yet, many clinicians have adopted the no-touch technique. Therefore we devised a prospective controlled trial to test the effect of the no-touch technique on the occurrence of metastases after operation. 236 patients entered the trial between 1979 until 1982. Patients with Dukes D tumor were excluded. The no-touch technique was executed in 117 patients and 119 patients were operated following the conventional technique. The essential difference between the two operations is the early ligation of the vascular pedicle and mesenterial structures in the no-touch technique whereas in the conventional technique the colon segment with the tumor is mobilised first. It appeared that significantly less liver metastases did occur in those patients with a sigmoid cancer operated by the no-touch technique (Table I).

Table I.   Number of liver metastases and
            site of primary tumor.

Localisation of tumor	No-touch	Conventional
right colon	4	5
transverse colon	2	2
sigmoid	3	10
rectosigmoid	5	5

The two groups were comparable for Dukes staging and other
aspects as sex and age. The Turnbull modification of Dukes
staging was used. In the no-touch group were 26 patients
with Dukes A,54 patients with Dukes B and 37 patients with
Dukes C. In the conventional group 30 patients had Dukes A
cancer, 53 patients Dukes B and 36 patients Dukes C. So far
14 liver metastases were detected in patients operated with
the no-touch technique and 22 liver metastases in the
conventional group. These results seem to indicate that a
significant process of tumor spread occurs during operation
which can be prevented by special operation techniques.
Other tumor recurrences occurred in 15 patients in the
no-touch group and 12 patients in those patients operated
in the conventional way. One would expect a more profound
effect of the no-touch technique in those patients with
tumors that show angio-invasive growth and hence have a
higher incidence and potential of tumor dissemination. Such
a relation between venous tumor invasion and patient's
survival has been described (8), and the 5-year survival
appeared to be 73% when a venous invasion was not present
and 33% when extramural veins were invaded. We have
investigated in the prospective trial whether the no-touch
operation was of special benefit in those patients with
angio-invasive tumor growth. In patients without angio-
invasive growing tumor, liver metastases and other
recurrences did not differ in the two experimental groups
(Table II).

Table II.   No angio-invasive growth.

	liver metastases	all recurrences
Conventional surgery	21.5%	30.7%
No-touch surgery	17.5%	30.2%

On the other hand a significant difference in the number of liver metastases was found when angio-invasive tumor growth was present; 33% of the patients in the conventional group developed liver metastases and 12% of the patients after the no-touch operation (Table III).

Table III.   Angio-invasive growth.

	liver metastases	all recurrences
Conventional surgery	33.3%	58.3%
No-touch surgery	12.0%	44.0%

These results do provide indirect proof for the theory that tumor spread during operation can induce metastases which can be prevented by relatively simple methods.

An alternative explanation is that the no-touch isolation technique did not prevent dissemination of cancer cells, but rather the spreading of certain factors from the primary tumor that do influence the growth of metastases already present in the liver. Experimental studies performed in the rat do support such a theory. We have investigated the effect of removal of the primary tumor on experimental metastasis in WAG rats bearing a transplantable isogeneic basal cell carcinoma. 20 rats were subcutaneously injected with basal cell carcinoma on day 0. On day 21 1×10^5 cancer cells were injected intravenously followed by excision of the subcutaneous tumor in the experimental group and by a sham operation in the control group on day 25.

The number of lung metastases provoked by intravenous injection of tumor cells was counted on day 35. In the 10 controls, 5-43 lung nodules were counted with a mean of 22 whereas 27-84 lung nodules were counted in the experimental group with a mean of 63, which is a significant difference ($p < 0.01$). Thus excision of the primary tumor did enhance the formation of lung metastases, suggesting that factors present in the primary tumor can influence tumor growth.

In summary there is evidence for significant occurrence of metastases in the perioperative period either by dissemination of cancer cells or by growth promoting factors. Efforts to reduce the number or growth of metastases during operation may be worthwhile and should be studied more extensively.

REFERENCES

1. Paget S. 1889. The distribution of secondary growth in cancer of the breast. Lancet i: 571-573.
2. Baldwin RW, Barker CR. 1967. Demonstration of tumour-specific humoral antibody against aminoazo dye-induced rat hepatoma. Br J Cancer 21: 793-801.
3. Kaplan HS, Murphy ED. 1949. The effect of local roentgen irradiation on the biological behavior of a transplantable murine carcinoma. I: Increased frequency of pulmonary metastases. J. Natl Cancer Inst (9): 407-413.
4. Schatten WE. 1958. An experimental study of postoperative tumor metastases. I: Growth of pulmonary metastases following total removal of primary leg tumor. Cancer (11): 455-459.
5. Gorelik E, Segal S, Feldman M. 1978. Growth of a local tumor exerts a specific inhibitory effect on progression of lung metastases. Int J Cancer (21): 617-625.
6. Gorelik E, Segal S, Feldman M. 1981. On the mechanism of tumor concomitant immunity. Int J Cancer (27): 847-856.
7. Griffiths JD, McKinna JA, Rowbotham HD, Tsolakidis P, Salsbury AJ. 1973. Carcinoma of the colon and rectum: circulating malignant cells and five-year survival. Cancer 31: 226-236.
8. Talbot IC, Ritchie S, Leighton MH, Hughes AO, Bussey HJR, Morson BC. 1980. The clinical significance of invasion of veins by rectal cancer. Br J Surg 67: 439-442.
9. Turnbull RB Jr, Kyle K, Watson FR, Spratt J. 1967. Cancer of the colon: the influence of the no-touch isolation technique on survival rates. Ann Surg 166: 420-427.

62

10. Marquet RL, Schellekens H, Dijkema R, Westbroek DL, Jeekel J, 1983. The biology of the interferon system. Elsevier Science Publishers B.V.
11. Tartter PI, Burrows L, Gruenstein S, Slater G, Papatestas AE. 1983. Early colon cancer recurrence is associated with perioperative blood transfusion. Suppl. J Exp Clin Cancer Res (2): 32-33.

DIAGNOSIS AND STAGING OF LIVER METASTASES

THE DETECTION OF LIVER METASTASES BY LABORATORY TESTS

M. MARGARET KEMENY, M.D.

1. INTRODUCTION

The early diagnosis and treatment of metastatic cancer to the liver remains one of the most challenging problems in clinical oncology. The liver is the major site of metastases for all the gastrointestinal malignancies and for many of the extra-abdominal cancers as well. With the advent of newer techniques for treatment of hepatic metastases such as implantable pumps for continuous regional perfusion and hepatic wedge resections, the need for early and accurate diagnosis of these lesions becomes more important. Clearly, imaging tests such as the computerized axial tomography (CAT) scans and probably NMR in the future, will help delineate the hepatic lesions in ways biochemical laboratory tests would fail. There still remains a need for biochemical tests that could predictably indicate the presence of hepatic metastases so that an imaging study could be used for correlation. Since biochemical tests can be done easily and frequently with no risk or major cost to the patient, they are more practical as screening tools than the imaging studies. There have been numerous reports on the use of various biochemical laboratory tests to detect hepatic metastases. Many scientific groups have been searching for the one test that will provide this information. However, as of this time there is no single test that stands above the others for detecting hepatic metastases. Basically, the conventional liver function tests with the addition of carcinoembryonic antigen (CEA) are still the most useful biochemical parameters for detecting hepatic metastases. This chapter will review studies on conventional liver function tests, the CEA and other biochemical liver parameters. The data re-emphasizes the strengths and failures of these tests and adds some new data to re-establish these points.

2. CONVENTIONAL BIOCHEMICAL LIVER FUNCTION TESTS

The conventional liver function tests that appear on the chemistry panels in most hospitals include alkaline phosphatase (AP), bilirubin (bili), lactic dehydrogenase (LDH), serum glutamic oxalacetic transaminase (SGOT) and serum glutamic pyruvic transaminase (SGPT). Many studies have been done to access the relative sensitivities and specificicities of these separate liver function tests.

In a NIH prospective analysis of laboratory tests done in 1982 to detect hepatic metastases, 80 patients with primary tumors were studied with standard liver function tests as well as carcinoembryonic antigen (CEA), leucine aminopeptidase (LAP), gamma-glutamyl transpeptidase (GGTP), 5' nucleotidase (5N) and alphafetoprotein (AFP). Serum bilirubin was dropped from evaluation because of the very low number of abnormal values in patients with liver metastases. If one considered the accuracy of the tests – that is the number of tests that correctly identified the presence or absence of a metastasis divided by the total number of tests – SGPT and LDH were the most accurate at 65 and 64% respectively. AP had a 63% accuracy with SGOT at 61%. None of these differences were statistically significant. If two of the tests were combined the

sensitivity (true positive ratio) would rise but the
specificity (true negative ratio) would become worse, and
overall the accuracy decreased. Thus, LDH and AP together
had an accuracy of 61% for detecting liver metastases while
the accuracy of LDH alone was 64%. The conclusions of this
study were that the conventional biochemical liver function
tests were not significantly different from one another and
that they were moderately, but not extremely sensitive to
the presence of hepatic metastatic disease[1].

In a study done in 1963 of 159 patients who died of
cancer, the ability of several liver function tests to
determine the presence of liver metastases was evaluated.
The bili, AP, bromsulphathalein retention (BSP), SGOT and
other examinations which have become obsolete were included.
All patients had laboratory tests drawn within two weeks of
their death and all had autopsies. The AP was the most
reliable test with a sensivity of 54% and an accuracy of
72%[2]. In a more recent study from France, AP, GGTP, LDH,
SGOT and SGPT were compared in 116 patients with known
gastrointestinal cancer. Again the AP had the highest
sensitivity (73%) and specificity (90%)[3]. Other reports
have had similar results such as a 1972 study comparing AP,
SGOT, SGPT and bili where AP was the most accurate
(sensitivity 58% and specificity 89.2%)[4]. A retrospective
study done in 1979 determined the usefulness of AP in
detecting hepatic metastases in patients with metastatic
breast cancer. In this study all patients with abnormal
liver scans, who went on to have deteriorating hepatic
function had abnormal AP at the time of the study. They
concluded that AP was a good indicator of liver metastases
in breast cancer patients[5]. A study done in 1982 compared
biochemical liver function tests (AP, SGOT, LDH, bili) to

TABLE I
ALKALINE PHOSPHATASE

AUTHOR	YEAR	TYPE OF STUDY	SENSITIVITY	SPECIFICITY	ACCURACY
Yesner	1963	Autopsy	$\frac{40}{74}$ 54%	$\frac{66}{73}$ 85%	$\frac{85}{106}$ 72%
Huguier	1981	Prospective	NG*73%	NG 90%	NG
Castagna	1972	Retrospective	$\frac{29}{50}$ 58%	$\frac{45}{51}$ 88.2%	NG
Rutenburg	1963	Retrospective	$\frac{99}{158}$ 63%	NG	NG
Tartter	1980	Retrospective	$\frac{43}{56}$ 77%	$\frac{217}{327}$ 66%	NG
Sugarbaker	1977	Retrospective	NG 71%	NG 60%	NG
Cederqvist	1972	Retrospective	$\frac{20}{69}$ 29%	$\frac{221}{243}$ 91%	77%
Tempero	1982	Retrospective	$\frac{35}{44}$ 80%	NG	NG
Kemeny	1982	Prospective	$\frac{15}{32}$ 47%	$\frac{35}{47}$ 74%	$\frac{50}{79}$ 63%

*NG = Not given

liver scans. The biochemical tests taken together were more sensitive than the liver scans (85% vs 65%). However, the accuracies of the biochemical tests and the liver scan were equivalent(73% vs 74%). The LDH and AP were the most sensitive of the tests (84 and 80% respectively)[6].

Two other studies concentrated on liver metastases from breast cancer or gastric cancer. The report on patients with gastric cancer and liver metastases was out of Denmark in 1972, and compared the five standard liver function tests. The sensitivity of all the tests were quite low. LDH was most sensitive at 32% (8/25), SGOT 30% (15/50), AP 29% (20/69) and SGPT 12% (3/25). Overall accuracy was higher at 75%, 77%, 77% and 79% respectively[7]. The study by Sugarbaker et al., on breast cancer metastatic to the liver, compared AP, LDH and SGOT. SGOT and LDH were more sensitive at 74% with AP at 71%, but AP was more specific at 60%, LDH 42% and SGOT 69% [8]. (Table I)

In a recent study at the City of Hope National Medical Center (unpublished), we have investigated the usefulness of the liver function tests to detect the presence of liver metastases and the extent of these metastases. Sixty patients were entered on a prospective protocol for the treatment of hepatic metastases. All had hepatic metastases proven pathologically at laparotomy. All patients had a full liver chemistry panel and a CEA level drawn before laparotomy. The results of the data revealed that SGOT, SGPT, bilirubin and prothrombin time were not diagnostic of liver metastases. The three tests that did change significantly from normal were the AP, LDH and CEA.

The median level of the LDH was 271 IU/L (normal levels of LDH are within 108-225 IU/L) with a sensitivity of 58%. The median level of CEA was 91 (normal level of CEA is less than 2.5 ng/ml) with a sensitivity of 83%. The AP had a

median level of 122 IU/L (normal levels 45-110 IU/L) with a
sensitivity of 61%.

**PREOPERATIVE LEVELS OF AP, LDH AND CEA IN 60 PATIENTS
WITH HEPATIC METASTASES FROM COLORECTAL CANCER**

	CEA <2.5ng/ml	LDH 108-222IU/L	AP 45-110IU/L
All Patients (Median)	91	271	122
Resectable Patients (Median)	56	207	103
Unresectable Patients (Median)	287	339	150

The group of 60 patients were divided within the
protocol by the amount of disease in their liver. Those
with less disease were in what was called the "resectable"
group, and those with more disease were in the unresectable
group. The last group were those patients with metastatic
disease outside the liver, as well as liver metastases.

In the "resectable" group the median AP was 103 with 9
of 22 (41%) patients having values above normal. The median
CEA was 56 with 17 of 22 (77%) having abnormal levels. The
median LDH was 207 IU/L with a sensitivity of 27%. Only
three patients in this group had all three values elevated
(13%), while 86% had either AP or CEA elevated, 81% had
either LDH or CEA elevated, and 50% had either AP or LDH
elevated. Twenty out of 22 patients had one of the three
values elevated.

In those patients with more hepatic disease the median
value of AP went up to 150, with 19 out of 26 (73%) patients

having abnormal values. The median value of the CEA was 287 with 23 out of 26 (88%) having elevated values. The median level of the LDH was 339 with 19 out of 26 (73%) having elevated levels. Fourteen of the 26 patients had either the AP or the CEA elevated, twenty-five of the 26 had either the LDH or the CEA elevated, (96%) and 22 of the 26 had either the AP or LDH elevated (85%). All of the patients had one value elevated. The mean values of the AP, LDH and CEA for the unresectable group were 313, 685 and 1858 respectively. These were all significantly higher than the values for the resectable group. (135, 224 and 6). Figure 1 is a three dimensional graphic depiction of the differences in levels of AP, LDH and CEA in the resectable and non resectable groups.

In the third group patients had both liver metastases and extrahepatic metastases. In this group of 13 patients one patient had normal values for LDH, AP and CEA. The other twelve patients all had at least two abnormal values. The mean values for the three tests were not as high in this group as in those patients with "unresectable" liver disease.

SENSITIVITY OF AP, LDH AND CEA IN 60 PATIENTS WITH HEPATIC METASTASES FROM COLORECTAL CANCER

SENSITIVITY	CEA	LDH	AP
All Patients	83%	58%	61%
Resectable Patients	77%	27%	41%
Unresectable Patients	88%	73%	73%

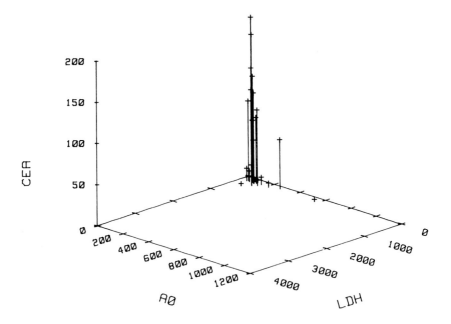

RESECTABLE LIVER METASTASES

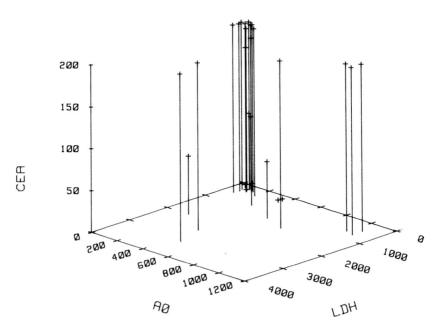

NON-RESECTABLE LIVER METASTASES

In summary, there is no one biochemical liver function test in the conventional screening panels that is significantly superior to the others. It does seem, however, that AP and LDH are more useful than SGOT, SGPT and bilirubin. However, the accuracy of these two tests is not high enough to be useful as screening tests for liver metastases. The greater the intrahepatic spread of the metastases the more likely the abnormality of these biochemical tests.

3. OTHER BIOCHEMICAL LIVER FUNCTION TESTS

There are several other biochemical tests which have been thought to be more specific than the standard liver function tests for detecting liver metastases. These include gamma glutamyl transpeptidase (GGTP), leucine aminopeptidase (LAP) and 5' nucleotidase (5N). In our study from the NIH these liver function tests were studied along with the standard biochemical tests. The GGTP was the most sensitive at 69%, with LAP at 31% and 5N at 28%. The specificities were reversed with 5N at 77%, LAP at 76 and GGTP at 45. The overall accuracies were 53% for GGTP, 57% for LAP and 5N. None of these three tests were superior to the standard biochemical liver function tests.

A study in 1961 compared LAP, 5N, and AP in patients with metastasic carcinoma to the liver. Of the 36 patients with metastases 32 had elevations of LAP and 34 had elevations in 5N and AP. This difference was not significant[9]. A more recent study compared AP and GGTP for detecting liver metastases. The sensitivities were respectively 42% and 47%. No significant difference was found between the two tests[3]. An earlier study of the same two enzymes drew the same negative conclusions[10].

Another study compared LAP and AP in 158 patients with liver metastases. Eighty-two percent had an elevated LAP and 63% had an elevated AP. The authors concluded LAP was a more sensitive test than AP for detecting liver metastases[11].

In a study from Scotland, serum enzymes were evaluated in patients with colorectal carcinoma. LDH, AP, GGTP, and 5N were compared and again the differences were not significant. The sensitivities of the tests all ranged from 42 to 58%[12].

Taking all the reports into account, it again seems clear that no one biochemical test is far superior to any other and that none of the tests are good screening tools for detecting patients with liver metastases.

4. AFP

Alphafetoprotein (AFP) is a protein that is normally found in the serum of newborns and fetuses, while it is absent or below 10 ng/ml in the serum of the normal adult. In 1963, AFP was discovered in mouse hepatomas and in human hepatocellular carcinomas. In 1965, Tatarinov found AFP in the serum of patients with hepatocellular carcinoma[13]. Further studies of patients with various liver diseases indicated that AFP was specific for hepatocellular carcinomas, and it did not rise in patients with cholangio-carcinoma or cirrhosis. Again, as with CEA, a radio-immunoassay made AFP a useful and sensitive test for the presence of hepatocellular carcinoma. However, as further studies were completed, it was clear that not all cases of hepatocellular carcinoma had elevated AFP and that some other tumors did produce AFP (embryonal and teratocarcinoma, lung, colon, stomach and pancreatic cancers)[14]. Also, the AFP levels were effected by the geographic location of the hepatoma patients - 80% of Africans with hepatomas had elevated AFP levels while only 30% of Americans with hepatomas had elevated AFP values[14].

An NIH study of AFP levels in over 400 patients with gastrointestinal carcinomas was done in 1945. Elevated AFP levels were seen in 24% of the 45 patients with pancreatic cancer, 25% of the 8 patients with biliary tract cancer, 15% of the 95 patients with gastric cancer, 3% of the 191 patients with colon cancer, none of the 14 patients with esophageal or small bowel cancer and 70% of the 73 patients with primary liver cancer. Thus, there was a degree of non specificity of the AFP levels, although the highest rate of correlation was still seen in the hepatocellular carcinoma. This study also explored the metastatic involvement of the liver in these patients with increased AFP levels. In the 14 patients with gastric carcinoma and elevated AFP levels, 8 had liver metastases (57%); 3 of the 5 patients with colon carcinoma had liver metastases. From this study it could be concluded that only small percentages of patients with carcinomas other than hepatocellular cancer will have elevated AFP levels, and that somewhere between 50-75% of these patients will have liver metastases; so that aside from   patients with hepatocellular carcinoma the serum AFP was not a good test of hepatic metastases in patients with carcinoma[15]. These conclusions are supported by our study from the NIH which was a prospective analysis of laboratory tests including AFP to detect hepatic lesions. Two abnormal values of AFP were recorded from the entire group of 80 patients with malignances. Thus, AFP was not even evaluated as a parameter for hepatic metastases because of its obvious poor correlation with any metastatic disease[1].

5. CEA

In 1965 carcinoembryonic antigen (CEA) was first
demonstrated in extracts from cancer of the colon by Gold
and Freedman. Since then it has been widely studied as the
hoped for tumor marker that could predict the presence of,
if not all cancers, at least colon cancers. A radioimmune-
assay was developed that was sensitive enough to pick up
levels below 1 nanogram per milliliter. The plasma
concentration of 0-2.5 ng/ml was considered to be the normal
range in 97% of the healthy non smoking population[16].
However, it soon became clear that not all colon cancers
produced CEA, and that there were numerous benign conditions
that caused elevations of CEA.

Because CEA was not elevated in all patients with colon
cancer its promise as the screening indicator for colon
carcinoma never materialized. In fact, in a 1982 review of
collected cases of CEA levels in patients with carcinoma, it
was clear that in localized carcinoma CEA was often within
normal limits. In over 1,000 cases of localized colon
cancer, 77% had normal CEA levels between 0 - 5 ng/ml.
However, in patients with metastatic colon cancer only 16%
had normal levels of CEA. The picture with gastric cancer
was similar with normal CEA levels in 72% of patients with
localized cancer and 21% of patients with metastatic
disease. Eighty-five percent of patients with localized
breast cancer and 44% of patients with localized pancreatic
cancer had normal CEA values, while only 28% of patients
with metastatic breast cancer and 22% of patients with
metastatic pancreatic cancer had normal values[17].
(Table II) These figures all pointed to the fact that CEA
was not a perfect screening tool. However, it might be more
useful at assessing metastatic disease.

The specific ability of CEA to detect liver metastases

TABLE II

CEA LEVELS IN PATIENTS WITH LOCALIZED OR METASTATIC CANCER*

CEA Level ng/ml	Colorectal Cancer		Gastric Cancer		Pancreatic Cancer		Breast Cancer	
	Localized	Metastatic	Localized	Metastatic	Localized	Metastatic	Localized	Metastatic
	(n=1081)	(n=205)	(n=43)	(n=43)	(n=78)	(n=119)	(n=604)	(n=575)
0-5	77%	16%	72%	21%	44%	22%	85%	28%
> 5	23%	84%	28%	79%	56%	78%	22%	72%

*From Beatty J.D., and Terz J.J., Value of Carcinoembryonic Antigen in Clinical Medicine

has been studied by many groups including our own. A recent
study from Scotland looked at the value of CEA in detecting
asymptomatic disseminated colorectal cancer. Of 50 patients
followed, 13 developed liver metastases. Eight of these
patients had an elevated CEA level prior to death. Thus,
38% had false negative CEA values[18]. The limited extent
of the hepatic metastases may have had an impact on this
high false negative figure.

A double blind study by McCartney and Hoffer in 1976
was directed at assessing the value of CEA and liver scans
for detecting hepatic metastases. Thirty-two of the 57
patients with liver metastases (56%) had elevated CEA levels
(i.e. levels greater than 9 ng/ml). Of the eighteen
patients who had elevated CEA levels, but no liver
metastases, 14 had cancer elsewhere[19]. All of the
patients with positive liver scans and elevated CEA values
had liver metastases. Thus, these authors concluded that
CEA should be used in conjunction with a liver scan for
more accurate hepatic metastatic evaluations.

In a study from Memorial Hospital by Wanebo et. al.,
358 patients with colorectal cancer were evaluated with
preoperative CEA levels. Of the 31 patients with Duke's D
disease, 65% had elevated CEA levels, while elevated levels
were seen in only 44% of patients with Duke's C disease, 25%
of patients with Duke's B disease and 49% of patients with
Duke's A disease. Most of the patients with Duke's D
disease had liver metastases (exact number is not given).
The study goes on to follow 155 patients with CEA levels
after their primary surgery. Of the 52 patients who then
developed liver metastases, 92% had CEA values above 5
ng/ml[20]. A more recent study from Mt. Sinai
compared CEA and alkaline phosphatase values as screening
parameters for liver metastases from colorectal primary

tumors. Twenty-one of the twenty-six patients with liver metastases had elevated CEA levels (greater than 5 ng/ml), a sensitivity of 81%. There were 46 (24%) false positive values in the 190 patients with no liver metastases[21].

Minton and Martin have published many reports on the use of CEA as an indicator of tumor recurrence. In their prospective study, 18 patients had second look procedures because of elevated CEA values, with 4 patients having liver metastases. Their conclusion was that patients with elevated CEA values who have had previous colon resections should have second look laparotomies. They did not address the sensitivity of the laboratory test to detect metastases[22].

A study done in Poland in 1981 reviewed 340 patients with colorectal carcinoma. Ninety of these patients developed liver metastases which were divided into four stages: 1. metastases in one lobe with less than 50% of the liver involved; II. metastases in both lobes with less than 50% of the liver involved; III. metastases in one or both lobes with more than 50% of the liver involved. IV. liver metastases plus intra-abdominal spread to lymph nodes, peritoneum, extra-abdominal metastases, or a non-resectable colonic lesion. Sixty-six of the 90 patients with liver metastases had plasma CEA levels drawn, and 49 (74%) had elevated values. They also reported that the levels of CEA directly correlated with the stage of liver involvement[23].

A study by Sugarbaker, et. al., concentrated on levels of CEA in metastatic breast cancer. When hepatic metastases were present 76% of the patients had an elevated CEA value, while only 25% of the patients with no metastases had a falsely elevated CEA. In this study the levels of CEA were more sensitive than alkaline phosphatase levels (71% true positive) and more specific (40% false positive)[8].

In our study from the NIH, which was a prospective analysis of the ability of laboratory tests to detect hepatic lesions in patients with malignancies, CEA was the most sensitive single test at 70% (16/23). All these patients had levels above 2.5 ng/ml. The specificity of CEA was much lower, with 17 normal values of CEA in the 32 patients without liver metastases. If those patients with colorectal primary tumors were analyzed separately the sensitivity of the CEA was up to 86% with a specificity of 60% and an accuracy of 79%. For these patients the CEA was the single most accurate test[1].

CEA LEVELS IN PATIENTS WITH LIVER METASTASES

		Elevated CEA	(>2.5ng/ml)
Finlay	1982	8/13	62%
McCartney	1976	32/57*	56%
Wanebo	1978	48/52**	92%
Tartter	1980	21/26**	81%
Szymendera	1982	49/67	73%
Sugarbaker	1977	22/29	76%
Kemeny	1982	16/23	70%

*CEA > 9 ng/ml
**CEA > 5 ng/ml

In the study completed at the City of Hope, only patients with colorectal cancer and liver metastases seen on previous laparotomy, CAT scan or liver scan were evaluated. All sixty-one of the patients had biopsy proven metastases on laparotomy. Fifty-one patients (83%) had CEA levels above 2.5 ng/ml. The median value for the group was 91 ng/ml. These patients were divided into three groups according to the extent of their metastases with Group I being resectable disease. Group II had unresectable hepatic disease and Group III had hepatic disease of any extent with extra hepatic metastases. Of the 22 patients in Group I, 17 (77%) had levels of CEA greater than 2.5 ng/ml and the median CEA value was 56 ng/ml. In group II, patients with unresectable disease, 23 of the 26 patients (88%) had CEA values of greater than 2.5 ng/ml with a median level of 287 ng/ml. In Group III, 11 of 13 patients (85%) patients had elevated CEA levels with a median value of 35 ng/ml.

In summary, of all these reports, CEA seems to be one of the most sensitive indicators of hepatic metastases, especially in patients with colorectal carcinoma. However, patients can be found with extensive hepatic disease who do not have abnormal CEA levels. Also, the level of CEA seems to be higher in patients with more extensive disease, but again a very high CEA does not definitely signify the size or extent of liver metastases.

CONCLUSION:

Conventional laboratory liver function tests including AP,LDH, SGOT, SGPT are accurate in the range of 60% for detecting liver metastases. AP and LDH have been shown to be superior in some studies, however, no one test is significantly superior to the others in repeated studies.

AFP is useful for detection of hepatocellular carcinoma but not useful to detect hepatic metastases from other primary carcinomas.

CEA is the most accurate laboratory test for detecting liver metastases in patients with colorectal primaries. In patients with liver metastases from other primaries CEA is no more useful than AP.

In new studies done at the City of Hope, the levels of AP, CEA and LDH were shown to increase significantly as the amount of hepatic disease increased.

In summary, the standard liver function tests and the CEA are the mainstay of the diagnostic armamentarium for detection of hepatic metastatic disease.

REFERENCES

1. Kemeny MM, Sugarbaker PH, Smith TJ, Edwards BK, Shawker T, Vermess M, Jones AE. 1982. A prospective analysis of laboratory tests and imaging studies to detect hepatic lesions. Ann Surg 195; 163-167.

2. Yesner R, Conn HO. 1963. Liver function tests and needle biopsy in the diagnosis of metastatic cancer of the liver. Ann Intern Med 59; 62-73.

3. Huguier M, Lacaine F. 1981. Hepatic metastases in gastrointestinal cancer. Arch Surg 116; 399-401.

4. Castagna J, Benfield JR, Yamada H, Johnson DE. 1972. The reliability of liver scans and function tests in detecting metastases. Surgery, Gyn and Obst 134; 463-466.

5. White DR, Maloney JJ, Muss HB, Vance RP, Barnes P, Howard V, Rhyne L, Cowan RJ. 1979. Serum alkaline phosphatase determination. JAMA 242; 1147-1149.

6. Tempero MA, Petersen RJ, Zetterman RK, Lemon HM, Gurney J. 1982. Detection of liver metastatic liver disease. JAMA 248; 1329-1332.

7. Cederqvist, C and Nielsen J. 1972. Value of liver function tests in the diagnosis of hepatic metastases in patients with gastric cancer. 1972. Acta Chir Scand 138; 604-608.

8. Sugarbaker PH, Beard JO, Drum DE. 1977. Detection of hepatic metastases from cancer of the breast. Am J Surg 133; 531-534.

9. Kowlessar OD, Haeffner LJ, Riley EM, Sleisenger MH. 1961. Comparative study of serum leucine aminopeptidase 5-nucleotidase and non-specific alkaline phosphatase in diseases affecting the pancreas, hepatobiliary tree and bones. Am Jour Med 31; 231-237.

10. Baden H, Andersen B, Augustenborg G, Hanel HK. 1971. Diagnostic value of gamma-glutamyl transpeptidase and alkaline phosphatase in liver metastases. Surg, Gyn & Obstet 133; 769-773.

11. Rutenburg AM, Banks BM, Pineda EP, Goldbarg JA. 1964. A comparison of serum aminopeptidase and alkaline phosphatase in the detection of hepatobiliary disease in anicteric patients. Ann Intern Med 61; 50-55.

12. Beck PR, Belfield A, Spooner RJ, Blumgart LH, Wood CB. 1979. Serum enzymes in colorectal cancer. Cancer 43; 1772-1776.

13. Tatarinov YS. 1979. Fetoprotein in the laboratory testing for cancer. Gann 70; 133-139.

14. Sugarbaker PH, Dunnick NR, Sugarbaker EV. 1982. Diagnosis and staging in Principles and Practice of Oncology. J.B. Lippincott Company, Philadelphia.

15. McIntire KR, Waldmann TA, Moertel CG, Go VLW. 1975. Serum fetoprotein in patients with neoplasms of the gastrointestinal tract. Cancer Research 35; 991-996.

16. Shively JE, Beatty JD. Carcinoembryonic antigen - related antigens molecular biology and clinical significance. (In Print) CRC Press, Boca Ratan, Florida.

17. Beatty, JD, Terz JJ. 1982. Value of carcinoembryonic antigen in clinical medicine. Progress in Clinical Cancer, Vol VIII.

18. Finlay IG, McArdle CS. 1983. Role of carcinoembryonic antigen in detection of asymptomatic disseminated disease in colorectal carcinoma. Br Med J 286; 1242-1244.

19. McCartney WH, Hoffer PB. 1976. Carcinoembryonic antigen assay in hepatic metastases detection. JAMA 236; 1023-1027.

20. Wanebo JH, Rao B, Pinsky CM, Hoffman RG, Stearns M, Schwartz MK, Oettgen H. 1978. Preoperative carcino-embryonic antigen level as a prognostic indicator in colorectal cancer. New Eng Jr Med 299; 448-451.

21. Tartter PI, Slater G, Gelernt I, Aufses AH. 1981. Screening for liver metastases from colorectal cancer with carcinoembryonic antigen and alkaline phosphatase. Ann Surg 193; 357-360.

22. Minton JP, Martin EW. 1978. The use of serial CEA determinations to predict recurrence of colon cancer and when to do a second-look operation. Cancer 42: 1422-1427.

23. Szymednera JJ, Wilczynska JE, Nowacki MP, Kaminska JA, Szawlowski AW. 1982. Serial CEA assays and liver scintigraphy for the detection of hepatic metastases from colorectal carcinoma. Dis Col & Rect 25:191-197.

RADIONUCLIDE IMAGING FOR THE DETECTION OF LIVER METASTASES

V. RALPH MCCREADY & ERNEST K.J. PAUWELS

1. INTRODUCTION

The diagnosis of early metastatic involvement of the liver remains one of the most difficult problems of diagnosis by imaging techniques. Although the newer physical techniques of ultrasound, CT and NMR have offered great promise, in fact they all suffer inherent limitations which result in a significant percentage of tumours not being detected. Fundamentally the ability to detect small lesions relies upon good contrast between the abnormality and the surrounding normal tissue. In the case of radionuclide imaging the contrast is rather low because the abnormality (without radioactivity) is surrounded by normal uptake of radionuclide by the reticulo endothelial system. This limits the smallest lesion detectable to about 2 cm superficially and of the order of 5 cm at depth. Ultrasound inherently has high resolution but apart from the fact that it is often difficult to image the total volume of liver tissue, contrast between tumour and surrounding normal parenchyma is often low making the confident diagnosis of tumours difficult. Similar arguments apply to CT scanning and possibly in the future to NMR imaging. In both ultrasound and CT various techniques have been suggested to improve the contrast but as with isotope imaging it is usually the appearance of the normal tissue which is enhanced. Thus none of the currently available techniques offer 100% diagnostic rate. Radionuclide imaging has the advantage of being easy to carry out, atraumatic to the patient and relatively inexpensive. It therefore still holds the first position in most diagnostic staging protocols, the more sophisticated and time consuming tests being carried out should the initial scan be otherwise than totally normal in appearance.

2. PLANAR LIVER SCINTIGRAPHY

Planar liver scintigrams are taken 20 minutes following the injection of approximately 40-80 MBq of Technetium 99m labelled colloid. Images are usually taken erect although the decrease in liver movement does not improve accuracy (Harauz & Bronskill, 1979). The uptake in normal liver parenchyma is related to the relative blood flow between liver, spleen and bone marrow and to the size of the colloid. The rate and degree of uptake is altered by the presence of space occupying lesions or diffuse disease (Geslien, Pinsky et al, 1976) redistributing the colloid to the spleen and bone marrow. However, before using this feature as a diagnostic aid it is necessary to know the normal distribution of the colloid of the particular radiopharmaceutical being employed (Adams, Horton, Selim, 1980).

All types of space occupying lesions within the liver produce similar appearances. The appearances therefore give little clue to the differential diagnosis. Single lesions are more likely to be abscesses or haemangiomas (Front, Royal et al, 1981; Engel, Marks et al, 1983). Since the latter can mimic metastases labelled red cells with tomography are useful in confirming the vascular nature of the lesion. Multiple lesions favour a diagnosis of metastases although polycystic disease should be excluded by ultrasound where the cysts have a characteristic appearance. Attempts have been made to use other radiopharmaceuticals to differentiate between neoplastic and other diseases. Gallium 67 has proved useful in confirming neoplastic involvement of the liver (Kew, Geddes & Levin, 1974) and has been of particular value in finding hepatomas in patients with cirrhosis and for differentiating cystic from solid disease. False positive scans have been reported (Douglas, Zambartas et al, 1981). Care has to be taken since it also is taken up in both bacterial and fungal abscesses (Errasti, Gomez-Escolar et al, 1981). Some workers have found images of the vascularity of lesions a valuable aid to diagnosis (Stadalnik, DeNardo et al, 1975). The inclusion of this technique in liver examinations has been found to raise space occupying lesion detection from 85% to 100% in one series (Sarper, Fajman et al, 1981). Using a similar approach but carrying out vascular and gallium 67 studies in addition to colloid imaging has been shown to provide more information regarding etiology of liver disease (Muller-Brand, Benz et al, 1977), although it must be remembered that when ultrasound is available it gives a quicker and more accurate diagnosis. Anecdotally particular tumours have shown increased concentration of colloid (in hepatomas), of bone imaging agents (in liver tumours) (Stevens & Clark, 1977; Garcia, Yeh & Benua, 1977; Ghaed & Marsden, 1978) and pyridoxylidene compounds (in hepatomas) (Ueno & Haseda, 1980; Utz, Lull et al, 1980). However images taken with ^{99m}Tc-HIDA alone have proved to be no more accurate than those with colloids (Schulze, Stritzke & Stolzenbach, 1981). The combination of the two however has successfully diagnosed Caroli's disease (Georgio, Alevizaki & Proukakis, 1983) preoperatively.

2.1 Accuracy of liver scintigraphy

The difficulty in determining the accuracy of liver scintigraphy or any other test lies in the problem of confirming the presence or absence of liver involvement. Series quoting accuracies often rely on clinical follow up, which has been shown to be inaccurate since tumour doubling times have a wide variation. Biopsies can miss lesions due to the random sampling nature. Laparotomy has also been shown to be inefficient, missing deep lesions (Goligher, 1941). Even palpation at post mortem has been shown to miss more than 10% of lesions found when the liver is sectioned (Ozarda & Pickren, 1962). In this situation all figures of sensitivity are open to doubt. However typical of the figures quoted are 77.3% accuracy (Lunia, Parthasarathy et al, 1975), confirmed by laparotomy, biopsy and autopsy within 40 days of imaging. In another series with short interval autopsy 81% of liver involved by metastases were correctly diagnosed with a 15% false positive and 21% false negative rate (Ostfeld & Meyer, 1981). The accuracy of detection relates to the types of disease. Gut secondaries from gut neoplasms tend to be single, well defined and more easily seen. In such situations up to 88% of lesions from colonic carcinoma have been identified (Drum & Beard, 1976) while only 67% of metastases from breast carcinoma were detected. However when other criteria such as liver size and irregularity of colloid distribution are included the sensitivity has increased to 90% (Galli, Maini et al, 1982).

In series which compare radioisotope imaging with other techniques the relative accuracy of isotope imaging is sometimes higher, sometimes lower (Biello, Levitt et al, 1978; Grossman, Wistow et al, 1977).

Overall in the routine clinical situation there is probably little to choose although when the tumours are visible, ultrasound and CT imaging have the advantage of giving a more accurate differential diagnosis.

3. NEW DEVELOPMENTS

The accuracy and differential diagnosis of metastatic liver lesions using radionuclide methods is likely to improve over the next few years. While the resolution of planar imaging devices has probably reached its maximum, new developments in single photon emission computerised tomography and positron emission tomography are likely to increase the detail produced on the diagnostic images. This is basically due to the improved contrast between the "cold" lesion and the surrounding normal tissue found when tomography is used. Recently substantial progress has been made in developing tumour specific radiopharmaceuticals. Current results indicate that new developments in radiolabelled antibodies should enable radioactivity to be concentrated in the tumour rather than the normal surrounding tissue. The improved contrast found in this situation greatly improves the resolution increasing the chances of detecting small lesions deep inside the liver.

3.1. Single photon emission computerised tomography

This technique can be employed with many current routine imaging systems and technetium 99m labelled colloids. The detector is rotated around the patient taking a series of images which can then be reconstructed to produce cross sectional distributions of radioactivity. The quality of the end image depends upon the time spent in accumulating counts, the number of angles, the type of filter and the method of reconstruction. It can be difficult to differentiate between small metastases and the mottle produced by the reconstruction technique. Filtering smoothes the image but decreases the resolution. However with experience interpretation becomes easier. There no doubt that the tomographic technique detects smaller lesions and in addition gives positional information. However even with the extra information it can be difficult to differentiate between normal vascular and other anatomical structures and space occupying lesions. The addition of SPECT to planar imaging improves the accuracy of diagnosis and at least one series has shown the accuracy of detection to be comparable with that of CT.

3.2 Positron emission tomography

Up until now PET has been used mainly for metabolic studies generally limited to those involving the brain. However two factors are likely to change this situation. The Gelenium 68/Gallium 68 generator with a half life of 275 days enables the production of positron emitting radionuclides distant from cyclotron facilities. Gallium 68 can be made into a colloidal preparation which will localise in the liver (Kumar, Miller et al, 1981). Cheaper detectors are now being used in clinical trials (Ott, Bateman et al, 1983). These devices can be used either for tomography or for planar imaging. In either case the results should be much better than those obtained from low energy single photon techniques, because the higher energy of positron emitters produces less scatter, less complications with attenuation and higher sensitivity. The theoretical improvement in resolution is of the order of 50% and the increase in sensitivity is of the order of 500% (Ott, Bateman et al, 1983). Clinical studies on small organs have confirmed these predictions and it seems reasonable to assume that similar improvements can be found in liver imaging.

3.3 Antibody imaging

Bone scintigraphy has demonstrated clearly how good uptake of a radiopharmaceutical in an abnormality can result in the detection of very small lesions. Radiolabelled antibody imaging offers the possibility of demonstrating abnormalities by specific concentration of radioactivity in the lesion in a similar way to bone scintigraphy. In clinical studies carried out to date the uptake in tumours has been poor resulting in the necessity of a blood background subtraction technique to correct for circulating antibody in the blood. This technique often produces false positives and in general offers a sensitivity less than that found with other diagnostic methods. Nevertheless liver secondaries have been demonstrated successfully (Green, Begent et al, 1984). However a recent antibody (M8) produced by the Ludwig Institute of Cancer Research in Sutton, UK, has been used to demonstrate secondaries from breast carcinoma in bone prior to them becoming visible on bone scintigraphy (Rainsbury, Westwood et al, 1983). The concentration of this antibody is high enough to avoid the need for blood background subtraction and the complications it produces. So far this antibody has been less successful in soft tissue abnormalities but the initial results in bone secondary detection would suggest that given the correct antibody this approach offers a method for the detection of very small and early lesions.

4. CONCLUSION

At present liver scintigraphy continues to offer an easy technique for detecting hepatic metastases with an accuracy in the clinical situation approaching that of ultrasound and CT (McCready, 1981). The differential diagnosis using radionuclide techniques remains a problem. However the disease specificity of antibody imaging is encouraging. Emission tomographic techniques do help in the detection of smaller lesions but also produce problems in the differential diagnosis between normal and abnormal structures. The recent advances in positron emission tomography are very encouraging. The combination of this together with a positron labelled antibody specific to human tumours are now feasible and offer the chance of using radionuclide imaging of the liver as a screening method with greatly improved sensitivity and specificity.

REFERENCES

Adams, F.G., Horton, P.W., Selim, S.M., 1980. Clinical comparison of three liver scanning agents. European Journal of Nuclear Medicine 5, 237-239

Biello, D.R., Levitt, R.G., Siegel, B.A., Sagel, S.S., Stanley, R.T. 1978. Computed tomography of radionuclide imaging: a comparative evaluation. Radiology 127, 159

Douglas, J.G., Zambartas, C.N., Sumerline, M.C., Finlayson, N.D.C., 1981. ^{75}Se Selenomethionine in the diagnosis of hepatocellular carcinoma. Report of a false positive scan. European Journal of Nuclear Medicine 6, 91-92

Drum, D.E., Beard, J.M., 1976. Scintigraphic criteria for hepatic metastases from cancer of the colon and breast. Journal of Nuclear Medicine 17, 677-680

Engel, M.A., Marks, D.S., Sandler, M.A., Shetty, P., 1983. Differentiation of focal intrahepatic lesions with ^{99m}Tc-red blood cell imaging. Radiology 146, 777-782

Errasti, C.A., Gomez-Escolar, I.A., de Zarate, P.G., Angulo, J.M., 1981. Scintigraphic evaluation of the liver in fasciola hepatica with radiocolloid and ^{67}Ga-citrate. European Journal of Nuclear Medicine 6, 57-58

Front, D., Royal, H.D., Israel, O., Parker, J.A., Kolodny, G.M., 1981. Scintigraphy of hepatic hemangiomas: the value of Tc-99m-labeled red blood cells: concise communication. Journal of Nuclear Medicine 22, 684-687

Garcia, A.C., Yeh, S.D.J., Benua, R.S., 1977. Accumulation of bone-seeking radionuclides in liver metastasis from colon carcinoma. Clinical Nuclear Medicine 2, 265-269

Galli, G., Maini, C.L., Salvatori, M. Ausili Cefaro, G., 1982. The diagnostic application of radiocolloid liver scintigraphy in breast carcinoma. Nuclear Medicine 21, 140-144

Georgiou, E., Alevizaki, C., Proukakis, C., 1983. Preoperative scintigraphic evaluation of the liver and biliary tract in Caroli's disease. European Journal of Nuclear Medicine 8, 34-36

Geslien, G.E., Pinsky, S.M., Poth, R.K., Johnson, M.C., 1976. The sensitivity and specificity of ^{99m}Tc-sulfur colloid liver imaging in diffuse hepatocellular disease. Radiology 118, 115-119

Ghaed, N., Marsden, R.J., 1978. Accumulation of ^{99m}Tc-diphosphonate in hepatic neoplasm. Radiology 126, 192

Golicher, J.C., 1941. The operability of carcinoma of the rectum. British Medical Journal ii, 393

Green, A.J., Begent, R.H.J., Keep, P.A., Bagshawe, K.D., 1984. Analysis of radioimmunodetection of tumours by the subtraction technique. Journal of Nuclear Medicine 25, 96-100

Grossman, Z.D., Wistow, B.W., Bryan, P.J., Dinn, W.M., McAfee, J.G., Kieffer, S.A., 1977. Radionuclide imaging, computed tomography and gray-scale ultrasonography of the liver: a comparative study. Journal of Nuclear Medicine 18, 327-332

Harauz, G., Bronskill, M.J., 1979. Comparison of the liver's respiratory motion in the supine and upright positions: concise communication. Journal of Nuclear Medicine 20, 733-735

Kew, M.C., Geddes, E.W., Levin, J., 1974. False-negative ^{75}Se-selenomethionine scans in primary liver cancer. Journal of Nuclear Medicine 15, 234-236

Kumar, B., Miller, T.R., Siegel, B.A., Mathias, C.J., Markham, J., Ehrhardt, G.J., Welch, M.J., 1981. Positron tomographic imaging of the liver: ^{68}Ga iron hydroxide colloid. American Journal of Roentgenology 136, 685-690

Lunia, S., Parthasarathy, K.L., Bakshi, S., Bender, M.A., 1975. An evaluation of ^{99m}Tc-sulfur colloid liver scintiscans and their usefulness in metastatic workup: a review of 1,424 studies. Journal of Nuclear Medicine 16, 62-65

McCready, V.R., 1981. The role of radionuclide imaging in relation to other imaging modalities: thyroid, liver (biliary system), pancreas and bone. In Medical Radionuclide Imaging 1980, Vol. II, IAEA-SM-247/217, 635-656. International Atomic Energy Agency, Vienna.

Muller-Brand, J., Benz, U., Kyle, C.A., Boss, M., Fridrich, R., 1977. Triple radioisotope technique in etiologic evaluation of space-occupying lesions of the liver. European Journal of Nuclear Medicine 2, 231-238

Ostfeld, D.A., Meyer, J.E., 1981. Liver scanning in patients with short-interval autopsy correlation. Radiology 138, 671-673.

Ott, R.J., Bateman, J.E., Flesher, A.C., Flower, M.A., Leach, M.O., Webb, S., Khan, O., McCready, V.R., 1983. Preliminary clinical images from a prototype positron camera. British Journal of Radiology 56, 773-776

Ozarda, A., Pickren, J., 1962. The topographic distribution of liver metastases: its relation to surgical and isotope diagnoses. Journal of Nuclear Medicine 3, 149

Rainsbury, R.M., Westwood, J.H., Coombes, R.C., Neville, A.M., Ott, R.J., Kalirai, T.S., McCready, V.R., Gazet, J-C., 1983. Localisation of metastatic breast carcinoma by a monoclonal antibody chelate labelled with Indium 111. Lancet 934-938

Sarper, R., Fajman, W.A., Tarcan, Y.A., Nixon, D.W., 1981. Enhanced detection of metastatic liver disease by computerized flow scintigrams: concise communication. Journal of Nuclear Medicine 22, 318-321

Schulze, P-J., Stritzke, P., Stolzenbach, G., 1981. Liver imaging and detection of liver metastases with ^{99m}Tc-HIDA. Nuclear Medicine 20, 214-219

Stadalnik, R.C., DeNardo, S.J., DeNardo, G.L., Raventos, A., 1975. Critical evaluation of hepatic scintiangiography for neoplastic tumors of the liver. Journal of Nuclear Medicine 16, 595-601

Stevens, J.S., Clark, E.E., 1977. Liver metastasis of colon adenocarcinoma demonstrated on ^{99m}Tc-pyrophosphate bone scan. Clinical Nuclear Medicine 2, 270-271

Ueno, K., Haseda, Y., 1980. Concentration and clearance of Tc-99m-pyridoxylidene isoleucine by a hepatoma. Clinical Nuclear Medicine 5, 196-199

Utz, J.A., Lull, R.J., Anderson, J.H., Lambrecht, R.W., Brown, J.M., Henry, W., 1980. Hepatoma visualization with Tc-99m pyridoxylidene glutamate. Journal of Nuclear Medicine 21, 747-749

LIVER METASTASIS: THE VALUE OF DIAGNOSTIC ULTRASOUND

T.H. SHAWKER

There are three broad general indications for using ultrasound imaging
in the evaluation of a patient with suspected or known hepatic metastatic
disease. The first is in the initial diagnosis, either for detecting metastatic disease where there is a high degree of suspicion, or as part of
clinical staging in a patient with a known malignancy. The second general
indication might best be called "lesion substantiation." Ultrasound can
be used to substantiate or to refute the findings of an equivocal computerized tomography or nuclear medicine scan, or it can be used to add
additional information about the nature of a lesion, for instance, for
differentiating between solid tumor and liver cysts. Ultrasound can
also be used to accurately localize a lesion such as for distinguishing
between extra- and intrahepatic deposits or for locating a lesion to a
specific portion of the liver (1). Tissue substantiation of a lesion
can be accomplished by using an ultrasound-directed fine needle biopsy.
The third broad indication for using ultrasound is to follow the results of treatment. Ultrasound can be used for restaging patients at
suitable intervals during treatment, for accurately measuring the size
of metastatic nodules to determine therapeutic efficacy, and to detect
any complications that occur during the treatment program.

Typically, metastatic disease in the liver appears as one or more
focal, spherical solid lesions. Tumor nodules 2 cm in diameter or
larger can usually be detected with confidence; however, the detection
of smaller lesions depends upon the lesion location within the liver
and the echo amplitude of the lesion relative to the background
liver parenchyma. Metastatic tumor can be of low echo amplitute relative to the liver, probably the most common appearance (Figure 1)
or of high echo ampliture (Figure 2). The relationship of ultrasound
appearance to specific histological tumor type is tenuous (2). In

94

FIGURE 1.   Small, 1.7 diameter metastatic lesion in right lobe of liver
            (arrow).

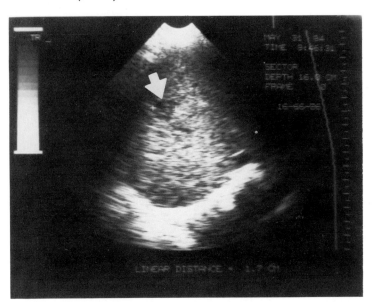

FIGURE 2.   One centimeter homogeneous high amplitude lesion.   This
            appearance (arrow) is identical to that of a benign heman-
            gioma.

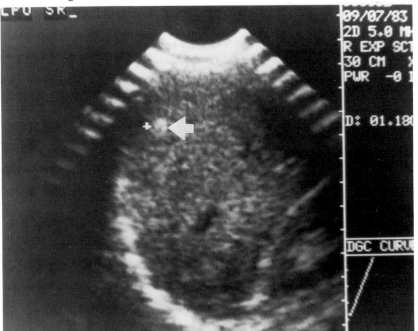

general, many sarcomas, some carcinomas and virtually all lymphomas
tend to give low echo amplitude lesions, while adenocarcinomas, particularly those arising from the colon and stomach, as well as metastatic pancreatic islet cell tumor, tend to give high echo amplitude
lesions (3-5). It has been suggested that there may be an approximate relationship to tumor vascularity for small lesions: high amplitude lesions tend to be hypervascular (6). In this instance, it
is hypothesized that the many small fluid-solid interfaces within
these hypervascular lesions is responsible for the high echo amplitude
seen on ultrasound imaging (6). Other tumor appearances that may be
encountered include target patterns (a central high echogenicity and
surrounding rim of low echo amplitude) metastatic tumor that is isoamplitude to the liver, nonfocal metastatic disease, and finally metastatic tumor that contains varying amounts of calcification and
fluid (Figure 3). Isoamplitude focal lesions and nonfocal involvement of the liver is probably the most difficult to detect. These
can be identified by using meticulous scanning technique and by pay-
ing particular and careful attention to any alteration in the parenchymal architecture of the liver. Displacement or loss of all or
part of normal intrahepatic vascular structures should be carefully
studied. Intralesion calcification may be seen in many varieties of
tumors, most notably in carcinoma of the colon, ovary, breast, and
stomach, as well as in melanoma, osteogenic sarcoma, neuroblastoma,
and islet cell pancreatic tumors (7). As with calcification occurring elsewhere in the body, ultrasound can readily detect calcification by demonstrating a high amplitude foci with a sharply marginated
posterior acoustic shadow (8). Intralesion fluid tends to be more a
sign of benign disease; however, fluid can occur within tumor as well.
This may be due to either tumor production of fluid, as in ovarian
carcinoma, or to the accumulation of fluid secondary to tumor cell
death with necrosis and hemorrhage (9). The distinction between a
fluid-filled malignancy and a simple liver cyst can be made by noting
that in tumors there is usually a solid echogenic rim surrounding
the fluid. Mural tumor nodules and irregular margins of the fluid
collection also suggest tumor as opposed to a liver cyst. A layer
of gravity dependent echos may be occasionally found within fluid
collections. In general, this tends to occur more often in benign

liver cysts and abscesses, but fluid-fluid levels may also occasionally be seen in necrotic liver metastases (10). In any given patient with liver metastasis, there is frequently a mixture of many types of lesions. It would not be unusual to find both high and low echo amplitude lesions occurring simultaneously in the liver of any given patient. Other features that may be encountered in a patient with metastatic disease of the liver are segmental biliary obstruction, gas within an infarcted tumor, and occasionally vascular invasion, although this last feature is more often seen in primary hepatoma than metastatic disease.

Sensitivity and specificity rates of 92% and 75-84% respectively have been reported for detecting focal hepatic lesions (11). In a prospective study performed in 1980-81, the relative ability of liver scintiscans, ultrasound, and computerized tomography to detect hepatic metastatic disease was examined (12). In this biopsy-proven study of 26 surgically detected metastatic cancers, no significant difference ($p < 0.1$) in sensitivity, specificity, or accuracy was found between the three imaging modalities. When laboratory tests were added to each of these three imaging studies, again, no significant difference was found in the detection rate (13). These studies with their reported efficacies validate the diagnostic value of ultrasound, but may not be currently true as ultrasound imaging has undergone considerable improvement in the past several years. The most significant changes that have occurred has been the switch from the use of the conventional articulated-arm static scanner to real-time scanners and the increasing use of higher frequency transducers. Small lesions are now being detected routinely and the number of less than statisfactory examinations is markedly diminished.

The detection of a focal lesion within the liver by ultrasound is, of course, not diagnostic of metastatic tumor. Primary hepatomas can mimic almost any ultrasound appearance of metastatic disease. Benign solid lesions also occur in the liver and are probably being detected with increasing frequency as liver scanning becomes more widespread. In general, benign solid lesions in the liver tend to be of high echo amplitude. These include cavernous hemangiomas, probably the most common benign lesion, liver cell adenomas, and focal nodule hyperplasia (14-16). Nontumor benign lesions that can occasionally be mistaken for

metastatic disease include abscesses, hematomas, and localized fatty
change within the liver (17). It is interesting that in one study
which examined the detection rate for high amplitude small hepatic
cavernous hemangiomas, lesions less than 10-15 mm in diameter were
detectable by ultrasound (15). These authors stated that ultrasound
was superior to CT scanning for the detection of these small lesions.
While this study was directed towards benign hemangiomas, the detection
rate found for these small lesions suggests that small high amplitude
metastatic deposits may be detected with similar accuracy.

Metastatic tumors should be localized in reference to the underlying
liver anatomy. In general, it is most useful to localize a focal liver
lesion to a particular liver segment. This can be done by noting the
relationship of the tumor to the anterior and posterior divisions of
the right portal vein or to the medial and lateral divisions of the
left portal vein, all of which course centrally within their respective
liver segments, and by locating a tumor in relationship to the three
hepatic veins which define the intersegmental fissures (18). Further
lesion substantiation or localization can be achieved by intraoperative
scanning (Figure 4). Makuuchi, et al. employed intraoperative ultrasound examination of the liver in 56 patients with both primary and
secondary liver tumors (19). They noted that intraoperative ultrasound
facilitated surgery by detecting unsuspected lesions, nonpalpable tumors,
daughter tumor nodules, multiple tumor foci, and tumor intravenous
thrombi. Accurate identification of the liver subsegment in which
tumor was present allowed the surgeon to better determine the extent
of his operation and to indicate the ligating points for the portal
and hepatic veins. The detection of small, previoulsy unsuspected,
metastatic lesions at the time of surgery is an important function
of intraoperative ultrasound since it may radically change the type
of treatment. For instance, in one example, unsuspected subcapsular
5 mm diameter liver metastases were found at the time of intraoperative
scanning (20).

Fine needle aspiration biopsy of suspect metastatic nodules can be
easily accomplished by using a real-time guided system. By visually
directing a needle into a focal lesion, one can achieve a considerable
improvement in diagnostic accuracy over the conventional Menghini liver
biopsy (21). Montali, et al. using real-time guided fine needle biopsy

98

FIGURE 3. A large high amplitude lesion (arrows) with a 1.5 cm area of
central fluid, presumably representing necrosis.

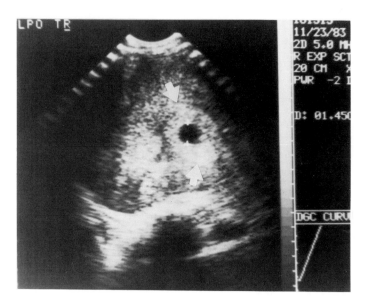

FIGURE 4. Intraoperative ultrasound scan with a 3 MHz sector transducer
visualizes a 5 cm metastatic lesion in the superior portion
of the right lobe.

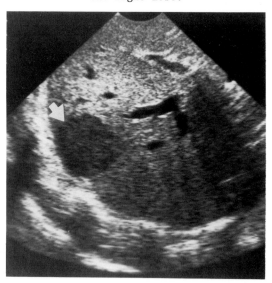

in 126 patients, aspirated cytological material from tumors ranging
in diameter from 2 to 9 cm (22). The true positive percentage from
this study was 92% (85/92) and the true negative percentage 100%
(34/34). There were no false positives. This procedure is indicated
especially when the patient has early or not widely disseminated
intrahepatic disease. In those instances where small focal lesions
or a solitary focal lesion is present there is a marked improvement
in diagnostic sensitivity and specificity over blind needle insertion.
The accuracy of fine needle aspiration using ultrasound control is as
accurate as peritoneoscopic directed liver biopsy but a less invasive
procedure.

The third broad category of use for diagnostic ultrasound in liver
metastasis is to follow therapy. Because of its unique ability to
scan in all imaging planes and therefore to find the largest diameter
of a mass, ultrasound is the most accurate imaging technique for
measuring the size of metastatic tumors. It is completely possible
for ultrasound to give the same degree of measurement accuracy to
tumor size as it currently does in other fields such as obstetrics
and cardiology. In those liver metastases that are spherical, change
in tumor size can be followed as a change in calculated volume from
a single measured diameter. Or, if the tumor is ellipsoid in shape
a calculated tumor volume can be derived from the three measured
diameters. Tumor volume doubling time and change in tumor size over
time can be calculated and exponential growth or exponential tumor
regression plotted (23,24). A knowledge of tumor growth rate makes
it possible to evaluate therapy in an individual patient, to detect
the onset of the therapeutic response or the beginning of therapeutic
failure with greater accuracy than with a less quantitative estimation.

What then is the current clinical value of liver ultrasound for the
examination of a liver metastases? At the moment, it appears that
ultrasound with state of the art equipment and operator expertise, is
as at least as accurate for deteting metastatic lesions as any other
imaging systems (12). Furthermore, in many instances, it can yield
additional information about focal lesions, for example to distinguish
between benign and malignant "cystic" masses, or to suggest tumor
origin based on echo amplitude pattern. Using the scanning plane
flexibility of real-time scanners, lesions can be very accurately

measured and related to the underlying liver segmental anatomy. Ultrasound is also the most simple method for performing an image-directed needle biopsy. Finally, and as the newest application, there is evidence that intraoperative ultrasound holds great future promise for detecting unsuspected metastatic lesions and to facilitate surgery. Considering, therefore, the numerous advantages of diagnostic ultrasound as well as its examining speed, less expense, and lack of patient morbidity, it is obvious that ultrasound is and will continue to be a valuable component in the clinical evaluation of liver metastatic disease.

REFERENCES

1. Graif M, Manor A, Itzchak Y: Sonographic differentiation of extra- and intrahepatic masses. Am J Roent 141:553-556, 1983.
2. Green B, Bree RL, Goldstein HM, Stanley C: Gray scale ultrasound evaluation of hepatic neoplasms: Patterns and correlations. Radiology 124:203-208, 1977.
3. Scheibel W, Gosink BB, Leopold GR: Gray scale echographic patterns of hepatic metastatic disease. Am J Roent 129:983-987, 1977.
4. Yoshida T, Okazaki N, Yoshino M, Matsue H, Kishi K: Ultrasonographic diagnosis of malignant hepatic tumors. Jpn J Clin Oncol 10:291-296, 1980.
5. Shawker TH, Doppman JL, Dunnick NR, McCarthy DM: Ultrasound investigation of pancreatic islet cell tumors. J Untraso nd Med 1:193-200, 1982.
6. Rubaltelli L, DelMaschio A, Candiani F, Miotto D: The role of vascularization in the formation of echographic patterns of hepatic metastates: Microangiographic and echographic study. Br J Radiology 53:1166-1168, 1980.
7. Schlang HA: Symptomatology of Metastatic Cancer, Medical Examination Publishing Co, Inc, Garden City, New York, 1981, pp 10-11.
8. Katragadda CS, Goldstein HM, Green B: Gray scale ultrasonography of calcified liver metastases. Am J Roent 129:591-593, 1977.
9. Paling MR, Shawker TH, Love IL: The sonographic appearance of metastatic malignant melanoma. J Ultrasound Med 1:75-78, 1982.
10. Baker DA, Morin ME: Gravity dependent layering in necrotic metastatic carcinoma to the liver. J Clin Ultrasound 5:282-283, 1977.
11. Plainfosse MCh, Bor Ph, Delalande JP: Diagnosis of hepatic metastases. Anatomoechographic correlations about 111 cases. In: Levi S (ed), Ultrasound and Cancer, Exerpta Medica, Amsterdam, 1982, pp 117-122.
12. Smith TJ, Kemeny MM, Sugarbaker PH, Jones AE, Vermess M, Shawker TH, Edwards BK: A prospective study of hepatic imaging in the detection of metastatic disease. Ann Surg 195:486-491, 1982.
13. Kemeny MM, Sugarbaker PH, Smith TJ, Edwards BK, Shawker TH, Vermess M, Jones AE: A prospective analysis of laboratory tests and imaging studies to detect hepatic lesions. Ann Surg 195:163-167, 1982.
14. Sandler MA, Petrocelli RD, Marks DS, Lopez R: Ultrasonic features and radionuclide correlations in liver cell adenoma and focal nodular hyperplasia. Radiology 135:393-397, 1980.
15. Itai Y, Ohtomo K, Araki T, Furui S, Iio M, Atomi Y: Computed tomo-

graphy and sonography of cavernous hemangioma of the liver. Am J
Roent 141:315-320, 1983.

16. Mirk P, Rubaltelli L, Bazzocchi M, Busilacchi P, Candiana F,
Ferrari F, Giuseppetti G, Maresca G, Rizzatto G, Volterrani L,
Zappasodi F: Ultrasonographic patterns in hepatic hemangiomas.
J Clin Ultrasound 10:373-378, 1982.

17. Newlin N, Silver TM, Stuck KJ, Sandler MA: Ultrasonic features
of pyogenic liver abscesses. Radiology 139:155-159, 1981.

18. Marks WM, Filly RA, Callen PW: Ultrasonic anatomy of the liver:
A review with new applications. J Clin Ultrasound 7:137-146,
1979.

19. Makuuchi M, Hasegawa H, Yamazaki S: Intraoperative ultrasonic
examination for hepatectomy. Jpn J Clin Oncol 11:367-390, 1981.

20. Plainfosse MC, Merran S: Work in progress: Intraoperative abdominal ultrasound. Radiology 147:829-832, 1983.

21. Rosenblatt R, Kutcher R, Moussouris HF, Schreiber K, Koss L:
Sonographically guided fine-needle aspiration of liver lesions.
JAMA 248:1639-1641, 1982.

22. Montali G, Solbiati L, Croce F, Ierace T, Ravetto C: Fine-needle
aspiration biopsy of liver focal lesions ultrasonically guided
with a real-time probe. Report on 126 cases. Br J Radiology 55:
717-723, 1982.

23. Paling MR, Shawker TH, Dwyer A: Ultrasonic evaluation of therapeutic response in tumors - Its value and implications. J Clin
Ultrasound 9:281, 1981.

24. Shawker TH: Monitoring response to therapy. In: Brascho DJ,
Shawker TH (eds), Abdominal Ultrasound in the Cancer Patient.
John Wiley & Sons, New York, 1980, pp 113-135.

EOE-13 AND OTHER CONTRAST AGENTS FOR COMPUTED TOMOGRAPHY OF THE LIVER

D.L. MILLER

1. INTRODUCTION

Except for the occasional patient with calcified hepatic metastases, there is relatively little difference in x-ray attenuation between metastases and normal liver parenchyma in most patients. Improvement in the computed tomographic (CT) detection of these metastases is dependent on the use of contrast agents to increase the difference in x-ray attenuation and improve visual contrast between the lesion and surrounding normal liver. These agents may selectively increase the attenuation of the normal liver or the metastasis, but ideally should not affect both. Should the x-ray attenuation of both increase, there will be no gain in visual contrast. Contrast agent research has been guided by this principle, and recent work has concentrated in two areas - improvement in the use of existing contrast agents and the development of new agents, such as EOE-13.

This review describes recent developments in the method of administration of available water-soluble contrast agents and discusses current work in the development of other, newer types of contrast agents, with particular emphasis on EOE-13.

2. WATER SOLUBLE (UROGRAPHIC) CONTRAST AGENTS

2.1 Pharmacokinetics

Several water soluble (urographic) contrast agents are currently available for clinical use. They have been used for many years and are associated with a low degree of toxicity (Shehadi, 1980). Diatrizoate and iothalamate salts are the most commonly used agents in the United States. All urographic-type water soluble contrast agents demonstrate essentially similar pharmacokinetics (Gardeur, 1980). They diffuse into the interstitial space within seconds after arterial or venous administration and an equilibrium phase is rapidly reached (Kormano, 1976; Newhouse, 1980;

Ono, 1980). In this phase, the iodine concentration of arterial and venous blood is essentially equal.

The maximum attenuation difference between tumor and liver is obtained during the non-equilibrium phase. When the equilibrium phase is reached, attenuation differences are minimal and metastases may actually be obscured (Burgener, 1981).

The timing of contrast administration and subsequent scanning has been extensively investigated in an attempt to determine the optimum method for scanning in the non-equilibrium phase. In a recent review, Clark and Matsui (Clark, 1983) defined seven different methods of CT scanning with water-soluble contrast agents. There is some overlap between categories, and not all will be discussed here.

2.2. Intravenous Infusion

The simplest, and probably the most common method of administration is by slow intravenous infusion. While some lesions may become more evident with this method, some lesions become isodense with surrounding liver and undetectable. If the infusion is sufficiently slow, the non-equilibrium phase may never be reached. In one series, known hepatic metastases were not visible in 13% of patients scanned with this technique (Moss, 1979). For this reason, most radiologists who employ this method also obtain CT scans before contrast agent administration. The detection rate for metastases using this combination is higher tham for either method alone (Moss, 1979). However, this doubles both the examination time and the radiation dose to the patient and increases the cost of the examination.

2.3. Intravenous Bolus Administration

Rapid administration of the contrast agent with immediate CT scanning permits imaging before the equilibrium phase of distribution is reached (Young, 1980). The difference in attenuation between tumor and liver is thus increased (Burgener, 1981) resulting in an improved contrast ratio and higher detection rates as compared to non-contrast CT (Berland, 1982; Foley, 1983) and intravenous contrast infusion (Moss, 1982; Burgener 1983b). The appearance of the metastases is variable and unpredictable; they may be of greater, lesser or the same attenuation as the surrounding liver (Marchal, 1980; Araki, 1980; Burgener 1983a).

The dose and rate of administration vary considerably from study to study, but do not appear to be important, as long as all scans are obtained within approximately one minute after contrast administration is complete. After a single intravenous bolus, contrast material opacifies the liver through the hepatic artery at 20-30 seconds and via the portal vein at 40-60 seconds after injection. Some investigators use several small (25-30 ml) bolus injections, while others prefer a single large (180cc) injection. Rapid hand injection of contrast material is the most common method, but rates as low as 1.5cc/sec and as high as 7cc/sec have been reported.

This method can also provide specific histologic diagnoses for hepatic hemangiomas, provided sequential scans are obtained through the lesion (Barnett, 1980; Itai, 1980). Metastases cannot be specifically diagnosed.

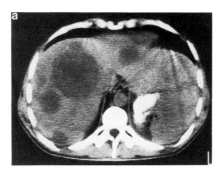 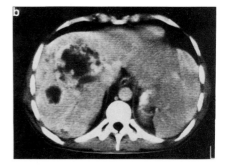

FIGURE 1. 30 year old man with a malignant pheochromocytoma. (a) A CT scan without contrast material demonstrates six metastases. (b) The administration of an intravenous bolus of water-soluble contrast material obscures several of the metastases.

There are four potential disadvantages to this method. For a screening examination, a third or fourth generation CT scanner is required to permit examination of the entire liver during the brief period of optimal contrast enhancement. A large dose of contrast material is necessary, and a physician must be present to administer it. The rapid intravenous administration of water soluble contrast agents produces nausea and vomiting in many patients, and technically inadequate scans can occur in as many as 27% of studies (Halvorsen, 1983). Finally, some metastases are obscured by this method (Fig. 1).

2.4. Intraarterial Adminstration

2.4.1. Computed tomographic arteriography Some investigators have utilized the existence of the liver's dual blood supply to further manipulate contrast agent administration. Hepatic metastases derive almost all of their blood supply from the hepatic artery, while normal liver receives only about 25% of its blood supply from this source (Healy, 1963). Injection of contrast material into the hepatic artery (computed tomographic arteriography) exploits this difference in blood supply to produce markedly increased attenuation in the metastasis as compared to surrounding liver (Prando, 1979; Freeny, 1983). This method is more sensitive than intravenous bolus administration (Cassel, 1982; Moss, 1982).

2.4.2. Arterial portography Portal venous blood may be selectively opacified by injection of a contrast agent into the superior mesenteric artery (arterial portography). A catheter is placed into the superior mesenteric artery and 50-70cc of contrast material is injected at a rate of 0.4-0.6 cc/sec, beginning 30 seconds prior to CT scanning and continuing during the entire scan. With this method, normal liver demonstrates increased attenuation while metastases are not enhanced. In one study, this method detected more metastases than any other imaging method in 13 of 17 patients (Matsui, 1983).

Both of these methods are extremely sensitive, but they are invasive and costly because an angiographic procedure is necessary prior to the CT scan. The morbidity associated with angiography and the requirement for hospital admission make these methods unsuitable for routine use. Computed tomographic arteriography may be employed if the patient has an indwelling catheter in place for hepatic artery infusion chemotherapy.

2.5. Delayed Scanning

Urographic contrast agents are excreted in the bile in patients with poor renal function. This process also occurs, although to a much lesser extent, in patients with normal renal function. It has been suggested recently that CT scanning be performed 3-6 hours after contrast agent administration, in order to permit opacification of the normal liver by contrast agent in the hepatocytes and biliary system (Rauschkolb, 1982). Very preliminary experience suggests that this method is promising (Fig.

2), but additional work is needed. It does appear that relatively large doses of contrast material are required.

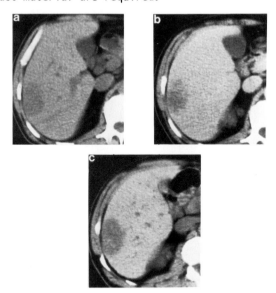

FIGURE 2. 62 year old man with carcinoma of the colon and a liver metastasis. There is faint central calcification in the metastasis. (a) A CT scan with contrast material shows the lesion. There is relatively little attenuation difference between the metastasis and the surrounding liver. (b) A CT scan during the intravenous bolus administration of water soluble contrast material demonstrates improved visualization, but the margins of the lesion are not clear. (c) A delayed CT scan, performed 6 hours following (b), and without further contrast material, shows the lesion to best advantage.

3. ORGAN-SPECIFIC CONTRAST AGENTS

Contrast agents may be specifically designed to opacify a particular organ or system in the body. Urographic contrast agents were originally designed to selectively opacify the cardiovascular system and the kidneys. In the development of organ-specific contrast agents directed at the liver, most work has been concentrated on excretion of contrast agent in the bile or phagocytosis of contrast agents by the reticuloendothelial cell system (RES) of the liver. Agents in both of these classes opacify normal liver but show little or no uptake in metastases, which are devoid of hepatocytes and Kupffer cells.

3.1. Biliary Contrast Agents

Several contrast agents exist which are exclusively or primarily excreted in bile. One of these, iodipamide (Cholografin, E.R. Squibb and Sons) has been used clinically for years. Unfortunately, its toxicity is considered too great for routine use in hepatic CT. Other contrast agents in this class have been developed, including iosefamate (Mallinckrodt, Inc.)(Koehler, 1979) and iosulamide (Sterling-Winthrop Research Institute) (Moss, 1981; Marincek, 1982). Experimental studies suggest that they may be effective clinically and may be less toxic than iodipamide (Nelson, 1980). However, these agents are excreted in the urine to a greater extent than iodipamide, and consequently are less effective for biliary opacification (Berk, 1981). No large-scale clinical trials have been performed with these agents.

3.2. Agents Directed at the Reticuloendothelial System

The theoretical basis and previous work on agents of this type have been extensively reviewed (Fischer, 1977). Intravenously administered particles of a specific size will be selectively phagocytosed by the liver and spleen (Laval-Jeantet, 1982). If these particles are made radiopaque they will selectively increase the x-ray attenuation of normal hepatic and splenic parenchyma, but not tumors within these organs (with the possible exception of RES-containing tumors such as focal nodular hyperplasia). Metastases will not be enhanced.

Many such preparations have been studied, all of which remain experimental at present. These include liposomes containing various contrast agents (Havron, 1981; Seltzer, 1983; Frey, 1983), heavy metals (Havron, 1980), iodinated starch (Cohen, 1981), and iodipamide ethyl ester (Violante, 1981). Several emulsions have also been examined, including perfluoroctylbromide (PFOB)(Mattery, 1982), various emulsions of iodinated oils prepared by French investigators (Laval-Jeantet, 1972; Lamarque, 1979) and EOE-13 (Grimes, 1979; Vermess, 1979). Of these RES contrast agents, only EOE-13 has been studied extensively in patients.

4. EOE-13

EOE-13 was developed by Michael Vermess, M.D. and colleagues at the National Institutes of Health (Vermess, 1979). It is an investigational agent and is not available for general clinical use. EOE-13 is an aqueous emulsion of an iodinated oil (Ethiodol, Savage Laboratories) with emulsifiers and a buffer, and is prepared by the Pharmaceutical Development Service of the National Institutes of Health. Details of its preparation have been described (Grimes, 1979).

Over 500 clinical examinations have been performed with EOE-13 in the United States, including approximately 300 examinations at the National Institutes of Health. The first 225 of these 300 studies have been reviewed recently (Miller, 1984c).

4.1. Patient Selection and Method of Administration

In clinical trials to date, all patients studied with EOE-13 have had histologically proven malignancy. Other criteria are that the patient should have normal or only slightly abnormal hepatic, renal, respiratory and hematopoietic function. In particular, patients with liver function tests more than 2 times the upper limit of normal have generally been excluded (Miller, 1984c).

We currently employ a dose of 0.25 ml/kg (50 mg iodine/kg), reduced by 1/5 to 1/3 in patients who have had a splenectomy or a major hepatic resection. For intravenous administration, EOE-13 is diluted with 100 ml of 5% dextrose in water to a final concentration of approximately 15% and infused into a peripheral vein over a period of 1 hour.

4.2. Opacification of the Liver and Spleen

Figure 3 shows attenuation data for pre-EOE-13 and post-EOE-13 CT studies in 103 examinations where both studies were performed on the same CT scanner. Thirty-five patients had hepatic metastases. The mean increases in attenuation are 32.5 Hounsfield units (HU) for the liver, 52.3 HU for the spleen, and 2.6 HU for hepatic and splenic tumor. The increases in attenuation for the liver and spleen are statistically significant ($p < 0.001$). The median increase in tumor attenuation was 1 HU and 90% of the tumors evaluated showed changes in attenuation of 8 HU or less (Miller, 1984). EOE-13 produces substantial contrast enhancement of the liver and spleen, but does not enhance tumor within these organs. The degree of contrast enhancement is greater than that produced by water-soluble contrast agents and biliary contrast agents, even though the administered dose of EOE-13 contains less iodine (Fig. 4). Enhancement persists for several hours, so that scanning may be performed without the time pressures associated with some of the methods used for water-soluble contrast agents.

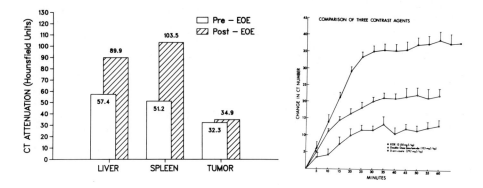

FIGURE 3. The mean CT attenuation for liver, spleen, and tumor in 103 examinations is shown both before and after the administration of EOE-13. FIGURE 4. Changes in CT attenuation of the liver in 6 dogs following 30 minute infusion of a water-soluble contrast agent (diatrizoate - lower curve), a biliary contrast agent (iosulamide - middle curve) and an RES contrast agent (EOE-13 - upper curve). EOE-13 produces the greatest increase in CT attenuation and also provides the lowest iodine dose. (Courtesy Dr. William Thompson, Durham, NC)

4.3 Efficacy

In a prospective comparison of CT without contrast material, CT with intravenous infusion of water-soluble contrast material and CT with EOE-13, Sugarbaker et al. demonstrated significantly greater sensitivity with EOE-13 for the detection of hepatic metastases. There was no loss of accuracy. The sensitivity of non-contrast CT was 40.6%, the sensitivity of CT with infusion of water-soluble contrast media was 33.6%, and the sensitivity of CT with EOE-13 was 76.7%. The size threshold for lesion detection was approximately one cm (Fig. 5)(Sugarbaker, 1984). In a comparison of EOE-13 CT and scintigraphy, Miller et al found a size threshold for EOE-13 of 1.0-1.5 cm (Miller, 1983). Lewis et al. feel that lesions 5mm in size can routinely be detected with EOE-13 (Lewis, 1982).

Studies are currently in progress comparing EOE-13 to intravenous bolus administration of water-soluble contrast agents and delayed scanning.

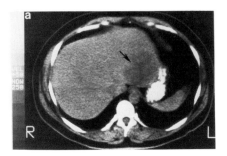 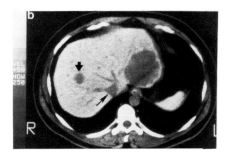

FIGURE 5. 48 year old man with colon carcinoma. (a) The CT scan without contrast material shows a lesion in the left hepatic lobe (arrow), proven at surgery to be an hemangioma. (b) The CT scan after EOE-13 administration shows better definition of the hemangioma. In addition, a previously unsuspected metastasis is identified (broad arrow). The inferior vena cava is also well seen (long arrow). (Reproduced with permission from JAMA 1984;251:707-708.)

4.4 Toxicity

4.4.1 Side Effects

There have been no deaths associated with the use of EOE-13. No permanent morbidity has been observed, with some patients followed for as long as 4 years after examination. Some patients have received 5 separate studies with EOE-13 during the course of their illness. Late complications that could be attributed to EOE-13 have not been observed. Table 1 summarizes the most frequent side effects encountered with EOE-13 in the first 225 examinations performed at the National Institutes of Health. Because of the high incidence of fever and chills in the first 31 patients, subsequent patients were given an intravenous bolus of hydrocortisone 100 mg (Solu-Cortef, UpJohn, Inc.) just prior to the EOE-13 infusion (Vermess, 1982). This significantly reduces the incidence of fever and rigor ($p < 0.001$) and also reduces the incidence of headache ($p = 0.9$). It has no other effect.

4.4.2 <u>Complications</u> Complications occurred in 8 of the 225 examinations (3.6%). None were life threatening. The most serious were three patients who experienced marked deterioration of liver function within 24 hours of EOE-13 infusion. These patients recovered completely within 10 days. This data is reviewed is more detail elsewhere (Vermess, 1982; Miller, 1984c).

4.4.3 <u>Histopathology and Analysis of Laboratory Studies</u> Pathologic specimens of liver, spleen or lymph nodes were available for 78 patients in the 225 NIH examinations. Nonspecific changes were often seen in the liver, of the type frequently seen in cancer patients. There were no pathologic alterations in any specimen specifically attributable to EOE-13. Analysis of serum chemistry and hematology values at 2 hours and 24 hours post-infusion showed no clinically significant changes compared to pre-infusion baseline values.

5. CT EVALUATION OF HEPATIC ARTERY INFUSION CHEMOTHERAPY WITH EOE-13
5.1. Nature of the Problem

Patients receiving hepatic artery infusion therapy require periodic radiologic studies to confirm that the diseased portions of the liver are being perfused. This must be done in order to assure that all metastases are receiving the chemotherapeutic agent. Angiography with water soluble contrast media was initially used for this purpose, but the flow rates required for adequate vessel opacification do not reproduce the perfusion pattern produced by the much slower flow rates used for drug infusion (Kaplan, 1978; Rodari, 1981).

At present, the only successful method for imaging hepatic perfusion patterns has been administration of ^{99m}Tc-labeled particles through the infusion catheter (Kaplan, 1978; Bledin, 1982). These embolize the arteriolar bed of the hepatic artery and remain in place. This method has several disadvantages. Hepatic metastases in the perfused area are poorly visualized. Hepatic metastases outside the perfused area are not visualized at all. Spatial resolution is poor. The ideal method would permit visualization of the entire liver, all metastases, and the perfusion pattern simultaneously, and would have high spatial resolution.

5.2 Rationale for the Use of EOE-13

Computed tomography is an ideal imaging method for this application. It visualizes the entire liver and provides excellent spatial resolution. For visualization of perfusion patterns, a contrast agent is required that will be removed by the liver and fixed in place on the first pass and that will provide sufficient enhancement to be visible on CT. RES agents fit this description, as they are phagocytosed and remain in place for some time after administration. EOE-13, as the only agent available for clinical use, was selected for an initial clinical study. It has been shown that direct infusion of EOE-13 into the hepatic artery entails no greater risk than intravenous administration (Miller, 1984b).

5.3 Clinical Study With EOE-13

5.3.1 Patients and Methods The methodology has been described in detail elsewhere (Miller, 1984a; Miller, unpublished). Briefly, the study was performed in 5 patients with liver metastases from carcinoma of the colon. All 5 patients were receiving hepatic artery infusion chemotherapy through a subcutaneously implanted pump (Model 400, Infusaid Corp.). EOE-13 was injected through the side port of the pump at a rate of 0.66 ml/min, using a dose ranging from 1/4 to 1/2 the usual intravenous dose. CT scanning was then performed. All 5 patients also underwent scintigraphy with arterial injection of ^{99m}Tc-macroaggregated albumin.

5.3.2 Results The perfusion pattern identified by CT correlated exactly with the areas of radionuclide uptake in all 5 patients. The anatomic location of the perfused portion of the liver was more clearly seen with EOE-13 CT in all four patients with partial hepatic perfusion. Metastases were visualized in all of the EOE-13 studies, with adequate visualization in both perfused and nonperfused portions of the liver. With scintigraphy, metastases were not adequately visualized in any patient (Fig. 6).

Two of the five patients had vague abdominal pain associated with the EOE-13 study. These patients had the smallest relative volumes of perfusion, and the discomfort may have been associated with saturation of a portion of the liver by EOE-13. None of the patients had laboratory or clinical evidence of hepatic toxicity.

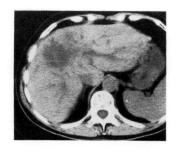
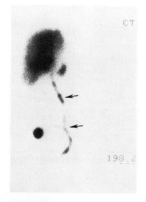
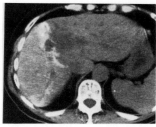

FIGURE 6. Sixty-year-old man with colon carcinoma receiving hepatic
artery infusion chemotherapy. (a) A baseline CT scan demonstrates a large
metastasis at the junction of the right and left lobes of the liver. (b) A
scintigram was obtained seven months later, with the injection of
99mTc-macroaggregated albumin through the infusion catheter (arrows). Only
the right lobe of the liver is perfused. The metastasis is not seen.
(c) A CT scan was performed after the injection of EOE-13 through the
infusion catheter. This study was obtained within one week of (b). The
perfusion pattern and the metastasis are clearly seen, and incomplete
perfusion of the metastasis is demonstrated.

5.3.3 Discussion   It is essential to demonstrate the perfusion status of
all hepatic metastases. A non-perfused lesion would not be expected to
respond to arterial chemotherapy. One patient in this study had 2
metastases; the EOE-13 CT showed that one was perfused and the other was
not. The perfused lesion regressed, but the unperfused lesion enlarged
(Miller, unpublished).

In patients receiving hepatic artery infusion chemotherapy, CT with
intraarterially administered EOE-13 provides visualization of all hepatic
metastases, the hepatic perfusion pattern, and the perfusion status of each
metastasis. No other single study provides all of this information, and
some of it is obtainable in no other way. CT with intraarterially
administered EOE-13 does not detect extrahepatic sites of perfusion, and
for this scintigraphy is required.

6. SUMMARY

Improvement in the detection of hepatic metastases with computed tomography requires the use of contrast agents to increase the difference in x-ray attenuation between the metastasis and normal liver. Current research is directed at improving the use of existing contrast agents and at developing new agents.

Water-soluble (urographic) contrast agents are currently available for general clinical use. The most effective methods of administration require angiographic techniques to deliver these agents into the hepatic artery or the superior mesenteric artery. These techniques are not suitable for screening examinations. Currently, intravenous bolus administration appears to be the best method for screening examinations. Delayed scanning may also prove to be highly effective.

Organ-specific contrast agents are under active development. These agents are designed to be excreted in the bile by the hepatocytes or phagocytosed by the RES cells of the liver. Of the many agents investigated to date, only EOE-13 has been used successfully in a large clinical trial.

EOE-13 is an investigational RES contrast agent, and is an emulsion of an iodinated oil. In clinical trials in the United States, it has produced substantial enhancement of the liver and spleen without enhancement of tumor in these organs. EOE-13 increases the sensitivity of CT examinations for the detection of metastatic disease in the liver. The complication rate is 3.6%. EOE-13 also appears to be useful for the evaluation of hepatic artery infusion chemotherapy.

REFERENCES
1. Araki T, Itai Y, Furui S, Tasaka A (1980). Dynamic CT densitometry of hepatic tumors. AJR 135:1037-1043.
2. Barnett PH, Zerhouni EA, White RI Jr., Siegelman SS (1980). Computed tomography in the diagnosis of cavernous hemangioma of the liver. AJR 134:439-447.
3. Berk RN, Barnhart JL, Nazareno G, Witt BL (1981). The potential of iosulamide meglumine as a contrast material for intravenous cholangiography: an experimental study in dogs. Invest Radiol 16: 240-244.

4. Berland LL, Lawson TL, Foley WD, Melrose BL, Chintapalli KN, Taylor AJ (1982). Comparison of pre- and post-contrast CT in hepatic masses. AJR 138:853-858.
5. Bledin AG, Kantarjian HM, Kim EE et al. (1982). ^{99m}Tc-labeled macroaggregated albumin in intrahepatic arterial chemotherapy. AJR 139:711-715.
6. Burgener FA, Hamlin DJ (1981). Contrast enhancement in abdominal CT: bolus vs. infusion. AJR 137:351-358.
7. Burgener FA, Hamlin DJ (1983a). Contrast enhancement of focal hepatic lesions in CT: effect of size and histology. AJR 140:297-301.
8. Burgener FA, Hamlin DJ (1983b). Contrast enhancement of hepatic tumors in CT: comparison between bolus and infusion techniques. AJR 140: 291-295.
9. Cassel DM, Young SW, Turner R (1982). Contrast enhancement: dynamic CT measurements and a mathematical model. Invest Radiol 17:82-89.
10. Clark RA, Matsui O (1983). CT of liver tumors. Semin Roentgenol 18: 149-162.
11. Cohen Z, Seltzer SE, Davis MA, Hamson RN (1981). Iodinated starch particles: new contrast material for computed tomography of the liver. J Comput Assist Tomogr 5:843-846.
12. Fischer HW (1977). Improvement in radiographic contrast media through the development of colloidal or particulate media: an analysis. J Theor Biol 67:653-670.
13. Foley WD, Berland LL, Lawson TL, Smith DF, Thorsen MK (1983). Contrast enhancement technique for dynamic hepatic computed tomographic scanning. Radiology 147:797-803.
14. Freeny DC, Marks WM (1983). Computed tomographic arteriography of the liver. Radiology 148:193-197.
15. Frey GD, Heim RC, Jendrasiak GL (1983). The hepatic uptake of radiocontrast agents incorporated into lipid aggregates: CT scanning studies. [Abstract] Radiology 149(P):248.
16. Gardeur D, Lautrou J, Millard JC, Berger N, Metzger J (1980). Pharmacokinetics of contrast media: experimental results in dog and man with CT implications. J Comput Assist Tomogr 4:178-185.
17. Grimes G, Vermess M, Galleli JF, Girton M, Chatterji DC (1979). Formulation and evaluation of ethiodized oil emulsion for intravenous hepatography. J Pharm Sci 68:52-56.
18. Halvorsen RA, Foster W, Roberts L, Gibbons R, Thompson WM (1983). Bolus versus infusion enhancement for CT of the liver. [Abstract] Radiology 149(P):212.
19. Havron A, Davis MA, Seltzer SE, Paskins-Hurlburt AJ, Hessel SJ (1980). Heavy metal particulate contrast materials for computed tomography of the liver. J Comput Assist Tomogr 4:642-648.
20. Havron A, Seltzer SE, Davis MA, Shulkin P (1981). Radiopaque liposomes: a promising new contrast material for computed tomography of the spleen. Radiology 140:507-511.
21. Healy JE Jr., Sheena KS (1963). Vascular patterns in metastatic liver tumors. Surg Forum 14:121-122.
22. Kaplan WD, D'Orsi CJ, Ensminger WD, Smith EH, Levin DC (1978). Intraarterial radionuclide infusion: a new technique to assess chemotherapy perfusion patterns. Cancer Treat Rep 62:699-703.
23. Koehler RE, Stanley RJ, Evens RG (1979). Iosefamate meglumine: an iodinated contrast agent for hepatic computed tomography scanning. Radiology 132:115-118.

24. Kormano M, Dean PB (1976). Extravascular contrast material: the major component of contrast enhancement. Radiology 121:379-382.
25. Itai Y, Furui S, Araki T, Yashiro N, Tasaka A (1980). Computed tomography of cavernous hemangioma of the liver. Radiology 137: 149-155.
26. Laval-Jeantet AM, Laval-Jeantet M, Bergot C (1982). Effect of particle size on the tissue distribution of iodized emulsified fat following intravenous administration. Invest Radiol 17:617-620.
27. Lewis E, AufderHeide JF, Bernardino ME, Barnes PA, Thomas JL (1982). Detection of hepatic metastases with Ethiodized Oil Emulsion 13. J Comput Assist Tomogr 6:1108-1114.
28. Marchal GJ, Baert AL, Wilms GE (1980). CT of noncystic liver lesions: bolus enhancement. AJR 135:57-65.
29. Marincek B, Young SW, Enzmann DR (1982). Time-density evaluation of the liver after iosulamide meglumine: a tissue-specific CT contrast agent. Invest Radiol 17:90-94.
30. Matsui O, Kadoya M, Suzuki M, et al (1983). Work in Progress: Dynamic sequential computed tomography during arterial portography in the detection of hepatic neoplasms. Radiology 146:721-727.
31. Mattrey RF, Long DM, Multer F, Mitten R, Higgins CB (1982). Perfluoroctylbromide: a reticuloendothelial-specific and tumor-imaging agent for computed tomography. Radiology 145:755-758.
32. Miller DL, Rosenbaum RC, Sugarbaker PH, Vermess M, Willis M, Doppman JL (1983). Detection of hepatic metastsases: comparison of EOE-13 computed tomography and scintigraphy. AJR 141:931-935.
33. Miller DL, Schneider PD, Willis M, Vermess M, Doppman JL (1984a). Intraarterial administration of EOE-13 for the CT evaluation of hepatic artery infusion chemotherapy. J Comput Assist Tomogr 8:332-334.
34. Miller DL, Girton M, Vermess M, Doppman JL (1984b). Direct infusion of EOE-13 into the hepatic artery: experimental evaluation in monkeys. Invest Radiol (In press).
35. Miller DL, Vermess M, Doppman JL, et al(1984c). CT of the liver and spleen with EOE-13: review of 225 examinations. AJR (In press).
36. Miller DL, Schneider PD, Gianola FJ, Willis M, Vermess M, Doppman JL. Intraarterial EOE-13 administration for the assessment of hepatic artery infusion chemotherapy. Unpublished.
37. Moss AA, Schrumpf J, Schnyder P, Korobkin M, Shimshak RR (1979). Computed tomography of focal hepatic lesions: a blind clinical evaluation of the effect of contrast enhancement. Radiology 131: 427-430.
38. Moss AA, Brito AC (1981). Computed tomography of the liver in rhesus monkeys following iosefamate meglumine administration. Radiology 141: 123-127.
39. Moss AA, Dean PB, Axel L, Goldberg HI, Glazer GM, Friedman MA (1982). Dynamic CT of hepatic masses with intravenous and intraarterial contrast material. AJR 138:847-852.
40. Nelson JA, White GL Jr., Nakashima EN (1980). Iosulamide: human tolerance study of a new intravenous cholangiographic drug. Invest Radiol 15:511-516.
41. Newhouse JH, Murphy RX Jr. (1981). Tissue distribution of soluble contrast: effect of dose variation and changes with time. AJR 136: 463-467.

42. Ono N, Martinez CR, Fara JW, Hodges FJ III (1980). Diatrizoate distribution in dogs as a function of administration rate and time following intravenous injection. J Comput Assist Tomogr 4:174-177.
43. Prando A, Wallace S, Bernardino ME, Lindell MM Jr. (1979). Computed tomographic arteriography of the liver. Radiology 130:697-701.
44. Rauschkolb EN, Steinberg RM, Sandler CM, Toombs BD, Wheatley KJ, Gibbs BJ. Delayed computed tomography of the liver following intravenous contrast. Presented at the 68th Annual Meeting of the Radiology Society of North America, November 1982.
45. Rodari A, Bonfanti G, Garbagnati F, Marolda R, Millela M, Buraggi GL (1981). Microsphere angiography in hepatic artery infusion for cancer. Eur J Nucl Med 6:473-476.
46. Seltzer SE, Shulkin PM, Adams DF, et al. (1983). Liposomes carrying hepatobiliary contrast agent: new materials for reticuloendothelial tissue opacification on CT images. [Abstract] Radiology 149(P):211.
47. Shehadi WH, Toniolo G (1980). Adverse reactions to contrast media: a report from the Committee on Safety of Contrast Media of the International Society of Radiology. Radiology 1980;137:299-302.
48. Sugarbaker PH, Vermess M, Doppman JL, Miller DL, Simon R (1984). Improved detection of focal lesions with computerized tomographic examination of the liver using ethiodized oil emulsion (EOE-13) liver contrast. Cancer (In press).
49. Vermess M, Chatterji DC, Doppman JL, Grimes G, Adamson RH (1979). Development and experimental evaluation of a contrast medium for computed tomographic examination of the liver and spleen. J Comput Assist Tomogr 3:25-31.
50. Vermess M, Doppman JL, Sugarbaker PH, et al. (1982). Computed tomography of the liver and spleen with intravenous lipoid contrast material: review of 60 examinations. AJR 138:1063-1071.
51. Violante MR, Mare K, Fischer HW (1981). Biodistribution of a particulate hepatolienographic CT contrast agent: a study of iodipamide ethyl ester in the rat. Invest Radiol 16:40-45.
52. Young SW, Turner RJ, Castellino RA (1980). A strategy for the contrast enhancement of malignant tumors using dynamic computed tomography and intravascular pharmacokinetics. Radiology 137:137-147.

NUCLEAR MAGNETIC RESONANCE IMAGING OF THE LIVER: CURRENT STATUS AND
FUTURE POSSIBILITIES

M. VERMESS

While in the first 50 years following the discovery of x-rays little
advance has been made in imaging hepatic lesions, the three decades
following this has brought an abundance of liver imaging modalities.
In approximate chronological order the newer imaging techniques utilized
for demonstrating liver lesions are radionuclide scanning, angiography,
sonography and, the latest and probably most important development,
computed tomography. A great deal of time is spend nowadays on discussions concerning the proper order and combination of these examinations to exclude or investigate hepatic lesions. In other words, to
determine the proper algorithm for hepatic imaging. The multitude of
examinations in these algorithms for liver imaging clearly indicates
that not one modality is perfect and, despite the rapid progression of
the new techniques, we still lack the technique which can be considered
as the ultimate in diagnostic imaging of the liver. The comparable
accuracy of the three most commonly used imaging modalities is shown
in Figure 1.

Most recently, however, an entirely new imaging modality surfaced
into the already confusing gamut of imaging techniques, nuclear magnetic resonance (NMR). This new technique, just as ultrasound, is
not based on x-ray attenuation. Images are created by the response
of the atomic nuclei to rapid changes in the magnetic field direction
caused by specific radiofrequency waves. Since all medical NMR imaging
to date is based on the hydrogen atoms, the radiofrequency are tailored
to the specific frequency of the hydrogen nucleus (proton) in a given
magnetic field. Thus, NMR essentially depicts the hydrogen distribution
of a given biological specimen.

Early reports indicate that NMR is capable to demonstrate primary and

FIGURE 1. Sensitivity, specificity and accuracy of the three most commonly used liver imaging studies for the detection of hepatic metastases. The liver spleen scan was the most sensitive (true positive percentage of 80%). The ultrasound was found to be the most specific (false positive percentage of 4%). However, the accuracy of the CT scan was the greatest at 84%. None of these differences were found to be statistically significant. From Smith TJ, Kemeny MM, Sugarbaker PH, et al: A prospective study of hepatic imaging in the detection of metastatic disease. Ann Surg 195:486-491, 1982.

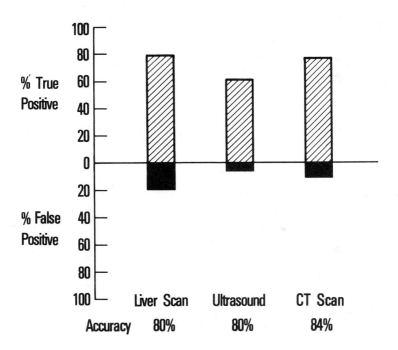

secondary liver tumors (1,2). Moss and colleagues, in their review of
the NMR appearance of liver tumors, felt that NMR and CT detected
hepatic lesions equally well but the internal architecture and the
relationship of lesion to the hepatic vasculature were better seen
on NMR (3). As demonstrated in Figure 2, NMR is a promising modality
to evaluate parenchymal liver disease (4,5). NMR has shown itself to
be extremely valuable in the evaluation of increased iron disease
states of the liver such as primary hemochromatosis and transfusional
hemosiderosis. NMR is particularly promising in the diagnosis of
primary hepatocellular carcinoma. Computed tomography, particularly
with dynamic bolus contrast enhancement, has brought about a very
significant advance in the diagnosis of hepatomas. Prior to study
with NMR it was usually quite difficult to determine the correct extent
of this tumor by CT because these tumors rarely occur in otherwise
normal livers. The differentiation between the abnormal area due to
cirrhosis and the abnormal area representing tumor is unreliable.
The differentiation of the tumor from the surrounding abnormal liver
parenchyma and thus the definition of the actual size of the tumor
is usually more obvious on the NMR image (6). It is fair to say, then,
that in studying iron overload of the liver and primary hepatocellular
carcinomas, NMR is of great promise.

Since even the fastest NMR imaging takes more than 30 seconds to
obtain, respiratory motion is probably the most significant handicap
to NMR imaging of the liver. It is not realistic to believe that the
NMR imaging time could be significantly reduced, thus the answer to
this physiological motion is respiratory gating. Considerable effort
is being exerted by the NMR manufacturing companies to design a
practical cardiac and respiratory gating system. Until the time this
has been achieved, it is unlikely that NMR will exceed computed tomography in sensitivity for the demonstration of small hepatic lesions
such as metastases.

A very significant advantage of NMR imaging is the capability of
imaging in any desired plane. An area where the advantage of this is
already clearly shown is the differentiation of retroperitoneal tumors
protruding into the liver parenchyma from bonifide liver lesions. This
can be extremely difficult on computed tomography.

Naturally, we are looking forward to the chemical analysis of liver

FIGURE 2. NMR image of the normal liver. Note visualization of the aorta and inferior vena cava. There is good demonstration of portal venous branches without injection of contrast media.

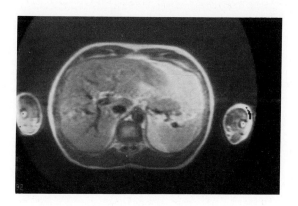

parenchyma by NMR spectroscopy simultaneously with the imaging. If accomplished, this would realize the so called "bloodless biopsy" where we could noninvasively analyze the liver tissue or lesions within the liver by NMR spectroscopy. This could give us information about the metabolic processes as well as the physiological and pathological status of the liver and lesions within the liver. At this time, this is only a hope but not an unrealistic one. NMR imaging and NMR analysis of biological specimens are very rapidly advancing fields, anything written today will probably be outdated tomorrow. It is very probable, however, that NMR will become a very significant addition to existing imaging modalities, even if it would not necessarily replace them.

REFERENCES

1. Margulis AR, Moss AA, Crooks LE, Kaufman L: Nuclear magnetic resonance in the diagnosis of tumors of the liver. Sem Roentgenol 18:123-126, 1983.
2. Doyle FH, Pennock JM, Banks LM, et al: Nuclear magnetic resonance imaging of the liver: Initial experience. AJR 138:193-200, 1982.
3. Moss AA, Goldberg HI, Stark DB: Hepatic tumors: Magnetic resonance and CT appearance. Radiology 150:141-147, 1984.
4. Stark DD, Goldberg HI, Moss AA, Bass NM: Chronic liver disease: Evaluation by Magnetic resonance. Radiology 150:149-151, 1984.
5. Stark DD, Bass NM, Moss AA, et al: Nuclear magnetic resonance imaging of experimentally induced liver disease. Radiology 148: 743-751, 1983.
6. Vermess M: Nuclear magnetic resonance imaging of the liver in primary hepatocellular carcinoma (manuscript in preparation).

RADIOLABELED ANTIBODIES FOR THE DETECTION OF CANCER: NEW APPROACHES TO IMPROVE THE SENSITIVITY AND SPECIFICITY OF IMMUNOSCINTIGRAPHY.

J.-P. MACH, J.-Ph. GROB, F. BUCHEGGER, V. von FLIEDNER, S. CARREL, J. PETTAVEL, A. BISCHOF-DELALOYE and B. DELALOYE.
Ludwig Institute for Cancer Research, 1066 Epalinges, Switzerland and Department of Surgery and Division of Nuclear Medicine, CHUV, 1011 Lausanne, Switzerland.

1. INTRODUCTION

Paul Ehrlich's concept of "magic bullet" for the cure of diseases has been revitalized by the development of the monoclonal antibody (Mab) technology allowing the production in unlimited amounts of antibodies of perfect homogeneity and specificity directed against various tumor markers. This chapter will review one aspect of the magic bullet concept, the use of radiolabeled antibodies as tracer for tumor detection by immunoscintigraphy. We shall critically consider the results obtained in this attractive field, from our early experimental results with ^{131}I labeled polyclonal antibodies against carcinoembryonic antigen (CEA) up to the most recent clinical results obtained with ^{123}I labeled fragments of anti-CEA Mab. Special emphasis will be given to the difficulties encountered in the detection of liver metastases when using intact anti-CEA antibodies and to the improvement obtained when we used ^{123}I labeled Mab fragments and single photon emisssion computerized tomography (SPECT) for their localization in three dimensions.

2. EXPERIMENTAL RESULTS WITH POLYCLONAL ANTIBODIES

Research on tumor localization of radiolabeled antibodies was initiated almost 30 years ago by Pressman (1) and Bale (2), who showed that labeled antibodies against Wagner osteosarcoma or Walker carcinoma cells were concentrated in vivo by these tumors.

In 1974, we introduced into this field the model of nude mice bearing grafts of human colon carcinoma and the use of affinity purified antibodies against carcinoembryonic antigen (CEA) (3). We showed that purified ^{131}I-labeled goat anti-CEA antibodies could reach up to a 9 times higher concentration in the tumor than in the liver, while the concentration of control normal IgG in the tumor was never higher than 2.3 times that in the liver. We observed, however, great variations in the degree of specific tumor localisation by the same preparation of labeled antibodies, when colon carcinoma grafts derived from different patients were tested. This is probably due to the fact that human tumors keep their initial histologic properties and degree of differentiation after transplantation into nude mice and these two factors appear to affect the ease with which circulating antibodies gain access to the CEA present in tumors. The detection of ^{131}I-labeled antibodies in tumors by external scanning also gave variable results. With colon carcinoma grafts from certain donors we obtained scans with good tumor localisation, whereas with colon carcinoma grafts from other donors the antibody uptake was not sufficient to give satisfactory scanning images. In this context we think that results in the nude mouse model are a good reflection of the clinical reality observed in patients.

Independently, Goldenberg et al. (4) showed specific tumor localization and detection by external scanning with ^{131}I-labeled IgG fractions of anti-CEA serum, using two human carcinomas which had been serially transplanted into hamsters for several years. Using the same experimental model Hoffer et al. (5) also demonstrated tumor localization with radiolabeled IgG anti-CEA by external scanning.

3. CLINICAL RESULTS WITH POLYCLONAL ANTI-CEA ANTIBODIES

The first detection of carcinoma in patients obtained by external scanning following injection of purified ^{131}I-labeled anti-CEA antibodies was reported by Goldenberg et al. (6,7). They claimed that almost all the CEA producing tumors could be detected by this method and that there was no false positive results. However, our experience, using highly purified goat anti-CEA antibodies and the same blood pool subtraction technology as Goldenberg was that only 42% of CEA producing tumors (22 out of 53 tested) could be detected by this method (8-9). Furthermore, we found that in several patients the labeled anti-CEA antibodies localized non-specifically in the reticuloendothelium particularly in the liver. Despite the use of the subtraction technology, these non-specific uptakes were difficult to differentiate from the specific uptakes corresponding to liver metastases. The discrepancy of results between the group of Goldenberg and our own is unlikely to be due to a difference in the quality of the anti-CEA antibodies used, since we showed by direct measurement of the radioactivity in tumors resected after injection that our antibodies were capable of excellent tumor localization (8). Furthermore, in a few patients scheduled for tumor resection, we injected simultaneously 1 mg of goat anti-CEA antibodies labeled with 1 mCi of ^{131}I and 1 mg of control normal goat IgG labeled with 0.2 mCi of ^{125}I. By this paired labeled method adapted to the patient situation, we could demonstrate that the antibody uptake was 4 times higher than that of control normal IgG (8).

These results were very encouraging in terms of specificity of tumor localization. However, the direct measurement of radioactivity in tumors also showed that only 0.05-0.2% of the injected radioactivity (0.5-2 μCi out of 1000 μCi) were recovered in the resected tumors 3-8 days after injection (8). This information is important if one is considering the use of ^{131}I labeled antibody for therapy (10).

4. MONOCLONAL ANTI-CEA ANTIBODIES USED IN PHOTOSCANNING

The obvious advantage of monoclonal antibodies (Mab) are their homogeneity and their specificity for the immunizing antigen. Another advantage of Mab is that they each react with a single antigenic determinant and thus should not be able to form large immune complexes with the antigen (provided that the antigenic determinant is not repetitive).

The first Mab used for immunoscintigraphy in patients was Mab 23 anti-CEA (11). Already in 1981, the well characterized Mab 23 (12) was injected intravenously to 26 patients with large bowel carcinomas and 2 patients with pancreatic carcinomas. Each patient received 0.3 mg of purified Mab labeled with 1-1.5 mCi of ^{131}I. The patient's premedication included lugol 5% iodine solution, promethazine and prednisolone, as previously described (8,9). The patients had no personal history of allergy. They were also tested with an intracutaneous injection of normal mouse IgG and found to have no hypersensitivity against this protein. None of the patients showed any sign of discomfort during or after the injection of labeled mouse antibodies. The patients were studied by static external photoscanning 24, 36, 48 and 72 h after injection. In 14 of the 28 patients (50%) a radioactive spot corresponding to the tumor was detected 36-48 h after injection. In 6 patients the scans were doubtful and in the remaining 8 patients they were entirely negative (11).

The results were slighly better than those obtained with polyclonal anti-CEA antibodies (8,9). Namely there was less background radioactivity in the liver, but the method was not yet considered as clinically useful in comparison with the most modern other methods of tumor diagnosis.

5. DETECTION OF COLORECTAL CARCINOMA BY TOMOSCINTIGRAPHY

A logical approach to improve tumor detection by immunoscintigraphy is the use of tomoscintigraphy. As we have seen, static photoscanning is limited in part by the presence of radiolabeled antibodies or free ^{131}I released from them, in the circulation, the reticuloendothelial system, the stomach, intestine and urinary bladder. Increased radioactivity in these compartments may give false positive results. Specific tumor sites may be masked by non-specific radioactivity. These problems cannot be entirely resolved by the presently available subtraction methods using ^{99m}Tc labeled HSA and free ^{99m}TcO$_4^-$. Axial transverse tomoscintigraphy is a method initially developed by Kuhl and Edwards in 1973 (13) with the potential to resolve some of these problems. This method, also called single photon emission computerized tomography (SPECT), corresponds to the application of the tomographic technique used in transmission computerized axial tomography (CT-scan) to scintigraphic data. Mathematical techniques similar to those used in positron and X-ray tomographies allows the reconstruction of transverse sections as well as frontal, saggital or oblique sections of patients. In collaboration with Ch. Berche and J.-D. Lumbroso from the Institut Gustave Roussy in Villejuif, we have shown that tomoscintigraphy can improve the sensivity and specificity of tumor detection by radiolabeled anti-CEA Mabs (11,14). With this methods 15 out of 16 carcinoma tumor sites studied (including 10 colorectal carcinomas, 1 stomach, 1 pancreas and 4 medullary thyroid carcinomas) were detectable. These results were encouraging in term of sensitivity. However, it should be noted that numerous non-specific radioactive spots, sometimes as intense as the tumors, were observed. Thus, the problem of non-specific accumulation of antibodies remained, but the three dimensions localization of radioactive spots by tomoscintigraphy helped to discriminate specific tumor uptakes from the non-specific ones (14).

6. MAB FRAGMENTS TESTED IN EXPERIMENTAL ANIMALS

In order to further improve this method, we produced a series of 26 new hybridomas secreting anti-CEA antibodies and selected them first, <u>in vitro</u>, by criteria of high affinity for CEA (15) and low crossreactivity with glycoproteins present on the surface of granulocytes, termed NCA-55 and NCA-95 (16). Furthermore, $F(ab')_2$ and Fab fragments were prepared from three selected Mab and tested for their capacity to localize, <u>in vivo</u>, in human colon carcinoma heterotransplanted in nude mice (17). Groups of 4-7 mice were injected simultaneously with ^{131}I labeled Mab or fragments and with normal IgG or their corresponding fragment labelled with ^{125}I. The mice were dissected 2-5 days later. The results of antibody and normal IgG concentration per g of tumor and normal organ obtained with Mab 35 and expressed in percentage of the total radioactivity recovered for each isotope are shown in Figure 1 for Mab 35.

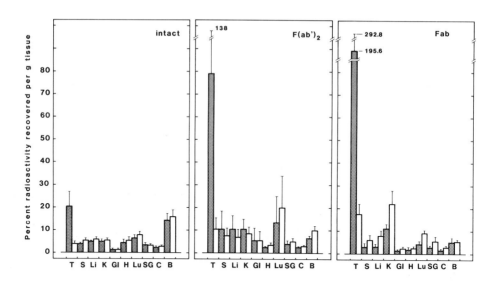

FIGURE 1. Distribution of Mab 35 or its fragments (shaded bars) and control IgG or fragments (open bars) injected simultaneously into nude mice bearing grafts of a human carcinoma. The vertical lines represent the standard deviations calculated from groups of four to seven animals per Mab or fragment. T, tumor; S, spleen; Li, liver; K, kidneys; GI, gastrointestinal tract; H, heart; Lu, lungs; SG, salivary glands; C, carcass and head; B, blood. (Reproduced with the permission of the J. Exp. Med) (17).

It is evident that the ratios of tumor to normal organs antibody concentration is increasing dramatically with the use of fragments. The ratios of tumor to normal organs antibody concentration (average from all normal organs) were 7 for intact Mab, 25 for $F(ab')_2$ and 85 for Fab. The specificity indices obtained by dividing the tumor to normal organs ratios obtained for antibody by the corresponding ratio obtained for control IgG were 3.4 for intact Mab, 8.2 for $F(ab')_2$ and 19 for Fab (17).

The scanning results obtained with these experimental animals paralleled those obtained by direct measurement of radioactivity. With intact Mab tumor grafts of 0.5-1 g gave contrasted positive scans only 3 days after injection, whereas fragments of Mab allowed the detection of smaller tumors at an earlier time. The best results were obtained with Fab fragments of Mab 35 which allowed the clear detection of a tumor graft of 0.1 g 48 h after injection (17).

7. DETECTION OF CARCINOMA USING ^{123}I LABELED MAB FRAGMENTS AND TOMOSCINTIGRAPHY

Based on the above experimental results, we tested a series of 23 patients with colorectal carcinoma after injection of $F(ab')2$ and Fab fragments of Mab 35 labeled with ^{123}I. This isotope, which has a very favorable energy of 159 keV and a relatively short physical half life of 13.2 hours, proved to be excellent for tomoscintigraphy. ^{123}I was prepared from the ^{127}I(p,5n) ^{123}Xe reaction by the Schweizerisches Institut für Reaktorforschung at Würenlingen, Switzerland. Using a Searle-Siemens double head rotating camera, tomographic studies of the pelvis and upper abdomen were performed in all patients at 6 h and 24 h after injection and in the majority of patients at 48 h. Other parts of the body such as thorax and bones were studied only when there was a clinical suspicion of tumor in these areas or when an abnormal radioactive uptake was detected on whole body scanning (systematically performed before the tomographic studies). No subtraction techniques were used, but additional scintigraphic studies of the liver with ^{99m}Tc sulfur colloid were regularly performed after the last ^{123}I analysis with the patient remaining in the same position. Sulfur colloid scintigraphy allowed to identify anatomical landmarks and in some cases to compare filling defects of ^{99m}Tc colloid with area of increased

^{123}I antibody unptake. A representative example of such a comparison is shown in figure 2.

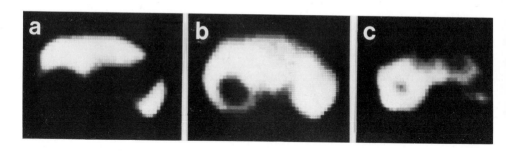

FIGURE 2. Transverse tomographic sections of the upper abdomen at the same level showing: Panel a, 99m-Tc sulfure colloid 30 min after injection; Panel b, 123-I labeled F(ab')2 fragments of Mab 35 anti-CEA, 6 h after injection; Panel c, some 123-I labeled fragment 48 h after injection.

These results were obtained in a 75 years old female patient, who had evidence of liver metastases from a right colon carcinoma by sonography. Figure 3 (Panel a) shows a tomographic transverse section of a ^{99m}Tc sulfur colloid scan demonstrating a large filling defect localized in the right posterior part of the liver. The patient was injected with 1.5 mg of F(ab')2 fragments from Mab 35 labeled with 3.5 mCi of ^{123}I. Six hours after injection, a transverse section (Panel b) taken at the same level as that of the sulfur colloid scan shows tracer uptake around the tumor as well as in normal liver and spleen, but a large filling defect in the center of the tumor. Forty-eight hours after the injection, a similar transverse section (Panel c) shows that the radiolabeled antibody fragment has penetrated deeply into the tumor and that only the center of the tumor (probably necrotic) is not filled up with radioactivity. The spleen and normal liver retain very small amounts of radioactivity, exept for an additional hot spot (localized on the right side of the major uptake on Panel c) corresponding probably to a second smaller liver metastasis, also detectable by a discrete notch on the ^{99m}Tc colloid section (Panel a).

The sensitivity of tumor detection was rather high. In the 13 patients injected with F(ab')2 fragments labeled with ^{123}I, 23 out of 28 tumor sites were detected by tomoscintigraphy. This includes 6/6 primary or recurrent localized carcinomas, 5/8 patients with liver metastases, 0/2 lung metastases (of less than 2 cm diameter) and 12/12 bone metastases (in 2 patients). In the 10 patients injected with Fab fragments, 30 out of 31 tumor sites were detected by tomoscintigraphy, including 6/7 primary or recurrent carcinomas, 6/6 patients with liver metastases and 18/18 bone metastases (in a single patient). We realize that this very high sensitivity is due in part to the selection of patients with known tumors and to the relatively large size of the tumors detected. The smallest primary tumor detected was a carcinomatous polyp of the rectum weighing 4.5 g and the smallest liver metastases detected had less than 3 cm in diameter as determined by the CT-scan.

8. DISCUSSION

The major advantage of the use of tomoscintigraphy and ^{123}I labeled Mab fragment consist in the high quality of the images which allows to distinguish tumor accumulation of radioactivity from physiological organ concentration and circulating radioactivity without the artifacts inherent to the subtraction technology. Our optimistic results in term of sensitivity should be confirmed in a prospective study in order to prove that such type of immunotomoscintigraphy can compete with the most modern morphological diagnostic methods such CT-scan and nuclear magnetic resonance. In any case, we think that for diagnostic purposes small fragments of Mab with high affinity for a relatively abundant tumor marker such as CEA represent the best tracer. If one consider the use of radiolabeled antibody for therapy, however, the strategy should be different, because the Fab fragment with its 50,000 molecular weight is too rapidly eliminated by the kidneys.

Only three groups have reported results of radioimmunotherapy. Order et al. (10) have used semi-purified polyclonal antibodies against CEA and ferritin labeled with therapeutic doses of ^{131}I to treat biliary tract carcinoma and hepatoma, respectively. The moderately optimistic results obtained, may be due to the fact that a high percentage of the injected polyclonal antibodies will always accumulate in the liver and therefore may have some usefulness against these two types of tumor. The specificity of the results however, remains difficult to evaluate. Larson et al. (18) have used intact and Fab fragments of Mab directed against the p-97 melanoma associated antigen in the treatment of this tumor. Despite the repeated injection of relatively high doses (100 mCi) of ^{131}I, the anti-tumor effect has been very modest. Recently, Epenetos et al. (personal communication, and in press in Lancet) reported on the intraperitoneal injection of Mab directed against the milk fat globule antigen, labeled with 18 mCi of ^{131}I in a patient with a peritoneal dissemination from an ovarian carcinoma. The apparent remission observed seems, however, too preliminary to conclude that it was due to the injected radiolabeled antibodies.

In conclusion, the detection of human cancer by radiolabeled antibodies has markedly improved thanks to the Mab selection and fragmentation as well as to the new nuclear medicine technology. We do not know yet, however, if the tumor uptakes of radioactivity which are useful for diagnosis may justify the use of larger amounts of antibody bound radioactivity for therapy.

REFERENCES

1. Pressman, D. and Korngold, L. The in vivo localization of anti-Wagner osteogenic sarcoma antibodies. Cancer 6:619-623, 1953.

2. Bale, W.F., Spar, I.L., Goodland, R.L. and Wolfe, D.E. In vivo and in vitro studies of labeled antibodies against rat kidney and Walker carcinoma. Proc. Soc. Exp. Biol. Med. 89:564-568, 1955.

3. Mach, J.-P., Carrel, S., Merenda, C., Sordat, B. and Cerottini, J.-C. In vivo localisation of radiolabeled antibodies to carcinoembryonic antigen in human colon carcinoma grafted into nude mice. Nature 248:704-706, 1974.

4. Goldenberg, D.M., Preston, D.F., Primus, F.J. and Hansen, H.J. Photoscan localization of GW-39 tumors in hamsters using radiolabeled anti-carcinoembryonic antigen immunoglobulin G. Cancer Res. 34:1-9, 1974.

5. Hoffer, P.B., Lathrop, K., Bekerman, G., Fang, V.S. and Refetoff, S. Use of 131-I-CEA antibody as a tumor scanning agent. J. Nucl. Med. 15:323-327, 1974.

6. Goldenberg, D.M., DeLand, F., Enishin, K., Bennett, S., Primus, F.J., van Nagell, J.R., Estes, N., DeSimone, P. and Rayburn, P. Use of radiolabeled antibodies to carcinoembryonic antigen for the detection and localization of diverse cancers by external photoscanning. N. Engl. J. Med. 298:1384-1388, 1978.

7. Goldenberg, D.M., Kim, E.D., DeLand, F.H., Bennett, S. and Primus, F.J. Radioimmunodetection of cancer with radioactive antibodies to carcinoembryonic antigen. Cancer Res. 40:2984-2992, 1980.

8. Mach, J.-P., Carrel, S., Forni, M., Ritschard, J., Donath, A. and Alberto, P. Tumor localization of radiolabeled antibodies against carcinomebryonic antigen in patients with carcinoma. N. Engl. J. Med. 303:5-10, 1980.

9. Mach, J.-P., Forni, M., Ritschard, J., Buchegger, F., Carrel, S., Widgren, S., Donath, A. and Alberto, P. Use and limitations of radiolabeled anti-CEA antibodies and their fragments for photoscanning detection of human colorectal carcinomas. Oncodevelop. Biol. Med. 1:49-69, 1980.

10. Order, S.E., Klein, J.L., Ettinger, D., Alderson, P., Siegleman, S. and Leichner, P. Use of isotopic immunoglobulin in therapy. Cancer Res. 40, 3002-3007, 1980.

11. Mach, J.-P., Buchegger, F., Forni, M., Ritschard, J., Berche, C., Lumbroso, J.D., Schreyer, M., Girardet, Ch., Accolla, R.S. and Carrel, S. Use of radiolabelled monoclonal anti-CEA antibodies for the detection of human carcinomas by external photoscanning and tomoscintigraphy. Immunology Today 2:239-249, 1981.

12. Accolla, R.S., Carrel, S. and Mach, J.-P. Monoclonal antibodies specific for carcinoembryonic antigen and produced by two hybrid cell lines. Proc. Natl. Acad. Sci (USA) 77:563-566, 1980.

13. Kuhl, D.E. and Edwards, R.D. Image separation radioisotope scanning. Radiology 80:653-662, 1963.

14. Berche, C., Mach, J.-P., Lumbroso, J.-D., Langlais, C., Aubry, F., Buchegger, F., Carrel, S., Rougier, P., Parmentier, C. and Tubiana, M. Tomoscintigraphy for detecting gastrointestinal and medullary thyroid cancers : First clinical results using radiolabelled monoclonal antibodies against carcinoembryonic antigen. Brit. Med. J. 285:1447-1451, 1982.

15. Haskell, C.M., Buchegger, F., Schreyer, M., Carrel, S. and Mach J.-P. Monoclonal antibodies to carcinoembryonic antigen : ionic strength as a factor in the selection of antibodies for immunoscintigraphy. Cancer Research 43:3857-3864,1983.

16. Buchegger, F, Schreyer, M., Carrel, S. and Mach, J.-P. Monoclonal antibody identify a CEA crossreacting antigen of 95 KD (NCA-95) distinct in antigenicity and tissue distribution from the previously described NCA of 55 KD. Int. J. Cancer. 33:643-649, 1984.

17. Buchegger, F., Haskell, C.M., Schreyer, M., Scazziga, B.R., Randin, S., Carrel, S. and Mach J.-P. Radiolabeled fragments of monoclonal anti-CEA antibodies for localization of human colon carcinoma grafted into nude mice. J. Exp. Med. 158:413-427, 1983.

18. Larson, S.M., Carrasquillo, J.A., Krohn, K.A., Brown, J.P., McGuffin, R.W., Ferens, J.M., Graham, M.M., Hill, L.D., Beaumier, P.L., Hellström, K.E., and Hellström, I. Localization of 131-I-labeled p97-specific Fab fragments in human melanoma as a basis for radiotherapy. The Journal of Clinical Investigation. 72:2101-2114, 1983.

PERITONEOSCOPY IN THE DIAGNOSIS OF LIVER METASTASES

F.C.A. DEN HARTOG JAGER, E. GORTZAK, J.J. BATTERMANN

1. INTRODUCTION

Peritoneoscopy or laparoscopy is direct inspection of the peritoneum and abdominal organs with a laparoscope introduced through a small incision in the abdominal wall after previous pneumoperitoneum. We use local anaesthesia, 1% xylocaine and mild sedation: ½ mg atropine i.m., 2 cc thalamonal i.m. and 10-20 mg diazepam i.m. or i.v.

The advantage of this invasive technique is the possibility to detect very small lesions on the liver surface and to take biopsies under direct vision with an accuracy of about 90% (1, 2, 3, 4, 5, 6).

2. LAPAROSCOPY AND LIVER SCINTIGRAPHY

In a study comparing laparoscopy and liver scintigraphy in patients with proven gastrointestinal cancer we found a sensitivity (true positive results) of 95% and a specificity (true negative results) of 100% for laparoscopy (7). This sensitivity is higher than usually found in the literature (80-90%) (8, 9), probably due to patient selection (G.I. patients in a late state) and the absence of concomitant liver disease. The radionuclide scan is non-invasive, reproducible, but less sensitive, with a lower specificity (50-82%). It does not give precise anatomic localisation and does not differentiate between solid tumor and cysts (10). Good results were obtained, when both methods were combined.

The rapid developments in other non-invasive techniques such as

computer tomography and ultrasonography (11, 12, 13, 14) give
rise to the following question: Is there a place for peritoneoscopy in the diagnosis of liver metastases in 1984?
There are only   few studies comparing laparoscopy and computer
tomograpy and ultrasound (15, 16, 17) available.

3. LAPAROSCOPY AND COMPUTER TOMOGRAPHY

A review of Mayo Clinic Experience (16) comparing computer
tomography (CT) and peritoneoscopy showed a higher sensitivity
of CT of 39% vs 62% for peritoneoscopy, with comparable specificity of respectively 94% and 96%.
In 97 patients 45 tissue proven lesions were found. Computer
tomography missed 4 metastases on the liver surface detected by
peritoneoscopy; peritoneoscopy failed in 16 cases where mainly
deep metastases were visible on CT.

4. LAPAROSCOPY AND ULTRASONOGRAPHY

A comparison of computer tomography with fine needle aspiration
and peritoneoscopy with liver biopsy in the staging of the liver
in 56 patients with small cell bronchogenic carcinoma suggested
ultrasonography to be superior. Metastatic disease was proven
with ultrasonography in 15 and with peritoneoscopy in 7 patients
(17).
Our experience is that the impact of these non-invasive techniques
is already clearly visible in clinical practice and we feel that
no other studies comparing incomparable techniques for incomparable patients are necessary. Fig. 1 shows that although more
new patients are seen each year in the Netherlands Cancer
Institute, the number of peritoneoscopies diminished with the
introduction of CT and ultrasound.

5. INDICATIONS FOR LAPAROSCOPY

The indications for laparoscopy diminish rapidly with increasing experience with CT and ultrasound. Laparoscopy is considered
when clinical suspicion of liver metastases, e.g. abnormal

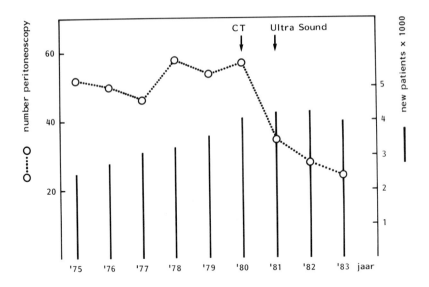

FIGURE 1. Diminishing number of peritoneoscopies with the introduction of CT and ultrasound.

laboratory data, complaints, hepatomegaly, is present and
screening with ultrasonography, CT or both procedures is inconclusive or contradictory. Consequences in therapeutic management
are prerequisite. Our indications in the past 3 years can be
divided into 4 categories:

A. DIAGNOSTIC.

In patients with clinical evidence of liver metastases of an
unknown primary tumor where CT and ultrasound are inconclusive
or pathology remains negative, laparoscopy with biopsy under
direct vision can save time and unnecessary investigations.
When considering surgery for a solitary liver metastasis, very
small secondaries elsewhere in the liver or on the peritoneum
may be detected with this method.

B. DIFFERENTIAL DIAGNOSIS

In patients with an established primary tumor, hepatomegaly
and/or abnormal laboratory data, the differential diagnosis with
liver metastases is not always easy, especially when other causes

for liver damage, e.g. alcohol, drugs, previous anaesthesia, chemo- or radiotherapy are present.

C. STAGING

Mutilating surgery aims for cure and is usually not performed when liver metastases are present. Laparoscopy can settle doubts in patients where amputation of an extremity, breast or rectum is planned or in patients where an extensive E.N.T. operation is considered, e.g. laryngectomy.

D. SAFETY

The last category is the high risk patient with coagulation disturbances, where we hope to be able to make a diagnosis either without taking a biopsy, as in liver cirrhosis or cystic liver, or to lessen the risk by avoiding necrotic, cystic or vascular areas. Also we can choose instead for brush cytology or small forceps biopsy and there is the possibility of haemostasis.

6. LAPAROSCOPY IN THE STAGING OF DISTAL ESOPHAGEAL OR CARDIA CARCINOMA. Our experience in a prospective study.

We used laparoscopy in the staging of patients with a distal esophageal or cardia carcinoma even when no clinical evidence of liver metastases was present. In these patients extensive thoraco-abdominal surgery was only performed with curative intent and laparoscopy was felt to be able to diminish the high number of unnecessary exploratory laparotomies. As survival,even in patients where operation was felt to be successful, was disappointing due to distant metastases, an attempt was made to improve the prognosis by adding pre- operative irradiation therapy. A prospective study was performed in 50 patients in the period January 1978 - December 1982. Patients with a distal esophageal or cardia carcinoma were se- lected for age, $\leqslant$ 70 years, and length of the tumor on endo- scopy, $\leqslant$ 6 cm. Patients with metastases on physical examination or chest X-ray were excluded. During the three week course of radiotherapy (30 Gy/3wk), exten- sive staging was performed, including laparoscopy. In the

beginning of the study liver scanning was used, later to be
replaced by computed tomography. All patients were seen by one
team, consisting of a surgeon, radiotherapist and gastro-
enterologist.

7. RESULTS

Laparoscopy was performed in 49 patients. On one patient with
a large abdominal aortic aneurysm, laparoscopy was not
performed; there were no liver metastases at surgery. Laparoscopy
was negative in 44 patients, dubious in 2 where negative biopsies
were found to be accurate at exploratory laparotomy, and positive
in three patients where multiple tiny liver metastases were seen.
Two of these patients had small peritoneal implants also.
Liver scintigraphy was performed in 34 patients; there were one
false positive and three false negative results. Computed
tomography in 27 patients gave one false positive and no false
negative results.   In 7 patients abnormal laboratory data
were found, all due to other disease!
Of 50 patients, 5 were not acceptable for anaesthesia due to
cardio-pulmonary problems.
One patient developed a positive lymph hnode during the irradiation period. Plus three patients with liver metastases found
at laparoscopy, only 41 patients went to surgery.
18 patients were found to be inoperable due to local irresec-
tability or lymph node metastases.
Although no additional patients with liver metastases were
found, we felt that laparoscopy (3/49 positive) was of very
limited value in the staging of these patients and we now omit
this step in the staging procedure.

8. IN CONCLUSION

In 1984 there is only occasionally on very strict indication
a place for laparoscopy in the detection of liver metastases:
after real time ultrasonography with fine needle biopsy,
after computer tomography or after both procedures combined.

REFERENCES

1. Bleiberg H, Rozencweig M, Mathieu M, Beyens M, Gompel C, Gérard A. The use of peritoneoscopy in the detection of liver metastases. Cancer 1978, 41:863-867.
2. Bleiberg H, LaMeir E, Lejeune F. Laparoscopy in the diagnosis of liver metastases in 80 cases of malignant melanoma. Endoscopy 1980, 12:215-218.
3. Liver Metastasis. Chapter 13. Riemann JF. 1982. GK Hall, Medical Publishers.
4. Lightdale C J. Laparoscopy and biopsy in malignant liver disease. Cancer 1982, 50:2672-2675.
5. Lightdale CJ, Clinical applications of laparoscopy in patients with malignant neoplasms. Gastrointest Endosc 1982, 28:99-102.
6. Margolis R, Hansen HH, Muggia FM, Kanhouwa S. Diagnosis of liver metastases in bronchogenic carcinoma. Cancer 1974, 34:1825-1829.
7. Lesmana L, Tijtgat GN, Grijm R. Diagnostiek van levermeta-stasen bij gastrointestinaal carcinoom. De waarde van laparo-scopie vergeleken met leverscintigrafie. Tijdschrift voor Gastro-enterologie 1982, 4:63-69.
8. Sauer R, Fahrländer H, Fridrich R. Comparison of the accuracy of liverscans and peritoneoscopy in benign and malignant primary and metastatic tumours of the liver. Scan J GE 1973, 8:389-394.
9. Boyd WP. Relative diagnostic accuracy of laparoscopy and liver scanning techniques. Gastrointest Endosc 1982, 28:104-106.
10. Clouse ME. Roentgenographic techniques for the diagnosis and management of liver tumours. Seminars in Oncology 1983, 10:159-175.
11. Snow JH, Goldstein HM, Wallace J. Comparison of scintigraphy, sonography, and computed tomography in the evaluation of hepatic neoplasms. AJR 1979, 132:915-918.
12. Alderson PO, Adams DF, McNeil BJ, Sanders R, Siegelman SS, Finberg HJ, Hessel SJ, Abrams HL. Computed tomography, ultrasound and scintigraphy of the liver in patients with colon or breast carcinoma: A prospective comparison. Radiology 1983, 149:225-230.
13. Shinagawa T, Ohto M, Kimura K, Tsunetomi S, Morita M, Saisho H, Tsuchiya Y, Saotome N, Karasawa E, Miki M. Ueno T, Okuda K. Diagnosis and clinical features of small hepatocellular carcinoma with emphasis on the utility of real-time ultra-sonography. Gastro-enterology 1984, 86:495-502.
14. Sheu JCh, Sung JL, Chen DS, Yu JY, Wang TH, Su CT, Tsang YM. Ultrasonography of small hepatic tumors using high-resolution linear-array real-time instruments. Radiology 1984, 150:797-802.
15. Mansi C, Savarino V, Picciotto A, Testa R, Canepa A, Dodero M, Celle G. Comparison between laparoscopy, ultrasonograpy and computed tomography in widespread and localized liver diseases. Gastrointest Endosc 1982, 28:83-85.

16. Danielson KS, Sheedy PF, Stephens DH, Hattery RR, LaRusso NF. Computed tomography and peritoneoscopy for detection of liver metastases: Review of Mayo Clinic Experience.
17. Hansen SW, Jensen F, Petersen NT, Hansen HH. Staging procedures of the liver in small cell bronchogenic carcinoma. A prospective comparative trial of peritoneoscopy with liver biopsy versus ultrasonograpy with fine needle aspiration. ASCO Abstracts 1983, C-20.

HISTOPATHOLOGICAL AND CYTOPATHOLOGICAL ASPECTS OF FOCAL
LIVER LESIONS

D.J. RUITER, G.J. VAN STEENIS

INTRODUCTION
Focal liver lesions may be caused by tumor-like conditions,
primary benign tumors, primary malignant tumors and tumor
metastases. It is important to note that not only metastasis
but also other conditions may be multiple, thereby mimicking
metastases (1). This may occur in abscesses, hemangiomas,
hepatocellular adenomas and hepatocellular carcinomas. The
following discussion will be devoted to autopsy data available on liver metastases,staging of liver metastases, and to
the diagnostic cytological and histological aspects of this
problem.

AUTOPSY DATA.
Observations in 9700 autopsies of patients with a malignant
tumor by Pickren et al. indicate that the liver is the most
frequent site for blood-borne metastases (2). However, the
liver is the only site of metastasis in 0.8% of cases.
Single foci of liver metastasis were observed in only 6% of
cases. Multiple metastases were almost always present in
undifferentiated carcinoma, transitional cell carcinoma and
malignant lymphoma. The most common histological types of
liver metastases found were in order of decreasing frequency: adenocarcinoma, squamous cell carcinoma, and leukemia.
It was noted that the incidence of liver metastases declined
with increasing age of the patient. In reviewing the origin
of liver metastases, the same authors (2) found 643 cases of
leukemia, 635 of breast cancer, 593 of lower respiratory
tract cancer, 525 of malignant lymphomas and 383 of
colorectal cancer. The proportion of primary tumors that had
metastasized to the liver was 78% in ocular malignant
melanoma (14 cases), 75% in pancreatic cancer (148 cases),
61% in breast cancer (635 cases), 61% in gallbladder and

bile duct cancer (23 cases), 57% in colo-rectal cancer (158 cases). It should be noted that these figures are derived from an autopsy study, suggesting that the distribution of tumor foci might be different at an earlier stage of the disease.

STAGING

Assessment of the extent of the malignant disease is referred to as staging. To stage a malignant process the histological type of tumor and anatomic site of the primary must be determined. Also the pathologist should estimate the histological grade of the tumor. Important in the staging of hepatic metastasis (3) are: 1) the percentage of liver involved, 2) the localisation of the tumor deposits, 3) the original stage of the primary cancer, 4) the level of carcino-embryonal antigen in colo-rectal carcinoma, 5) the level of performance, 6) the histological type and grade of the primary cancer, 7) the degree of vascularity of the metastases and 8) the serum albumin level (4). The degree of vascularity of liver metastases is of importance, because it influences tumor growth and has consequences for diagnostic and therapeutic perfusion procedures. It can be assessed radiologically and pathologically, the latter by gross casting procedures and histology. Visualisation of endothelial cells in tissue sections is possible with histochemical or immunohistochemical techniques (5). All these clinical and pathological features should be noted before the patients prognosis can be most knowledgeably assessed.

ASPIRATION CYTOLOGY

For the confirmation of liver-malignancy the cytological approach has been very useful (10,12,13,14,22,23). The method is simple, the trouble for the patient is minimal, it is safe and a definitive diagnosis is available within minutes (16). Also the technique may short cut many diagnostic procedures and be very economical.

The procedure should be kept as simple as possible. Random samples are taken if the liver is full of tumor or if on palpation one can feel hepatomegaly or tumor. The cytology needle should be guided by ultrasound if the target is small or far away (7). The laparoscope is used if a more extensive inventarisation is wanted. Also laparoscopy allows staging of other intra-abdominal sites for cancer.

The risk of this procedure is low and complications are minimal. However, Bile-leakage (19) and bleeding (15) are reported in the literature (6). Dangerous intra-abdominal bleeding (18) is a risk that we have encountered on two occasions in patients with extensive intra-abdominal tumor growth (not in this series). Our policy now is to perform aspiration cytology only after exclusion of bleeding and coagulation disorders (9).

The morphology of the cells aspirated nearly always allows one to determine if a lesion is benign or malignant, especially if examination of the primary tumor is also possible. As a rule, the contrast between normal liver cells and tumor cells is great (Fig. 1). The difference between reactively altered liver cells and well differentiated hepatocellular carcinoma may be more difficult (13) (Fig. 2).

The results of our clinical study at University Hospital Leiden are summarized here. We have examined the follow-up of all the patients having a liver-puncture for cytology during the past 10 years. Of the total of 208 patients, cytologic reports showed 57% malignant tumor, 39% benign lesions and 4% uncertain. For comparison with the cytological diagnosis we used: autopsy, histological biopsy, or clinical course. No sufficient data were present in 36 cases.

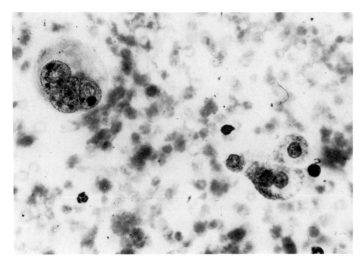

Fig. 1. Note the contrast between normal liver cells to the right and the big tumor cell to the left. Less differentiated hepato-cellular carcinoma, Giemsa stain, X 500.

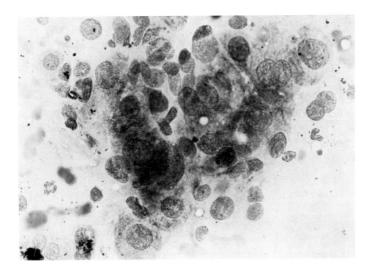

Fig. 2. Cytological aspect of well-differentiated hepato-cellular carcinoma. Normal liver cells among others at the left lower border. In the center a cluster of tumor cells, more and less caricatures of normal liver cells, Giemsa stain, X 500.

This results in the following figures (table 1 and 2).

Table 1. Comparison of cytological diagnosis with reference in cases reported malignant by cytology.

Reference	Number of cases reported malig- nant by cytology	Number of cases proven malignant by comparison with reference
Autopsy	23	23
Biopsy	13	13
Clinical course	74	74

Table 2. Comparison of cytological diagnosis with reference in cases reported benign by cytology.

Reference	Number of cases reported benign by cytology	Number of cases proven benign by comparison with reference
Autopsy	11	4
Biopsy	15	11
Clinical course	36	29

There were no false positive results in this series but, a negative answer had a very limited value. Based on review of the slides it was not thought to be caused by misinterpretation but because the liver lesion was not missed during the puncture. This is supported by the fact that we could reduce these figures in 19 histologically proven malignancies to 8 by repeating the puncture. More sophisticated ultra-sound guiding may further improve our results (17,22). The pathologic classification of the metastatic lesion can be usually assessed by cytology, especially if the primary tumor is known. In case of an unknown primary tumor aspiration cytology can alsmost invariably differentiate between adenocarcinoma, sarcoma and lymphoma.

HISTOPATHOLOGY.

Histopathological examination is warranted if cytological examination has not resulted in a diagnosis. This may be the case both in a focal liver lesion of unknown origin and one with a known primary tumor. In order to avoid sampling error guidance by means of ultrasonography or laparoscopy is advocated. An unequivocal diagnosis usually can be made histologically based on conventional hematoxylin and eosin stained paraffin sections. However, in about 15% of patients additional techniques such as immunohistochemistry or electron microscopy are necessary to establish an unequivocal diagnosis or to exclude diagnoses that have therapeutic implications (24). It is important that these techniques are employed step-wise on the basis of the differential diagnosis obtained by conventional histopathology (Fig. 3). All available information thus collected is integrated and an unequivocal diagnosis made by the pathologist is reported to the clinician.

Classification of poorly differentiated tumors is facilitated by demonstrating the type of cytoskeletal protein immunohistochemically (25,26). The presence of cytokeratin indicates epithelial and of vimentin usually indicates mesenchymal differentiation (Fig. 4). Malignant lymphomas and leukemias can be recognized by the presence of a common leukocytic antigen (27). Malignant melanomas may be detected by monoclonal antibodies directed against melanoma-associated antigens (Fig. 5) but, the ultimate proof for this diagnosis still is electron microscopy (28). For the discrimination between a primary hepatocellular carcinoma and liver metastasis of other origin immunohistochemical staining for alpha-fetoprotein or alpha-1-antitrypsin may be informative. The origin of tumor metastases can be also estimated by demonstrating the presence of thyreoglobulin, carcino-embryonal antigens, hormones or tumor type-associated antigens (24,27). The clinician must submit fresh tissue to the pathologist in

Fig. 3. Diagnostic work-up for focal liver lesions.

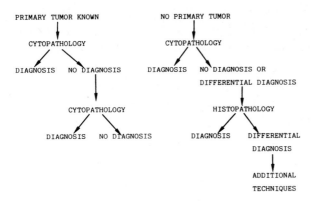

DIAGNOSTIC WORK-UP FOR FOCAL LIVER LESIONS

PRIMARY TUMOR KNOWN   NO PRIMARY TUMOR

       CYTOPATHOLOGY   CYTOPATHOLOGY

DIAGNOSIS   NO DIAGNOSIS   DIAGNOSIS   NO DIAGNOSIS OR

                               DIFFERENTIAL DIAGNOSIS

          CYTOPATHOLOGY   HISTOPATHOLOGY

     DIAGNOSIS   NO DIAGNOSIS   DIAGNOSIS   DIFFERENTIAL

                                   DIAGNOSIS

                                   ADDITIONAL

                                   TECHNIQUES

HISTOPATHOLOGICAL DIAGNOSIS OF "DIFFICULT" TUMORS

PROCEDURE (2)

PARAFFIN SECTIONS: DIFFERENTIAL DIAGNOSIS

               ADDITIONAL TECHNIQUE (1)

          DIAGNOSIS   DIFFERENTIAL

                        DIAGNOSIS

                  ADDITIONAL TECHNIQUE (2)

             DIAGNOSIS   DIFFERENTIAL

                       DIAGNOSIS

DIAGNOSIS WITH ADDITIONAL TECHNIQUES

POORLY DIFFERENTIATED MALIGNANT TUMOR

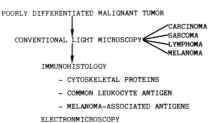

                                CARCINOMA

CONVENTIONAL LIGHT MICROSCOPY   SARCOMA

                                LYMPHOMA

                                MELANOMA

IMMUNOHISTOLOGY

    - CYTOSKELETAL PROTEINS

    - COMMON LEUKOCYTE ANTIGEN

    - MELANOMA-ASSOCIATED ANTIGENS

ELECTRONMICROSCOPY

    - DESMOSOMES

    - MELANOSOMES

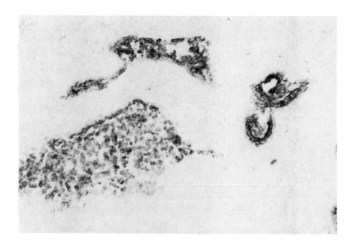

Fig. 4. Frozen section of poorly differentiated carcinoma showing marked staining for cytokeratin (x 160, counterstained with hematoxylin)

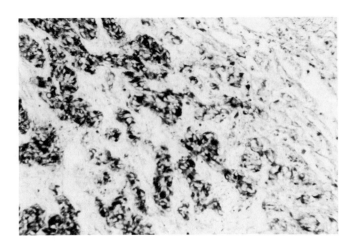

Fig. 5.
Paraffin section of melanoma metastasis reactive with a melanoma recognizing monoclonal antibody. Adjacent liver parenchymal cells do not stain. (X 160, counterstained with hematoxylin).

order to be able to preserve it for additional
histopathological diagnostic techniques.

SUMMARY.

Identification of the histologic type of a hepatic tumor
deposit is required for knowledgeable patient management.
Sometimes showing that a liver lesion is not malignant is
extremely important.
Aspiration cytology of the liver is an easy, rather safe,
quick and economic procedure. False positive results could
not be found in this series. If a lesion shows benign cytology, the accuracy of the test results is much less. One of
6 patients had a false negative result with a single puncture, 1 of 12 following repeat puncture. Biopsy may be
indicated when cytology does not result in a diagnosis and
clinical suspicion of a malignant process is high. Pathological grading of a hepatic tumor may also help determine
prognosis. The clinician must submit fresh tissue to the
pathologist in order to be able to preserve it for additional histopathological techniques, such as immunohistochemistry and electronmicroscopy, that are needed to establish a diagnosis in difficult cases.

REFERENCES

1. Harkins LA, Yap HY, Burdar AU, Blumenschein GR: Benign
   versus malignant hepatic lesions. A diagnostic dilemma
   with breast cancer patients. Cancer 1983; 52:
   1308-1311.

2. Pickren JW, Tsukada Y, Lane WW: Liver metastasis:
   Analysis of autopsy data. In: Liver Metastasis. GK Hall
   Med. Publ., Boston, 1982; pp.2-18.

3. Bengmark S, Jeppson B: Staging of liver metastasis. In:
   Liver metastasis. GK Hall Med. Publ. Boston, 1982; pp.
   268-274.

4. Weiss L, Gilberg HA: Introduction. In: Liver metastasis. GK Hall Med. Publ. Boston, 1982; pp. XVI-XXXI.

5. Mukai K, Rosai J, Burgdorf WHC: Localisation of factor VII-related antigen in vascular endothelial cells using an immunoperoxidase method. Am.J. Surg. Pathol. 1980; 4: 273-277.

6. Frable WJ: Thin-needle aspiration biopsy, vol. 14 in the series major problems in pathology. Philadelphia: Saunders, 1983; 232-240.

7. Hurwitz AL, Gueller R, Pugay P: Fine needle aspiration of malignant hepatic nodules for cytodiagnosis. J.A.M.A. 1974; 229: 814-815.

8. Kline TS: Handbook of fine needle aspiration biopsy cytology. St. Louis: Mosby Company 1981; 264-273.

9. Johansen S and Myren J: Fine needle aspiration biopsy smears in diagnosis of liver diseases. Scand. J. Gastroenterol. 1971;6: 585-588.

10. Koss LG: Diagnostic cytology 3e ed. Philadelphia: Lippincott, 1979; 863-871.

11. Jacobsen G, Gammelgaard J, Fuglo M: Coarse needle biopsy versus fine needle aspiration biopsy in the diagnosis of focal lesions of the liver. Acta Cytol. 1983; 27: 152-156.

12. Linsk JA, Franzen S: Clinical aspriation cytology. Philadelphia: Lippincott 1983; 182-190.

13. Lopes Cardozo P: Atlas of clinical cytology. Aalsmeer: Gerlings printing 1976; 383-391.

14. Lundqvust A: Fine needle aspiration biopsy for cyto-diagnosis of malignant tumour in the liver. Acta Med. Scand. 1970; 188: 465-470.

15. Lundqvist A: Fine needle aspiration biopsy of the liver. Acta Med. Scand. (Suppl.) 1971; 520: 1-28.

16. Mossler J, Barton TK, McClintock SC, Johnston WW: Cytologic detection of hepatic metastases. Acta Cytol. 1980; 24: 325-327.

17. Porter B, Karp W, Forsberg L: Percutaneous cyto-diagnosis of abdominal masses by ultrasound guided fine needle aspiration biopsy. Acta Radiol. Diagnosis 1981; 22: 663-668.

18. Riska H, Friman C: Fatality after fine needle aspiration biopsy of liver. Br. Med. J. 1975; 1: 517.

19. Schulz TB: Fine needle biopsy of the liver complicated with bile peritonitis. Acta Med. Scand. 1976; 199: 141-142.

20. Schwerk WB, Schmitz-Moormann P: Ultrasonically guided fine needle biopsies in neoplastic liver disease. Cancer 1981; 48: 1469-1477.

21. Soderstrom N: Fine needle aspiration biopsy. New York, Grune and Stratton 1966.

22. Zajicek J: Aspiration biopsy cytology in the seris monographs in clinical ctyology. Basel:Karger, 1974, 167-193 (by Wasastjerna).

23. Mackay B, Ordonez NG: The role of the pathologist in the evaluation of poorly differentiated tumors. Seminars Oncol. 1982; 9: 396-415.

24. Gabbiani G, Kapanci Y, Barazzone P, Frank WW: Immuno-chemical identification of intermediate sized filaments in human neoplastic cells: a diagnostic aid for the surgical pathologist. Am. J. Pathol.1981; 104: 206-216.

25. Muyen GNP van, Ruiter DJ, Ponec M, Huiskens-van der Mey C, Warnaar SO: Monoclonal antibodies with different specificities against cytokeratins. Am. J. Pathol. 1984;114: 9-17.

26. Damjanov I, Knowles BB: Biology of disease. Monoclonal antibodies and tumor-associated antigens. Lab. Invest 1983; 48: 510-525.

27. Duinen SG van, Ruiter DJ, Hageman Ph, Vennegoor C, Dickersin GR, Scheffer E, Rumke Ph: Immunohistochemical and histochemical tols in the diagnosis of amelanotic melanoma. Cancer 1984; 53: 1566-1573.

SCREENING FOR LIVER METASTASIS IN DAILY PRACTICE

F.J. Cleton

The detection of a liver metastasis means a poor prognosis for any cancer patient. The consequences of diagnostic procedures should therefore be carefully considered before any attempt at screening is made.

Three questions will be dealt with in this paper:

1. Which patient should be screened?
2. What is optimal screening?
3. What happens to a patient after a liver metastasis is detected?

The first question concerns two kinds of patients. In one the screening is part of a staging procedure and in the second it is part of a follow-up strategy. There are several examples in clinical oncology in which there is a need to exclude liver metastasis prior to treatment. In some patients extensive surgical procedures are considered, that may involve important mutilation. In patients scheduled for pelvic exenteration or limb amputation, the exclusion of metastases in the liver and in the lung can be crucial. Medical oncologists and radiotherapists often require accurate staging in the treatment of malignant lymphoma, when a choice between radio- therapy, chemotherapy or a combination of these two modalities has to be made. In such important decisions involving curative treatment, few physicians will rely on imaging techniques and routine liver chemistry. Often a surgical inspection of the abdominal cavity and palpation of the liver will be asked for.

In several forms of experimental aggressive treatment, for instance high dose chemotherapy followed by autologous bone marrow transplantation in moderately sensitive tumours, a careful staging of the liver will usually be performed. In modern protocols for the treatment of small cell lung cancer, accurate staging of the liver is required to determine a complete remission status. Only patients in complete remission will be considered for prophylactic brain irradiation and consolidation or maintenance chemotherapy.

It is customary for most oncologists to screen patients for liver metastases during follow-up after treatment of the primary tumour. The value of such screening can be questioned in many clinical situations. In patients treated according to an investigational protocol, it can be important to detect the first sign of liver metastases. Most protocols require tests of liver chemistry for this purpose. It is well known that such tests are less sensitive than the modern imaging techniques. The scientific value of this screening is often questionable. In patients who do not take part in a clinical study, the problem is even more complex. Cases of liver-only involvement, where liver metastases are the main object of treatment, occur in few tumour types such as colo-rectal cancer and of course primary liver cancer. Most tumours that spread to the liver, such as breast cancer and lung cancer, usually metastasize at the same time to other sites (Table 1 and 2).

TABLE 1. TUMOURS METASTASIS IN LIVER ONLY

- Colo-rectal adenocarcinoma
- Carcinoid
- Leiomyosarcoma of the gut wall

TABLE 2. TUMOURS METASTASIS IN- AND OUTSIDE THE LIVER

Lung	melanoma
Oesophagus	lymphoma
Breast	unknow origin

Most tumours in the upper G.I. tract including cancer of the oesophagus, the stomach and the pancreas, have a very poor prognosis when liver metastases are present. Surgical or

cytostatic treatment offers little or no benefit to the
patient. The discussion therefore will center on the colorectal tumours. The various therapeutic options will be
discussed in other sections of this course. Usually sophisticated surgery or experimental intensive chemotherapy is
required to obtain any therapeutic gain in the patient with
liver metastasis.

It is very problematic what the optimal screening
procedure should be. This varies among centers, but often
will include a history and physical examination, liver
chemistry, CEA assay, ultra-sound and in the doubtful cases,
a CT-scan. The costs of these investigations are considerable
and the benefit is often small. It is well known that many
of these tests lack sufficient sensitivity and specificity.
The figures that are reported from large centers often
concern investigations performed by experts and cannot be
expected in any small hospital. The damage in terms of
anxiety caused by false-positive results to many patients
should not be underestimated. A careful clinical staging is
always required, because the patient with advanced disease
outside the liver should not be submitted to aggressive and
high risk treatment. This is especially important in the
asymptomatic patients.

The extent of screening tests must depend on the possibilities of further treatment and on the level of scientific
interest and expertise in a center. For instance, in centers
where aggressive surgical treatment of liver metastases is
practized, early detection of small solitary tumour masses
is important, because survival is correlated with stage
(1, 2). Most surgeons maintain rigid criteria for the
resection of secondary liver tumours, accepting only solitary
metastasis with few satellite tumours in one lobe of the liver.
It is obvious that there should be absence of extra-hepatic
tumour and that the primary tumour should have been treated
radically. A similar argument applies to intra-arterial
chemotherapy.

The majority of patients presenting with symptomatic liver metastases will not be candidates for aggressive treatment. They may occasionally benefit from systemic chemotherapy with single agents. In the case of drug-resistance they may be considered for intra-arterial chemotherapy. Because in all controlled series no increase in survival was established, the treatment remains palliative. In the asymptomatic patient a 'wait and see' approach is often indicated.

REFERENCES

1. Bengmark S, Jönsson PE. 1982. Surgical treatment of liver metastases. In: Liver metastasis (L. Weiss & HA. Gilbert eds.). G.K. Hall, Boston.
2. Foster JW. 1978. Survival after liver resection for secondary tumours. Am. J. Surg. 135: 389.

THE NECESSITY FOR STAGING LIVER METASTASES AND STANDARDIZING
TREATMENT-RESPONSE CRITERIA. THE CASE OF SECONDARIES OF COLO-RECTAL
ORIGIN.

J. PETTAVEL, S. LEYVRAZ, P. DOUGLAS

There are only two ways of assessing the cure of a disease :

a) for a non-lethal condition : complete and long lasting
disappearance of all symptoms and signs from a clinical, biological
and radiological standpoint;

b) for a lethal disease : the same survival as that of a
comparable group of people free of disease.

The oncological idea of disease free survival (DFS) corresponds
to survival in complete remission but can be identified with cure
only if the mortality curve joins that of a normal population of the
same age.

Increase in survival, especially if the survival is of very
short duration is extremely difficult to establish, moreso if the
natural history of the disease is not clearly understood.   The
accurate assessment of treatment results necessitates a clear
knowledge of the disease evolution without the administration of
treatment.   As long as the results of treatment of patients with
2-3 small metastases of colorectal cancer will be compared to the
results obtained in patients where 75-80% of the liver volume is
replaced by metastatic deposits, assessment of the results will be
extremely difficult to interpret. The overall median survival of
liver metastases from colorectal cancer is in the order of
5,2 months for Pestana, 1964 (16), 5 months for Jaffé, 1968 (11),
4 months for Watkins, 1968 (22) and 4,5 months for Pettavel,
1969 (18).   Apparently, the median survival periods as quoted above
are not a true indication of survival time as considerable
disparities exist in the extremes of each group.   To overcome

this problem, the author proposed in 1967 (17) a classification of liver metastases in four stages, bearing in mind :

a) the size of the metastases,

b) liver function (established by laboratory liver function tests),

c) clinical hepatomegaly.

Using this classification, we were able to attribute to each stage a prognostic index (measured by survival time without the administration of treatment). This study was based on the observation of 61 cases in whom laparotomy was carried out and in which clinical prognostic criteria were put together, namely hepatomegaly, laboratory liver tests and surgical findings namely number and size of the liver metastases.

Using the Lausanne classification of 1967, survival rate calculated according to the stage :

- stage I	12 cases	21,5 months
- stage II	15 cases	10,7 months
- stageIII	26 cases	4,7 months
- stage IV	30 cases	1,4 month.

In 1970 a prospective series was added to this study and confirmed the precedent results. It was not until 1970 when Nielsen's work was published (15) that we saw another study using prognostic stratification.

Metastases	Number of cases	Mean survival time (months)
few	24	18
several	14	9
numerous	27	5

In 1976, Wood (23) analysed the survival of 113 patients who were untreated for hepatic metastases from colorectal cancer. The percentage of patients who survived for 1 year after the diagnosis of hepatic metastases was 60% for solitary metastases, 27% for several metastases in one lobe, and 5,7% for widespread metastases in both lobes.

Metastases	Number of cases	Mean survival time (months)
solitary	15	16,7
several (one lobe)	11	10,6
widespread (both lobes)	87	3,1.

If Nielsen had already observed the difference in survival relating to the number of metastases, Wood certainly emphasized the importance of the number of metastases as an important prognostic factor in separating solitary metastases which are in themselves a separate group from multiple metastases and by studying their distribution in liver tissue (unilateral or bilateral).

We also studied the role of unilateral or bilateral liver metastases in the study in 1979 (20). In 451 cases which we had examined by laparotomy for liver metastases from cancer of the colon and rectum, we found 110 who had synchronous liver metastases. These metastases were bilateral and multiple in 72 cases (65%) and unilateral and multiple in 24 cases (20%). The median survival without treatment was to our surprise 4 months in both groups.

If we look only at the topography of the liver metastases we can see that in 38 patients out of 110, i.e. 35% of the collective, it would have been possible to practice a right hepatectomy or a left hepatectomy or perhaps 50% of the time segmentectomy or metastasectomy. When we look at the survival of the 38 patients, we see a distinct difference between the two groups that we could easily have separated according to the age limit of 70 years.

Patients who were older than 70 years (14 cases) had a median survival of 5 months while the patients which were younger than 70 years (24 cases) had a median survival of 14 months. The number of cases excluded the question of coincidence.

1. The extremities of survival (survival range) were in the older age group from 0 to 30 months (with 3 post operative deaths), and in the group younger than 70 years from 0 to 34 months (with only one post-operative death).

As far as the length of survival is concerned, the unilaterality of the lesions and age seem to be the most important factors.

2. The number of metastases so long as they are situated on one side does not seem to worsen the prognosis as much as if the lesions are bilateral and occurring in an older age group.

The following figures are used to illustrate our point :
lateral metastases, in patients less than 70 years (24 patients) : median survival : 14 months.
Lateral metastases in patients older than 70 years (14 patients) : median survival : 5 months.
Bilateral metastases in patients less than 70 years (47 patients) : median survival : 4,5 months.
Bilateral metastases in patients older than 70 years (25 patients) : median survival : 2 months.

Fortner (7) in 1984 presented an interesting series of 75 patients with colorectal hepatic metastases treated by surgical extraction of the metastases (favourable cases metastases situated in the inferior hepatic region, unilateral, and patients of relatively young age). He arrived at the conclusion that the only important prognostic factor which predicts survival of a patient who had had hepatic extraction of a metastasis is that all the visible hepatic metastasis should be removed by the surgeon. It is interesting to note that only 5% of his patients were older than 70 years of age. We found in this study an indirect confirmation of our study of 1979 referred to previously except that Fortner thinks that for a comparable stage of the primitive tumor and for a comparable percentage hepatic replacement (PHR) it is of little importance to state the presence of the number of the metastases in the liver, the important thing being that the surgeon removes all of these metastases. In a parallel series of 114 patients with hepatic metastases from colorectal cancer, and treated by arterial chemotherapy, Fortner had especially looked at the degree of hepatic invasion (Percent Hepatic Replacement) for each patient. The PHR ranged from 5 - 95% with a median of 60%. The PHR estimation is a relatively subjective appraisal as it reflects the personal opinion of the investigator. Fortner looked at a first group where the PHR was equal or less than 50%, a second group where the PHR

was between 55% and 85% and a third group where the PHR was greater
than 80%. The patients of the first group who showed no evidence
of lymphatic invasion and who did not receive previous chemotherapy
had a median survival of 17,8 months whereas the median survival
had fallen to 12 months for patients of the same group with adverse
prognostic factors or for those of the second group without these
adverse factors. Survival is very short for advanced cases.
Unfortunately, Fortner does not tell us about the survival of the
patients who had received no treatment whatsoever. It is our
opinion that invasion of the hepatic tissue by the tumor mass is
of the utmost importance and extra-hepatic invasion as well. We
will come back to this point later on.

Balch in his study in 1983 (2) insisted on the adverse
influence on survival because of the presence of extra-hepatic
metastases and of an elevated PHR index. The favourable prognostic
factors, according to Balch, were that the liver metastases be
unilateral, that the hepatic function be normal, i.e. bilirubin
less than 0,5 mg/%, and alkaline phosphatase less than 200 mg/%.

Lahr and Balch (12) published in 1983 a bio-statistical study
in which they examined among 22 variables the parameters which
influence survival in 175 patients with liver metastases due to
colorectal cancer. Some of these variable parameters play a very
important part.   Here are a few of the important variables :
increase in the alkaline phosphatase (P = 0,0004)
increase in the bilirubin level (P = 0,0005)
unilateral localization or bilateral localization of the liver
metastases (P = 0,002), and number of involved lymph glands
(P = 0,015).

On the other hand, the CEA value before treatment had no
prognostic value. This biostatistic study, utilizing multifactorial
analysis is certainly interesting, especially as 175 cases
studied were patients with hepatic metastases but an interpretation
of the study is surely not above criticism because 60% of the

patients had laparotomies which means that 4 times out of 10 the
appreciation of liver metastases was carried out only by
radioisotopic studies and ultrasonography examination. The PHR
seems however important for the evaluation of prognosis since the
median survival of the patients with a **solitary metastasis is**
11 months against 4 months for those with 5 or more liver metastases
(P = 0,0001). Similarly, unilateral metastases are associated with
a median survival of 12 months as compared to 5 months for bilateral
metastases (P = 0,0001). Whether the metastases are synchronous or
metachronous is of little importance as the Fortner study has also
pointed out. Serum bilirubin level shows an even better correlation
with survival as the median survival is only 2,5 months for those
patients who had a serum bilirubin level between 1 and 5 mg. A
level above   5 mg was associated with a median survival of
less than 30 days. Similarly, the patients who had a normal level
of alkaline phosphatase (less than 100 UI) had a survival longer
than those in which the alkaline phosphatase was higher than 200 UI
(median survival of 9,2 months as compared to 2,5 months with
P = 0,0001). However, one can be critical in pointing out in this
article that 43 patients out of 175 did not have excision of the
primary tumor (the patient population was then heterogeneous and
difficult to compare). One of the most interesting conclusions of
Lahr's study is that the multifactorial analysis seems to show that
chemotherapy is far less important in survival than the initial
level of alkaline phosphatase or that of bilirubin, the fact that
the primary tumor is dissected or not, or that the hepatic metastases
are uni- or bilateral, or the fact that few or many lymph glands
are involved with tumor.

One can look at Lahr's work in the following way :

alkaline phosphatase (IU)	bilirubin (mg)		
	0 to 0,5	0,5 to 1	1 to 5
0 to 100	14 months	5 months	4 months
100 to 200	7 "	6 "	2,5 "
greater than 200	3 "	3 "	1,5 "
	median survival (months)		

To recapitulate, we would like to point out that the classification of Lausanne (1976) is made up of 3 evaluative stages based on the presence or absence of hepatomegaly, the normality or increase in the alkaline phosphatase level and that the survival in different stages was established as follows (19)

Lausanne, staging (1976)

evaluative stage	hepatomegaly	elevation of alkaline phosphatase	survival time(months)
I	absent	no	15
II		one or the other	4,7
III	present	yes	1,4

The multifactorial analysis of Lahr, 1983 (12), as the analyses by Balch 1983 (2) and that of Fortner, 1984 (8) confirm that regardless of which way we look at these studies it is clearly the disturbance of the laboratory tests, especially that of the alkaline phosphatases and the PHR, whether it is appreciated by the surgeon (at laparotomy), the clinician (hepatomegaly) or by the radiologist (by transverse tomography, ultrasonography and isotopic scintigraphy) which permits one to evaluate the prognosis regardless of treatment and therefore establish a proper evaluative staging. Certain other prognostic factors are equally important but no single or other combined factors provide better reliability than alkaline phosphatase and bilirubin and the extension of tumor invasion in the liver. In the last 12 years, a number of authors

have proposed different classifications for liver metastases due
to colorectal cancer, based on the PHR but without looking at the
correlation with survival. The PHR was first appreciated by
surgeons, despite the different radiological investigations
and echographies. Almersjö in 1972 (1), Bengmark in 1974 (3),
El-Domeiri in 1978 (6), Dahl in 1981 (5), Bengtsson in 1981 (4)
and especially Gennari in 1982 (9) and finally Fortner in 1984 (8).
(This last author had attempted to create a correlation with
survival). Other authors, for example Grage in 1979 (10) were
primarily interested in the symptomatology provoked by the tumor.

The estimation of the PHR in percentage seems attractive in as
much as it appears precise and one can compare for example liver
invasion of less than 25%, from 25% to 50%, from 50% to 75% and
more than 75%. But surgeons must never forget what pathologists
have always emphasized, i.e. that the visual and touch examination
of the volume of the liver which has been replaced by tumor is
extremely subjective and must be accepted with caution in the
living patient. The PHR estimation has a certain value when it is
carried out always by the same doctor as in Fortner's study in
1984 (7, 8). The value becomes relative when the volume of the
liver invasion is looked at by two different practitioners.
Furthermore, little tumors which are situated on the right superior
posterior aspect of the liver are practically impalpable. It is
advisable to compare the PHR with computerised tomographies in which
dye has been injected. A comparative prospective study of PHR
surgical evaluation and three dimensional reconstruction from
transverse tomographies has never to our knowledge been undertaken.
It is for this reason that we proposed in Frankfurt in 1983 (2) a
classification where the limits of the 3 stages of the Percent
Hepatic Replacement are arbitrarily placed in order to separate
a very favourable stage, an intermediary stage in which the majority
of the cases are found, and an advanced stage. This classification

proposes three evaluative stages :

stage   I   : PHR less than 25%

stage   II   : PHR between 25% to 75%

stage   III   : PHR more than 75%.

In stage II (25% to 75% of PHR) we notice that a great majority
of the patients in whom we had proposed chemotherapy by hepatic
vascular infusion are listed and it is because of this that we
have introduced two stratification factors, namely :

F : pathological liver tests (bilirubin, alkaline phosphatase,
and to a lesser degree GOT, gamma-GT and serum albumin) and

S : the patient is symptomatic (important weight loss, loss of
appetite, nausea, serious pain, Karnowsky performance status< 60%)
Other complementary stratification factors with varying importance
might be introduced :

- previous chemotherapy

- single metastasis

The group with solitary metastasis, it seems to us, should be
treated by surgical excision before regional chemotherapy to the
remaining liver. Whether the metastases are synchronous or
metachronous in relation to the primary lesion seems to us to be
of little importance.

Lausanne classification (1983 - 1984)

Stage I   : PHR less than 25% with stratification F, S, FS

Stage II   : PHR from 25% to 75% with stratification F, S, FS

Stage III   : PHR more than 75% (all the patients with FS).

Determination of response in treatment of liver metastases

The Committee on Standardization of Reporting of Results of
Cancer Treatment representing the International Union against Cancer,
the World Health Organization and the principal anti-cancer centres
of the world published in 1981 under the authorship of Miller (14)
an excellent reappraisal showing what the criteria of minimum
response to be considered are, in order to judge the objective
response of a cancerous patient to a treatment (for all cancer

localizations).

These recommendations remain a reference but in the case of
the appreciation of the treatment of liver metastases and in
particular if we deal with a controlled clinical trial we think
that Miller's criteria (14) must be improved. It is evident that
objective response to treatment can be determined by clinical means,
by radiological examinations and biochemistry or by surgical
pathological restaging and that the method used must be very fully
described.

Miller proposed as a definition for Complete Response, the
disappearance of all signs of illness on two clinical observations
not less than four weeks apart. In the case of liver metastases,
we think that the disappearance of all the metastases must be
confirmed by computeri ed tomography or ultrasonography. In our
opinion, the interval between the two clinical observations must be
8 weeks instead of 4 weeks for liver metastases, otherwise the
artifacts can be wrongly interpreted and thereby falsify the
interpretation. We also think that the normal level of the CEA
is also of great importance and two readings spaced at an 8 week
interval must be carried out because of the specificity of the
carcino-embryonic antigen.   Normal X-rays, normal ultrasonographies
without a return to the normal level of the CEA seems to us to
exclude a complete response.

Conversely, we think that the partial regression (50%) of the
metastases on the computerized tomography scans can be accepted
as a complete response if no other new liver metastases appear
during the period of 6 months and if the CEA level remains normal
during 6 months. We know that certain metastases, after becoming
necrotic can form calcification within the metastatic bed or
perhaps can be completely replaced by fibrous tissue which gives
an abnormal radiological or ultrasonographic image even when
histological verification of the lesions shows that there are no
cancer cells whatsoever. We have already published an objective
document (19).

Partial response (PR) as stated by Miller is the reduction in size of 50% of the tumor volume on two separate clinical observations during a period of 4 weeks without the appearance of new liver metastatic lesions. We think that an 8 week interval is preferable to that of 4 weeks in the case of liver metastases. We also think that it is necessary to emphasize reduction in volume of 50% of the normal CEA levels for 8 weeks (for the same reasons as we have said above). This is because the true volume on the computered axial tomography is often not accurately measured. At times it is very difficult to establish.

The clinical stage which we will call stable disease or no change (NC) corresponds to regression of less than 50% of the volume of the liver metastases and a drop in the level of the carcino-embryonic antigen for less than 8 weeks.

Progressive Disease (PD) corresponds to any progression of the volume of the liver metastases of at least 25% as shown by Miller. The presence of extra-hepatic metastases makes it even more difficult to interpret the levels of carcino-embryonic antigen. We are perfectly conscious of this but we think that it is better to be extra-careful in a field where the chemotherapist is often happy to accept minimal response or worse yet subliminal response.

We would like to propose as a result the following definitions for response of chemotherapy treatment to liver metastases from colorectal cancer :

COMPLETE RESPONSE   – Disappearance of all metastases by CT[1] or Ultrasonography for 8 weeks and normalisation of CEA for 8 weeks

or Partial regression 50% of metastases by CT*) without appearance of new liver metastases for 6 months and normalization of CEA for 6 months

1) if possible after injection of contrast material and with mention of tomography intervals in centimeters.

     * some metastases get necrotic and calcified
      without diseappearing by CT or US.

PARTIAL RESPONSE - Regression of 50% of the larger surface
        of hepatic metastases for 8 weeks
        and 50% decrease of CEA for 8 weeks.

STABLE DISEASE   - Any regression of less than 50% of the
        larger surface of hepatic metastases and
        any decrease of CEA for less than 8 weeks

PROGRESSION   - Any progression of the volume of hepatic
        metastases of at least 25%

N.B. One shall not forget that extra-hepatic metastases make
   CEA determination invalid.

The measurement of hepatomegaly and its consecutive decrease
in volume after treatment are interesting. It must be carried out
according to the recommendations of Lokich 1983 (13) but they
appear too difficult to estimate clinically to be really feasible
in patients with scar tissue after operation and do not correspond
to the necessary strict criteria to appreciate complete response.

As for the length of survival, it is evident that it is always
necessary to emphasize if this survival is measured from the time
of the diagnosis of the initial disease from the time of diagnosis of
hepatic metastases, or from the time when chemotherapy treatment
was started.

The duration of objective response should always be quoted
as well as the interval leading to the resumption of the progression
of the disease.

To compare the median survivals is interesting but again it is
necessary to emphasize each time the evaluative stage of the disease
before treatment was started.

The quality of life during the period of survival must also be
emphasized.

CONCLUSION

It is 20 years now since we have been treating hepatic metastases
resulting from colorectal cancers by surgery or chemotherapy following
different therapeutic modalities with the help of many devices
(permanent or transitory ischemia, chemotherapeutic agents fixed
in microspheres to provide slow absorption which later on provoke
a relatively important ischemia, isolated chemotherapeutic
perfusions followed by slow perfusions, etc...). All the comparisons
of treatment results have been more or less vain because the authors
have never referred to standardized criteria either for the type of
patients treated or for the definition of the different responses
to treatment.

20 years have passed also since certain authors some of whom were
quoted above have studied different prognostic factors relating to
the presence of liver metastases in colorectal cancer (Percent
Hepatic Replacement, uni- or bilateral metastases, age, laboratory
tests, bilirubin and alkaline phosphatase levels), symptomatic
disease or not, concomitant cirrhosis of the liver, previous
chemotherapy, the period between the onset of the primary lesion
and that of the liver metastases and the extra-hepatic localisation
of metastases).

We have presented a prognostic classification based on a series
of patients who were not treated in 1967. We have updated the
study in 1976 and made it more complete;hence,the Lausanne
comprehensive classification 1983-1984.

This last classification takes into account all the major studies
to date and will serve as a comparable basis to compare further
clinically controlled trials. We have even tried to improve on
the definition of the criteria of response to treatment as applied
to liver metastases in colorectal cancers.

REFERENCES

1 - ALMERSJO O, BENGMARK B, HAFSTROM Lo. Liver Metastases found
by follow-up of patients operated on for colorectal cancer.
Cancer 1976 ; 37 : 1454-1457.

2 - BALCH CM, URIST MM, SOONG SJ, McGREGOR M. A prospective Phase
II Clinical Trial of Continuous FUDR Regional Chemotherapy for
Colorectal Metastases to the Liver Using a Totally Implantable
Drug Infusion Pump. Ann. Surg. 1983; 198 : 567-573.

3 - BENGMARK S, FREDLUND PE. Temporary dearterialization combined
with intra-arterial infusion of oncolytic drugs in the treatment
of liver tumors. In Ariel IM (ed) : Progress in clinical cancer
VII. New-York : Grune and Stratton, 1978 : 207-216.

4 - BENGTSSON G, CARLSON G, HAFSTROM L, JONSSON PE. Natural History
of patients with untreated liver metastases. Am. J. Surg. 1981;
141 : 586-589.

5 - DAHL EP, FREDLUND PE, BENGMARK S. Transient hepatic dearterialization followed by regional intra-arterial 5-Fluorouracil
infusion as treatment for liver tumors. Ann. Surg. 1981 ;
193 : 82-88.

6 - EL-DOMEIRI AA, MOJAB K. Intermittent occlusion of the hepatic
artery and infusion chemotherapy for carcinome of the liver.
Am. J. Surg. 1978 ; 135 : 771-775.

7 - FORTNER JG, SILVA JS, GOLBEY RB, COX EB, MACLEAN BJ. Multivariate
Analysis of a Personnal Series of 247 Consecutive Patients with
Liver Metastases from Colorectal Cancer. I. Treatment by
hepatic Resection. Ann. Surg. 1984 ; 199 : 306-316.

8 - FORTNER JG, SILVA JS, COX EB, GOLBEY RB, GALLOWITZ H, MACLEAN B.
Multivariate analysis of a personnal series of 247 patients with
liver metastases from colorectal cancer II. Treatment with intrahepatic chemotherapy. Ann. Surg. 1984 ; 199 : 317-324.

9 - GENNARI L, DOCI R, BOZZETTI F, VERONESI U. Proposal for clinical
classification of liver metastases. Tumori 1982 ; 68 : 1443-1449.

10 - GRACE TB, VASSILOPOULOS PP, SHINGLETON WW, JUBERT AV, ELIAS EG,
AUST JB, MOSS SE. Results of a prospective randomized study of
hepatic artery infusion with 5-Fluorouracil versus intravenous
5-Fluorouracil in patients with hepatic metastases from colorectal
cancer : a central oncology group study. Surgery 1979 ; 86 :
550-555.

11 - JAFFE BM, DONEGAN WL, WATSON F, SPRATT JS Jr. Factors influencing
survival in patients with untreated hepatic metastases. Surg.
Gynécol. Obstet 1968 ; 127 : 1-11.

12 - LAHR CJ, SOONG SJ, CLOUD G, SMITH JW, URIST MM, BALCH CM.
A multifactorial analysis of pronostic factors in patients with
liver metastases from colorectal carcinoma. J. Clin. Oncol. 1983;
1 : 720-726.

13 - LOKICH JJ. Determination of response in treatment of hepatic neoplasia. Seminars in Oncology 1983 ; 10 : 228-237.

14 - MILLER AB, HOOGSTRATEN B, STAQUET M, WINKLER A. Reporting results of cancer treatment. Cancer 1981 ; 47 : 207-214.

15 - NIELSEN J, BALSLEV I, JENSEN HE. Carcinoma of the colon with liver metastases. Acta Chir Scand 1971 ; 137 : 463-465.

16 - PESTANA C, REITEMEIER RJ, MOERTEL CG, JUDD ES, DOCKERTY MB. The natural history of carcinoma of the colon and rectum. Am J Surg 1964 ; 108 : 826-829.

17 - PETTAVEL J, MORGENTHALER F. Natural history of cancer metastatic to the liver and protracted arterial infusions. 5th International Congress of chemotherapy, Vienna, 1967.

18 - PETTAVEL J, MORGENTHALER F. Traitement chimiothérapique des métastases hépatiques en fonction de leur évolution spontanée. Schweiz. Med. Wschr. 1969 ; 130 : 773-777.

19 - PETTAVEL J. MORGENTHALER F. Protracted arterial chemotherapy of liver tumors : An experience of 107 cases over a 12 years period. In Ariel IM (ed) : Progress in clinical cancer VII. New-York : Grune and Stratton, 1978 : 217-223.

20 - PETTAVEL J, MEYER A. Indication selective à l'exérèse chirurgicale des métastases hépatiques. Schweiz. Med. Wschr. 1979 ; 109 : 794-796.

21 - PETTAVEL J. Intraarterielle chemotherapie bei Lebermetastasen. C. Hottenrott, ed., Verlag C. Bindermagel, 6360 FRIEDBERG I, 1983.

22 - WATKINS EJ, KHAZEI AM, NAHRA KS. Surgical basis for arterial infusion chemotherapy of disseminated carcinoma to the liver. Surg. Gynec. Obstet. 1970 ; 130 : 580-605.

23 - WOOD CB, GILLIS CR, BLUMGART LH. A retrospective study of the natural history of patients with liver metastases from colorectal cancer. Clinical Oncology 1976 ; 2 : 285-288.

TREATMENT OF LIVER METASTASES

Management of Hepatic Metastases: A General Overview

Philip S. Schein, M.D., F.R.C.P.

The importance of liver metastases as a source of morbidity and
mortality from tumors arising in the gastrointestinal tract, breast
and lung is well recognized. It has been estimated that 50% to 75%
of patients who die of cancer have hepatic metastases. In response,
many investigators have focused their attention on this aspect of
clinical management, and have attempted to define new therapeutic
strategies[1]. These have been directed not only to the patient
with overt metastatic disease, but also to the surgical adjuvant
setting in an attempt to eradicate microscopic disease that may be
present in liver at the time of diagnosis. Many modes of treatment
now being evaluated are not new, and in some instances they have
been the subject of investigation for over twenty years. The field
of therapeutic management of hepatic metastases has, however, become
increasingly more sophisticated in the past five years as our
understanding of the mechanisms of metastases and their management
have increased substantially. The ultimate question is whether
specific forms of treatment have been proven to reduce morbidity and
mortality. My presentation will set the stage for discussions that
follow which deal in much greater detail with the specific
modalities that have been developed for the management of this
problem.

The important role of surgery in the management of hepatic
metastases has not been fully appreciated by the non-surgical
specialist. Foster[2], as well as Wilson and Adson[3] have
demonstrated that a 5 to 10 year disease-free survival can be
achieved in approximately 25% of patients after resection of an

apparently solitary colon or rectal metastases. Even in patients with metachronous metastases, a 20 - 25% survival has been estimated. Important research questions relate to the salvage rate in cases with greater than one metastasis, as well as tumor size and location.

The measurement of plasma CEA concentrations can, in many cases, lead to the early detection of an isolated hepatic metastasis, which is subsequently confirmed with a CAT scan. Obviously, a patient being considered for definitive resection of a liver metastasis must undergo a complete pre-operative evaluation for detection of other potential sites of disease, as well as careful intra-abdominal exploration prior to liver resection. Nevertheless, the identification of such patients and the subsequent management of their liver metastases by surgical resection represents the most effective measure currently available for achieving long-term disease-free survival. It is obvious, however, that for the majority of patients additional treatment will be required in order to eradicate residual tumor that resides in a microscopic form in liver or in other sites assuming such therapy can be defined.

Surgery may have an additional role in patients with overt metastatic tumor, particularly in the setting of carcinoid syndrome. It is recognized that established hepatic metastases draw their predominant blood supply from the branches of the hepatic artery. Hepatic artery ligation or embolization may result in a dramatic, albeit transient, reduction of hepatic metastases which control the endocrine manifestations of a hormone-secreting neoplasm. Hepatic artery ligation has been combined with intra-arterial infusion of chemotherapeutic agents, although this technique has never been subjected to a carefully performed control trial, and there is no indication to date that a clear advantage is achieved.

Radiation therapy for hepatic metastases is largely limited to the palliation of symptoms in patients with advanced disease, and specifically for reducing pain resulting from the distension of

Glissons capsule[4]. Dramatic responses in tumor reduction can,
however, be achieved in some cases with the use of conventional
doses of 2000 to 3000 rads to the entire liver. Patients receiving
doses in excess of 3500 rads are placed at considerable risk for the
development of radiation hepatitis. The structures that are most
sensitive to the effects of radiation therapy are the hepatic
venules and a veno-occlusive disease, resembling the Budd-Chiari
syndrome with hepatomegaly and ascites, has been well documented.
More experimental approaches such as the injection of radioactive
microspheres into the hepatic artery or the administration of
specific radiolabelled antibodies to tumor associated antigens as
proposed by Order and colleagues, remain to validated. The
Gastrointestinal Tumor Study Group in the United States is currently
evaluating the role of whole liver irradiation and 5-FU as an
adjuvant therapy for resected adenocarcinoma of the colon. In this
study, patients with Dukes-C colon cancer have been randomized to
either observation following surgery or combined modality
treatment. The latter consists of 2100 rads delivered over a total
of 14 days, with 5-FU, 350 mg/m^2, given on days 1-3 during
radiation therapy, as well as two-and-half weeks after completion of
hepatic irradiation. This study was designed in August of 1979 and
had to be modified because of several episodes of serious
hematologic toxicity associated with the original 5-FU dose of 500
mg/m^2. To date, over 200 patients have been randomized.
Forty-five patients have developed distant metastases, 13 of which
have involved the liver. This study remains active and the data are
blinded in regard to treatment, and it is premature to determine
whether hepatic recurrence and survival will be influenced by this
approach. Isolated instances of persistently elevated transaminases
have been observed, though in general this has not been a
significant problem since the reduction of 5-FU dose. This does
serve to emphasize that the addition of chemotherapy to hepatic
irradiation can potentiate the toxicity of the latter modality, and
this factor must be taken into consideration in the design of
studies.

The limitations of standard intravenous chemotherapy of hepatic metastases from colorectal cancer are well recognized. As a consequence, a number of experimental approaches have been undertaken, with principal emphasis on intra-arterial chemotherapy. The rationale for hepatic and intra-arterial chemotherapy involves the direct drug delivery to tumor in the hope of increasing intracellular concentrations of the cytotoxic agent. The prolonged infusions insure a longer duration of effective drug concentration, with a potential of maximizing the number of sensitive cells exposed to the agent during critical phases of the cell cycle. For specific drugs, hepatic extraction and catabolism can result in reduced systemic toxicity. In our studies with intra-arterially administered Streptozotocin in patients with islet cell carcinoma and hepatic metastases, we were able to demonstrate a significant first pass uptake of the intact drug [5]. The result was reduced exposure of normal tissues, and the kidneys in particular, to an agent with known nephrotoxic properties. For colorectal cancers, the principal tumor for purposes of this discussion, the fluorinated pyrimidines and FUdR in particular represent the only established therapeutic option. It is estimated that 95% of FUdR is extracted by the liver before reaching the systemic circulation. The first pass uptake of 5-FU, in contrast, is more variable and ranges between 20% to 50%. As a consequence FUdR has been assumed to have a therapeutic advantage, which has never been proven. A strong conceptual argument can be made in favor of 5-FU because of the need to treat microscopic extra-hepatic tumor that is an important unexposed site of recurrence in patients undergoing hepatic perfusions with the deoxyribonucleoside.

There is considerable controversy in regard to the current position of intra-arterial chemotherapy for hepatic metastases from colorectal cancer because of disparity of clinical data, with responses ranging from 35 to 80%, as well as variable median survivals. The question is whether the potential morbidity and increased cost associated with this approach is outweighed by improved response rates and more importantly survival benefit relative to standard intravenous therapy. In this regard, the

Central Oncology Group has performed what remains the most
definitive randomized controlled trial of hepatic artery infusion of
5-FU vs. intravenous administration of the same drug for patients
with colorectal cancer [6]. Patients with hepatic metastases from
colorectal cancer either received 5-FU by continuous intra-arterial
infusion at a dose of 20 mg/kg daily for a period of 14 days. In
patients who tolerated the therapy, an additional 7 days at a
reduced dose of 10 mg/kg was subsequently delivered. The
alternative treatment arm was systemic 5-FU at a dose of 12 mg/kg
daily by IV push for a period of 4 days followed by one-half this
dose every other day for an additional 4 treatments. A total dose
of 5-FU in the systemic therapy group did not exceed 1000 mg/day in
any case. After the initial course of therapy, all patients were
placed on maintenance therapy with 5-FU; 15 mg/kg intravenously at
weekly intervals. A total of 74 patients were entered into this
trial, 16 of which were considered acceptable. The response rate
with intra-arterial infusion was 34% compared to 24% with
intravenous therapy; the difference was not significant. Durations
of response and survival were similarly not statistically different.
An analysis was performed to ensure that the study was well balanced
in regard to prognostic factors. With the exception of sex, there
appeared to be no significant differences. The investigators
concluded that considering the additional complications, morbidity
and cost, the failure of intra-hepatic arterial infusion to provide
a prolonged survival raised serious doubts as to its future role in
the management of metastatic colorectal cancer. The Central
Oncology Group study has been the subject of considerable debate and
criticism, though at the time the study was initiated, it was
considered an appropriately designed randomized trial. The
following points have been raised in addition to the relatively
brief exposure of the liver to intra-arterial therapy: 60% of the
patients had catheters inserted percutaneously, with the potential
problem of position for effective hepatic perfusion. The study
utilized arterialgraphic contrast or plane abdominal x-ray to
monitor the position of the catheter in contrast to current use of
macroaggregated albumin nuclide arteriography for ensuring optimal
drug distribution at low infusion rates. The values of liver

function tests were employed to determine treatment response and
failure; it is now recognized that intra-arterial chemotherapy can
cause an elevation of serum transaminases independent of effect on
tumor. In essence, the current approaches to hepatic artery
chemotherapy have become refined, in particularly with the advent of
the Infusaid implantable pump.

Clearly, the Infusaid pump represents a substantial technological
advance but the question remains, given the limited number of
chemotherapeutic agents effective colorectal cancer, whether this
technique is superior to conventional intravenous therapy.
Ensminger and colleagues have reported an 83% response rate in
patients with colorectal cancer in whom the tumor was confined to
the liver [7]. This was associated with a median duration of
survival from time of diagnosis of metastases of 21 weeks. This
apparent benefit was restricted to patients with metastases confined
to liver, and a highly selected cohort. Confirmatory data have been
provided by the studies of Balch and co-workers where an 88%
response rate and a 26-month median duration of survival have been
reported [8]. Nevertheless, there are investigators in several
institutions that have employed similar techniques and patient
selection who have failed to produce these promising results. For
example, Levin and co-workers [9] at the University of Chicago
have reported a 29% response rate, comparable to the results
achieved by Weiss and co-workers at the Sydney Farber Cancer Center
[10]. We are all awaiting the results of carefully performed
control trials to prove that the use of the Infusaid pump, with the
associated need for inter-operative catheter placement as well as
associated cost, is superior to conventional intravenous 5-FU. In
this regard, Kemeny and co-workers at Memorial Sloan-Kettering
Cancer Center have reported the initial results of their randomized
control trial which compares intra-hepatic vs. systemic continuous
infusions of 5-FUDR [11]. All patients in this study have had an
exploratory laparotomy with insertion of an hepatic artery catheter
in placement of an implantable Infusaid pump. Those patients
randomized to systemic therapy had an additional catheter placed in
a large central vein. And those patients in intra-hepatic arterial

arm, the pump was connected to the hepatic catheter. In the systemic arm, the venous catheter is connected to the pump and the hepatic catheter to an infus-a-port; if disease progressed, the venous catheter was removed and the hepatic catheter was connected to the pump by a minor surgical procedure. In her presentation at the 1984 ASCO meeting, Kemeny reported on results in 35 evaluable patients. A 41% response rate was achieved with intra-hepatic 5-FUdR compared with 33% with systemic treatment. Recurrence or progression in liver was found in 10 of 17 patients treated with intra-arterial chemotherapy compared to 9 of 18 with systemic FUdR. There were a larger number of patients who demonstrated tumor regression in extra-hepatic sites with the use of intra-arterial chemotherapy. Median survival at the time of presentation was not different, 10.7 months with intra-hepatic chemotherapy compared to 11.8 months with systemic FUdR. There was a substantial incidence of hepatic toxicity, as well as gastric ulceration. The overall conclusions were that at the time of analysis, response rates for intra-hepatic and systemic chemotherapy were similar and the development of extra-hepatic disease was observed more commonly with intra-hepatic infusions and rarely with systemic infusions, and that gastrointestinal toxicity was common with both forms of infusions with ulceration reported with intra-hepatic therapy and diarrhea with systemic treatment. Similar results were reported by the Cancer Research Institute at the University of California. 41% of patients treated with intra-arterial 5-FUdR have demonstrated a partial response compared to 20% with intravenous therapy [12]. The differences have not reached statistical significance. Of increasing concern are the increasing numbers of reports of biliary sclerosis found in association with FUdR-pump treatment.

Overall, it is important for these control trials and others recently initiated to come to completion prior to drawing a final conclusion about the overall role of the Infusaid pump for the treatment of patients with colorectal cancer whose sole site of metastatic disease is the liver. The present data do not suggest a major advice. Ultimately, it will be what can be put into the pump, rather than the technology itself, which will dictate the quality and duration of response. As we all are aware the chemotherapeutic armamentarium for colorectal cancer is extraordinarily limited. It is for this reason that I believe that greater emphasis should given to the management of tumors which are recognized as more drug sensitive, such as breast cancer and gastric carcinoma.

While the subject of this symposium is hepatic metastases, it must be recognized that the management of this important clinical problem cannot be examined in isolation of the more typical presentation, generalized systemic involvement. While the importance of liver metastases from cancer cannot be minimized as a cause of morbidity and mortality, it is unlikely that a therapy design to treat this specific problem alone will have a major impact on survival statistics of any major tumor other than primary hepatoma. In this context, the incidence of serious adverse reactions and costs must be important considerations in assessing the overall impact of the new therapy.

It is my personal philosophy that greater emphasis should be given to the development of therapies that can be administered simply, and on an outpatient basis. Treatment must not only effectively control known or suspected liver metastases, but it is essential that it also deal with extra-hepatic tumor which is present in the majority of cases. Ultimately this will require the development of more effective forms of systemic chemotherapy perhaps used in combination with selective surgical resections.

References

1. Ramming K.P., Sparks F.C., Eilber F.R., Morton D.L.:   Sem.
    Oncol. 4:71-80, 1977.

2. Foster J.H., Berman M.M.:   Major Problems in Clinical Surgery,
    Philadelphia. Saunders, 1977, pp. 207-245.

3. Wilson S.M., Adson M.A.:   Arch. Surg. 111:330-334, 1976.

4. Turek-Maischeider M., Kazem I. JAMA 232: 625, 1975.

5. Kahn R.C., Levy G.L., Rardner J.P., Gordon P., Schein P.S.:
    New Eng J Med. 292:941-945, 1975.

6. Grage T.B., Vassilopoulos P.P., Shingleton W.W., et al.
    Surgery 86:550-555, 1979.

7. Ensminger W., Niederhuber J., Gynes J., et al. Proc. Am. Soc.
    Clin. Oncol. 1:94, 1982.

8. Balch C.M., Urist M.M., Soong S. J., et al. Ann. Surg.
    198:567-573, 1983.

9. Levin B., Karl R., DuBrow R., et al. Clin. Res. 30:783A, 1982.

10. Weiss G.R., Garnick M.B., Osteen R.T., et al. J. Clin. Oncol.
    1:337-344, 1983.

11. Kemeny N., Daly J., Oderman P., et al. Proc. Am. Soc. Clin.
    Oncol. 3:C-551, 1984.

12. Stagg R., Friedman M., Lewis B., et al. Proc. Am. Soc. Clin.
    Oncol. 3:C-577, 1984.

ADJUVANT CHEMOTHERAPY FOR COLORECTAL CANCER.

I. TAYLOR

1. INTRODUCTION

Colorectal cancer is one of the commonest malignancies facing Western civilisation and its incidence appears to be increasing. Many recent surveys have indicated that the progress for this condition has not materially improved over the last 20 years. Surgery, the mainstay of therapy, is now safer than previously but once a patient has left hospital following resection his chances of remaining free of recurrent disease are probably no better now than they were 20 years ago.

One of the reasons for this is undoubtedly related to the metastatic potential of colorectal cancer. Even in patients in whom, following surgery, no obvious residual tumour is apparant, it is likely that small "micrometastases" are present because of lymphatic or portal venous dissemination. An attractive approach to this problem is the administration of cytotoxic drugs during, or for periods of time following resectional surgery, in an attempt to destroy residual foci of disease.

2. RATIONALE OF ADJUVANT CHEMOTHERAPY

All malignant tissues are made up largely of dividing cells which synthesize DNA at some point in their life cycle. The fraction of the tumour cell population which is in the division cycle at any time varies with the type of malignancy and the particular stage of its natural history. Small tumours have a relatively high growth fraction compared to large and bulky tumours. The various agents which have been used for colorectal cancer act by inhibition of cells which undergo DNA synthesis at some stage in their life cycle. 5-fluorouracil acts at the G and S phases of the cell cycle.

Smaller tumours with a high growth fraction, such as micrometastases have a higher proportion of cells in the proliferative phase at any particular time, accordingly a high cell kill is likely. Large bulky

tumours have a greater proportion of mobile cells in the resting phase.
Hence the earlier drugs are given during the course of a malignant
process the more successful they are likely to be. Indeed, marked
therapeutic activity may be seen against small tumour cell population
whereas the same drugs may be totally inactive against large burdens of
tumour. In addition adjuvant chemotherapy has been demonstrated to be
more successful when the main bulk of the primary tumour is removed.

Circulating cancer cells have been demonstrated both in systemic (1)
and portal venous blood (2), however, not all such cells give rise to
metastases. The majority of such circulating cancer cells will be
destroyed and these have no pathogenic potential. Some, however,
undoubtedly survive and may develop into metastases. Two factors may
enhance this process; firstly manipulating the bowel at operation and
secondly the added effect of operative stress has been shown experimentally to produce an increase in the incidence of metastases
(particularly liver metastases) by improving the chances of survival of
cells and allowing them to establish growth within the liver (3).
Similarly, the induction of anaesthesia increases the incidence of
circulating malignant cells (4).

Various cytotoxic agents have been applied in an experimental
situation to reduce the number of metastases. Any chemotherapeutic
treatment which has been established for advanced disease should be of
potential benefit for patients with minimal residual disease after surgery.
This concept is sound, but is dependant upon having an effective anticancer agent with a high order of activity and specificity against the
disease.

3. SELECTION OF PATIENTS

This is a most important aspect of adjuvant chemotherapy. For
effective adjuvant chemotherapy it is necessary to reduce the incidence
of recurrent disease and improve survival with the minimum of toxic
side effects. It should also be remembered that overall, approximately
50% of patients with colorectal cancer will be cured by surgery alone.
Accordingly if adjuvant chemotherapy were to be given to all patients,
unnecessary and potentially toxic treatment, would be given to 50%. In
other words, in an attempt to improve overall survival in approximately
half the patients,all patients would be subjected to cytotoxicity.

Patients with Dukes A tumours have an excellent prognosis (90%
5-year survival) and hence the burden induced by a programme of postoperative chemotherapy is probably unjustified since an improvement on
these survival figures is unlikely. On the other hand, patients with
local lymph node involvement (Dukes C) even without macroscopic tumour
remaining after surgery ("curative" resection) are known to have a poor
prognosis with a high likelihood of recurrence within two years. One
would clearly be prepared to accept a degree of toxicity from adjuvant
therapy in this group of patients if the prognosis could be improved.

Those patients in whom the cancer is advanced at the time of surgery,
e.g. extensive local spread with residual tumour remaining, should be
considered not for adjuvant therapy, but for entry into therapeutic
programmes for advanced disease. Patients with metastatic spread, e.g.
to the liver at the time of surgery, are unlikely to achieve the same
degree of benefit as patients with minimal residual disease and in
general should not be considered for adjuvant therapy.

It is the patient with little or no local disease remaining after
surgery and with no evidence of macroscopic metastases who should be
considered for adjuvant therapy. If one could recognize more accurately
a population of patients who are likely to benefit from adjuvant
chemotherapy then treatment would be both more logical and effective.
In addition, patients unlikely to respond would be spared the burden of
unnecessary and unpleasant toxicity.

4. EARLY CLINICAL TRIALS OF ADJUVANT THERAPY

4.1. Single Agents

The original studies were carried out using thio-tepa. Two large
cooperative studies were undertaken (5,6). Thio-tepa was given both
intraperitoneally and intravenously at the completion of operation and
continued systemically in the postoperative period. Over 1800 patients
were included in both studies but no beneficial treatment effect could
be demonstrated although with extensive analysis a significantly higher
survival rate for women randomised to receive a higher dose level was
found.

4.1.1. Fluorodeoxyuridine (FUDR). In this treatment regimen (7)
5FUDR was given on the first, second and third postoperative days,
followed by a second course between 35 - 40th postoperative days. No

demonstrable benefit could be shown either as a whole or for various subgroups in the 704 patients allocated randomly to treatment or control groups.

4.1.2. <u>Trials involving 5-fluorouracil (5FU)</u>. Numerous trials involving various dosages and routes of administration have been carried out with 5FU for advanced large bowel disease. Trials were commenced in the early 1970's to assess the positive benefit of 5FU for adjuvant therapy. Details of these studies for systemic 5FU and for intraluminal 5FU are given in Tables 1 and 2 respectively.

TABLE 1.   Trials of Systemic 5FU alone.

Regimen	Survival		
12 mg/kg	"curative resection"		
3rd postoperative week	5 yr. survival;	treatment	- 58.5%
(reference 19)		control	- 49.4%
		N.S.	
	"residual tumour"		
		treatment	- 18.2%
		control	- 13.5%
		N.S.	
12 mg/kg every 6 weeks	"curative resection"		
(1½ years)		treatment	- 48.9%
(reference 20)		control	- 44.2%
		N.S.	
	"palliative resection" - 2 yr. survival		
		treatment	- 30.8%
		control	- 25.0%
Age and weight	Dukes C		
dependant dose		treatment	- 57.5%
(Historical controls)		control	- 24.3%
(reference 21)			
12 mg/kg (4 days)	N.S.		
6 mg/kg alternate days			
12 mg/kg weekly for one year			
(reference 22)			

TABLE 2.   Intraluminal 5FU

Study	Regimen (intraluminal)	Results
Rousselot et al (1972) (8)	10 mg/kg	N.S.
Lawrence et al (1975) (23) (156 patients)	30 mg/kg+ oral 5FU for 1 year	N.S.
Grossi et al (1977) (24) (506 patients)	30 mg/kg+ IV 10 mg/kg for 2 days	Dukes C Rectal + serosal involvement Treatment 40% Control 13%

The technique of intraluminal adjuvant chemotherapy was initially proposed by Rousselot et al (8). The technique involved the direct injection of 5FU into the lumen of the colon at the time of surgery after tapes had been applied proximally and distally to the tumour. It was hoped that the topical introduction of 5FU would lessen or control some phases of tumour spread within the area of surgical manipulation. Topical absorption of the drug would allow absorption into the splanchnic, lymphatic and venous circulation so that cancer cells already disseminated into these areas at the time of surgery might be destroyed.

4.1.3.   Intraportal 5FU. It has been estimated that the liver contains metastases in about one-third to one-half of fatal cases of colorectal malignancy. Cedermark et al (9) reported 456 patients who died with colorectal cancer and liver metastases were present in 45% of cases.

Liver metastases develop by invasion of the tumour into the mesenteric venous circulation. As a result tumour cells embolize into the portal venous system. The majority of these tumour cells will be destroyed and thus have no pathogenic potential. Some, however, survive and develop into macroscopic metastases. If it is hoped to prevent or reduce the incidence of liver metastases measures directly involving the portal venous circulation will be required.

Sporadic clinical reports have appeared in the literature advocating intraportal injection of cytotoxic agents at the time of surgery for colorectal cancer. Morales et al (10) utilized nitrogen mustard whereas other surgeons (11) preferred a "no-touch isolation" technique during resection. Follow-up studies of 5-year survival using this technique yield impressive results.

A prospective randomized trial of adjuvant portal vein perfusion with 5FU has been initiated in an attempt to reduce the incidence of liver metastases (12). Patients without clinical or scan (99m Tc sulphur colloid or ultrasound) evidence of liver metastases were randomised into control or adjuvant perfusion groups. Access to the portal vein was via the obliterated umbilical vein. Initial results of this study have been encouraging and suggest that the incidence of liver metastases, particularly in patients with Dukes B colon cancer, can be reduced.

4.2. Combination Chemotherapy

Because of the general disappointment associated with single agent chemotherapy in colorectal cancer several studies using combination chemotherapy have been undertaken. In one study patients undergoing curative resection were randomised either to surgery alone or surgery and treatment with 5FU and MeCCNU (13). No significant overall difference was apparent related either to survival or disease free survival. The only subset demonstrating a survival benefit from chemotherapy were those patients with 1 - 4 positive lymph nodes present.

A further study performed by the South West Oncology group in the USA studied the efficacy of 5FU and MeCCnU with and without the addition of oral BCG. Subsequently a control arm was added. Analysis of the data following the addition of an untreated control group failed to disclose significant differences between any of the three treatment arms (14).

During the period 1975 - 1976 the Gastrointestinal tumour study group randomised 621 patients with colon cancer into four treatment arms 1) MeCCNU + 5FU, 2) Immunotherapy, 3) MeCCNU + 5FU + immunotherapy, 4) No further treatment. A preliminary analysis of the data demonstrated no significant difference in any of the treatment arms. However, analysis of the data according to subsets disclosed a prolonged time to recurrence for the group receiving combined chemoimmunotherapy in Dukes C tumours (15).

Other studies utilizing combination chemotherapy have been initiated but the results are not yet available.

4.3. Other Chemotherapeutic Agents

Razoxane has been used in an adjuvant setting for resectable Dukes B and C colorectal cancer. Although an initial report suggested possible benefit with few side-effects, these improvements were recognised in the first two years only.

Anticoagulation may have an important role in effecting the metastatic process. An antimetastatic effect has been established in experimental models (16,17,18). Heparin may interfere with fibrin formation and thus inhibit the development of tumour cell thrombus.

5. CONCLUSIONS

It is probable that any future benefit of adjuvant chemotherapy in colorectal cancer will depend upon both the development and testing of more potent and specific chemotherapeutic agents. These must be shown to be effective both in experimental models and in well-conducted clinical trials. In addition, perhaps further emphasis should be placed on multi-modal adjuvant therapy. For example, adjuvant local radio-therapy designed to avoid local recurrence could be combined with adjuvant cytotoxic liver perfusion to decrease the incidence of liver metastases.

REFERENCES

1. Roberts S, Watne A, McGrath R, McGrew E, Cole WH. 1958. Technique and results of isolation of cancer cells from the circulating blood. Archives of Surgery, 76, 334.
2. Engel HC. 1955. Cancer cells in circulating blood. Acta Chirurgica Scandinavica, suppl. 201.
3. Fisher B, Fisher ER. 1959. Experimental studies of factors influencing hepatic metastases. III Effect of surgical trauma with special reference to liver injury. Annals of Surgery, 150, 731.
4. Griffiths JD, McKinna J, Rowbottom HD. 1973. Carcinoma of the colon and rectum : Circulating malignant cells and 5 year survival. Cancer, 31, 226.
5. Veterans Administration Surgical Adjuvant Cancer Chemotherapy Group. Adjuvant use of HN (NSC-762) and Thio-tepa (NSL-6396) - Progress Report. Cancer Chemotherapy Reports 1965, 44, 27.

6. Dixon WJ, Longmire WP Jr., Holden WD. 1971. Use of Thio-tepa as an adjuvant to the surgical treatment of gastric and colorectal carcinoma : Ten year follow-up. Annals of Surgery, 173, 26.
7. Dwight RW, Humphreys WE, Higgins GA, Keehn RJ. 1973. FUDR as an adjuvant to surgery in cancer of the large bowel. Journal of Surgical Oncology, 5, 243.
8. Rousselot LM, Cole DR, Gross CE et al. 1972. Adjuvant chemotherapy with 5FU in surgery for colorectal cancer. Dis. Colon & Rectum, 15, 169-174.
9. Cedermark BJ, Schulz SS, Bakshi S, Parthasarathy L, Mittleman A, Evans S. 1977. The value of liver scan in the follow-up study of patients with adenocarcinoma of the colon and rectum. Surgery, Gynecology and Obstetrics, 144, 745.
10. Morales F, Bell M, McDonald GD, Cole WH. 1957. The prophylactic treatment of cancer at the time of operation. Annals of Surgery, 146, 588.
11. Turnbull RB. 1970. Cancer of the colon. Five to 40 year survival rates following resection utilizing the isolation technique. Annals of the Royal College of Surgeons of England, 40, 243.
12. Taylor I, Rowling JT, West C. 1979. Adjuvant liver perfusion for colorectal cancer. British Journal of Surgery, 66, 833.
13. Higgins GA et al. 1984. Efficacy of prolonged intermittent therapy with combined 5FU and Methy CCNU following resection of carcinoma of the large bowel. Cancer, 53, 1-8.
14. Panettiere FJ, Chen TT. 1981. Analysis of 626 patients entered on the SWOG large bowel adjuvant program in Adjuvant Therapy of Cancer III. Eds Salmon SE & Jones SE. Grune & Stratton. p. 339-346.
15. Lessner AE et al. 1982. Adjuvant therapy of colon cancer - A prospective randomised trial. Proceeds of American Society for Clinical Oncology, 1, 351.
16. Agostino D, Clifton EE. 1962. Decrease of metastases of carcino-sarcoma Walker 256 with irradiation and heparin or finbrinolytic agents. Radiology, 79, 848.
17. Mooney B, Serlin M, Taylor I. 1982. The effect of Warfarin on spontaneously metastasising colorectal cancer in the rat. Clin. Oncol., 8, 55-59.
18. Goeting N, Cooke T, Taylor I. 1983. Effect of non-anticoagulating Warfarin on induced colorectal cancer in the rat. Gut, 24, 466.
19. Higgins GA, Dwight RW, Smith JV, Keehn RJ. 1971. Fluorouracil as an adjuvant to surgery in carcinoma of the colon. Archives of Surgery, 102, 339.
20. Higgins GA, Humphrey E, Juler GL, LeVeen HH, McCaughan J, Keehn R. 1976. Adjuvant chemotherapy in the treatment of large bowel cancer. Cancer, 38, 1461.
21. Li MC, Ross ST. 1976. Chemoprophylaxis for patients with colorectal cancer. Journal of the American Medical Association, 235, 2825.
22. Grage T, Cornell G, Strawitz J, Jonas K, Frelick R, Metter G. 1975. Adjuvant therapy with 5FU after surgical resection of colorectal cancer. Proceedings of the American Society of Clinical Oncology, 16, 258.
23. Lawrence W, Terz JJ, Horsley S, Donaldson M, Lovett WL, Brown PW et al. 1975. Chemotherapy as an adjuvant to surgery for colorectal cancer. Annals of Surgery, 181, 616.
24. Grossi CE, Wolff WI, Nealon TF, Pasternack B, Ginzburg L, Rousselot LM. 1977. Intraluminal fluorouracil chemotherapy adjuvant to surgical procedure for resectable carcinoma of the colon and rectum. Surgery, Gynecology and Obstetrics, 145, 549.

SURGICAL THERAPY OF HEPATIC METASTASES

P.H. SUGARBAKER, R.T. OTTOW, D.A. AUGUST

Currently the only potentially curative therapy for the patient
with hepatic metastases is surgical resection of the cancer.
Therefore, this option should always be evaluated before other
treatment alternatives are pursued. In selected patients resection can be performed with a morbidity and mortality similar to
that of many surgical procedures that are routinely performed.
Survival of patients with resected intrahepatic malignancy is far
superior to the natural course of the disease. In this chapter
we first review the results reported to date with liver surgery
for metastatic malignancy. We then present the NIH experience with
hepatic resection for colorectal metastatic disease, including our
experience with adjuvant intraperitoneal 5-FU chemotherapy.

Evolution of Surgical Techniques: Early surgical experience with
the liver was limited to treatment of trauma. The first elective
hepatic resections were attempted toward the end of the 19th century,
largely by the German school of surgeons (Table 1) (1-12). Credit
for the first resection of an intrahepatic malignancy is probably due
Bruns (1). As reported by his pupil Garrè in 1888, Bruns excised a
metastatic lesion within the liver using cautery for hemostasis. In
1899 Keen described a patient with primary liver carcinoma in whom he
resected what he called the left lobe; in present day terminology this
resection would probably be termed a left lateral segmentectomy (2).
In this report Keen also reviewed 76 cases from the world literature
involving hepatic surgery for presumed neoplasms. In Germany in 1910
Wendel resected the true right lobe and the medial part of the left
lobe of the liver to remove an adenoma (4). This may have been the
first resection performed which involved a preliminary hilar dissection
and ligation of the relevant artery and duct. Lortat-Jacob and Robert

Table 1. Historical Perspective – Liver Surgery

Date	Author	Country	Comment
1888	Garrè (Bruns)	Germany	Metastatectomy
1899	Keen	USA	Left lateral segmentectomy
1908	Pringle	Great Britain	Temporary occlusion of the portal pedicle
1910	Wendel	Germany	Right lobectomy, partial hilar dissection
1952	Lortat-Jacob & Robert	France	Preliminary hilar ligation for anatomic lobectomy
1958	Lin	Taiwan	Finger fracture technique
1971	Storm and Longmire	USA	Liver clamp
1975	Starzl, et al.	USA	Right trisegmentectomy
1977	Foster and Berman	USA	Liver Tumor Survey, Suction dissection technique
1979	Hodgson and Aufses	USA	Ultrasonic dissector
1981	Fortner, et al.	USA	High voltage cautery
1982	Starzl, et al.	USA	Left trisegmentectomy

From Ottow RT, August DA, Sugarbaker PH. Surgical therapy of hepato-biliary tumors. In: Bottino JC, Opfell R, Muggia F (eds) Therapy of Neoplasms Confined to the Liver and Biliary Tract. Martinus-Nijhoff, Boston (in press).

in 1952 reported a complete dissection of the porta hepatis with ligation of the pertinent portal venous structures as well as the artery and duct (5). Others may in fact have preceeded them, but their description was the first to gain wide attention. In 1975 Starzl, et al. reported a series of 14 right trisegmentectomies accomplished without mortality (8). Starzl, et al. in 1982, were the first to describe the left trisegmentectomy (12).

Many techniques have been developed which attempt to overcome the problems of transecting this well perfused organ which lacks avascular planes. Preliminary hilar dissection has been noted above. In 1908 Pringle described the temporary occlusion of the portal pedicle (the Pringle maneuver) (3). Keen used his thumb to bluntly shell out a liver tumor (2). In 1958 Lin, et al. described and popularized the finger fracture method by which hepatic parenchyma is digitally fractured, (presumably) preserving the more resiliant blood vessels and ducts. Those vessels which are identified are individually ligated prior to their transection (6). Liver clamps were used as early as 1907 by Garrè (13). Their current use is based upon descriptions by Storm and Longmire (7) and by Lin (14). Deserving special mention is the parenchymal dissection technique pioneered by Foster utilizing the inner cannula of a Poole sucker (9). Also, as described below, the ultrasonic scalpel as first used by Hodgson and Aufses in hepatic surgery is finding increasing acceptance (10). In 1981 Fortner and colleagues directed renewed attention to the technique of transecting hepatic parenchyma using high voltage electrocautery (11).

In an effort to define the optimal transection technique and to observe microscopically the effect of each technique at the parenchymal level, Ottow and colleagues performed a comparative study (13). Four transection techniques were studied with the pig as the experimental animal. The suction dissection technique popularized by Foster (9) was selected as the representative of the blunt techniques. Electrocautery and ultrasonic dissection were employed as the second and third technique. As a control, to determine what happened if no special measure was taken to control hemorrhage, simple transection with a scalpel was used. The blood loss, the number of vessels identified prior to their division, the need for additional hemostatic sutures and the time needed for each procedure were quantitated.

The blood loss (Table 2) with the ultrasonic dissector was the lowest, but the differences with the other methods in clinical use were not statistically significant. These three methods differed significantly from the control method (p < .005).

With the cautery and the sharp method, it was not possible to isolate vessels and clip them prior to their transection, but they were identified only when they began to bleed (Table 3). With the suction and the ultrasonic dissection about the same number of vessels could be atraumatically dissected free of hepatic parenchyma (Table 3, Column A). However, significantly fewer sutures were needed to secure bleeding points during parenchymal dissection and after the specimen was removed (Table 3, Column B) when ultrasonic dissection was compared to suction dissection. The greatest control in isolating vessels was achieved with the ultrasonic dissector.

The total number of vessels needing surgical attention (Table 3, Column C) was the same for the suction and the sharp dissection. This concurs with the view that the suction dissection helps in isolating the vessels, but has no intrinsic hemostatic effect on small vessels. Both the ultrasonic dissector and the cautery exert a hemostatic effect on the small vessels at the parenchymal level as shown by the markedly and significantly lower total number of vessels needing a clip or a suture. In summary, the ultrasonic dissector was the only transection technique that combined the ability to isolate vessels prior to their division, with a hemostatic effect on small vessels. A prospective study to quantitate the blood loss in patients undergoing major hepatic resections using ultrasonic dissection and suction dissection is underway at the NIH.

Technique of Metastasectomy: Prior to beginning the parenchymal dissection the foramen of Winslow must be clearly identified. A non-crushing vascular clamp may be used to intermittently occlude the portal structures while dissecting through liver. Attempting to stay approximately 1 cm from each metastasis, they are removed with a clear margin. Inflow occlusion of the liver classically is limited to 15 minutes. This period can safely be extended, possibly up to 60 minutes. Following removal of the metastasis and clipping of the vessels in the surrounding liver, a Gelfoam plug is placed within the defect to encourage blood clotting. It is especially

Table 2. Blood Loss by Transection Method

Blood Loss im ml

	Range	Median
Ultrasonic (1)	6-124	58
Suction (2)	28-164	87
Cautery (3)	9-332	79
Sharp (4)	58-720	121

(1),(2) & (3) vs. (4)	All p's < .005
(1) vs. (2)	p = .075
(1) vs. (3)	p = .15
(2) vs. (3)	p = .78

From Ottow RT, Barbieri BS, Sugarbaker PH, Wesley RA. Liver transection. A controlled study of four different techniques in pigs
(submitted for publication).

Table 3. Effect of Blood Vessels by Transection Method

	A — Number of Vessels Identified and Clipped Prior to their Division		B — Vessels Disrupted Without Prior Identification		C — A + B	
	Range	Median	Range	Median	Range	Median
Ultrasonic (1)	0-12	7	0-5	2	1-12	10
Suction (2)	4-16	9	3-10	5	8-22	14
Cautery (3)			2-10	6	2-10	6
Sharp (4)			10-21	14	10-21	14

(2) vs. (3) p = .093

Five other pair wise comparisons: all p's ≤ .002.

(1) vs. (3) p = .049

(2) vs. (4) Not significant

Four other pair wise comparisons: all p's ≤ .002.

From Ottow RT, Barieri BS, Sugarbaker PH, Wesley RA. Liver transection. A controlled study of four different techniques in pigs (submitted for publication).

important to check for bile leaks upon removal of the Gelfoam; if noted they should be suture ligated. We have encountered bile leaks following metastatectomy of large tumor deposits in several patients. They may require postoperatively percutaneous external drainage for a prolonged period of time.

Postoperative Care: Liver resection is usually well tolerated, but complications do occur. Subphrenic abcess can often be managed in consultation with the interventional radiologist by percutaneous CT or ultrasound guided drainage. Some biliary fluid leaking postoperatively is not unusual; it usually stops spontaneously because the biliary network is a low pressure system. Postoperatively many patients show transient jaundice. The SGOT often shows a sharp peak just after resection; the alkaline phosphatase is often elevated for months, even years after resection. In the first postoperative week serum albumin levels may be depressed and prothrombin times are often elevated. Albumin should be given along with fresh frozen plasma when indicated. Parenteral Vitamin K given preoperatively may be helpful. In noncirrhotic patients regeneration starts in a matter of days and is complete in two to six months. Cirrhotic livers do not show regeneration.

Results of Surgical Treatment of Colorectal Cancer Metastases: Table 4 summarizes the experiences of ten groups with resection of colorectal hepatic metastases (9,14-22). Five year survival of 30-40% is a consistent finding among these reports. The results of Iwatsuki, et al. from Starzel's group showing an operative mortality of 5% and a five year actuarial survival of 52% are particularly impressive (20). However, the above data must be interpreted with caution because: 1) Five year survival does not equate with cure, because as many as 25% of five year survivors may ultimately die from recurrent disease; 2) These data refer to crude survival and therefore mortality might be from causes unrelated to the malignancy; and 3) In the more recent series a number of patients received adjuvant chemotherapy or radiation therapy in addition to surgery. Nevertheless, the benefit of resection is clear especially when contrasted with the near zero five year survival of patients with untreated hepatic metastases. Table 5 presents survival data of patients with potentially resectable tumors in whom the neoplasm

Table 4. Results of Hepatic Resection for Colorectal Cancer Metastases

Authors	Year	Number of Patients	Operative Mortality (%)	Survival %			
				1 yr.	3 yr.	5 yr.	10 yr.
Wilson & Adson	1976	40	0			42	29
Foster & Berman	1977	126	6			18	
Attiyeh, et al.	1978	25	4			40	28
Adson & Van Heerden	1980	34	6	82	41		
Bengmark, et al.	1982	39	5		23		
Rajpal, et al.	1982	34	12	85	40		
Thompson, et al.	1983	22	0	80	38	31	
Iwatsuki, et al.	1983	24	0	91	73	52	
Fortner, et al.	1984	65	9	89	57	40	
August, et al.	1984	33	0	94	53		

From August DA, Ottow RT, Sugarbaker PH. Clinical perspective of human colon cancer metastasis. Cancer Metast Rev (in press).

Table 5. Survival of Patients with Potentially Resectable Untreated Hepatic Metastases from Colorectal Cancer

Author	Lesions	Number Patients	Number Metastasis	Survival %				Comments
				1	2	3	5	
Wilson & Adson	Solitary	46		68	42	18	0	Mostly small lesions
	Multiple	14		25	0	0	0	
Wood, et al.	Solitary	15		60		13.3		
	Multiple, 1 lobe	11		27		9.9		
Blumgart & Allison	Solitary		15	38				Prospective study
	Multiple, 1 lobe		13	45				

From Ottow RT, August DA, Sugarbaker PH. Surgical therapy of hepatobiliary tumors. In: Bottino JC, Opfell R, Muggia F (eds) Therapy of Neoplasms Confined to the Liver and Biliary Tract. Martinus-Nijhoff, Boston (in press).

was not removed (14,23,24). Occasional two and three year survivors are noted but no five year survivors are reported. These data show that if resection is possible it should be attempted.

Unfortunately, although hepatic resection is clearly of benefit to some patients, a simple calculation makes clear that it has only a small impact on the overall problem of colorectal cancer. Of 100 patients with a colorectal cancer approximately 20 will have liver metastases at the time of operation for their primary; only five of the 20 will be resectable. Of the original 100 patients another five will develop resectable metachronous hepatic metastases, making for a potential of ten resections. Three or four resected patients will survive five years, but one of these will develop recurrent disease. Two or three of 100 patients with primary colorectal cancer can be cured by hepatic resection. This estimate, combined with the high incidence of colorectal cancer (approximately 120,000 patients per year in the U.S.) would suggest that nationwide 12,000 liver resections need to be performed annually, and that 3,600 patients would be cured by such a policy.

Data recently reported by August and colleagues suggests that early detection of hepatic metastases and prompt therapeutic intervention may be important to prevent secondary spread from liver lesions to regional lymph nodes. This may increase the proportion of colorectal cancer patients undergoing potentially curative hepatic resections (25). Lymph drainage from all portions of the liver merges into several major thoracoabdominal lymphatic pathways, including the internal mammary chian via trans-diaphragmatic connections, the posterior mediastinal chain through both trans-diaphragmatic and celiac connections, and the cisterna chyli via the portal pedicle. August, et al. described nine patients who underwent resection of colorectal cancers who subsequently developed hepatic metastases which proved unresectable at celiotomy because of portal or celiac lymph node metastases. This lymphatic spread likely arose via "remetastasis" from the liver metastases. This report highlights the clinical significance of hepatic lymphatic efferents as pathways for secondary metastasis of liver metastases. Delay in diagnosis because of inadequate surveillance may permit secondary spread from hepatic metastases resulting in an unresectable situation.

Surgical Treatment of Other Metastases: Favorable results have
been reported for Wilms' tumor, where chemotherapy and radiation
therapy are combined with resection, and with functioning endocrine
neoplasms. Foster reviewed 15 patients with hepatic metastases from
Wilms' tumors; two and five year survival was 62 and 44% respectively
(26). Martin, et al. reported a series of four complete resections
of carcinoid metastases and one partial resection (27). The palliated
patient remained symptom free 19 months; one completely resected patient died symptom free of a myocardial infarction six months after
resection, and the other three patients were alive and asympomatic 12-
45 months post resection. Results following resection of hepatic metastases from other primary tumors are less clear. Foster in his 1978
review concluded that hepatic resection for metastases of other tumors
should usually be discouraged (26).

The experience described in a recent report by Iwatsuki, et al.
seems more favorable (20). This study presented survival statistics
for 43 patients with liver metastases from various primaries, including 24 patients with colorectal cancer. Comparison of the
subgroup with colorectal primaries with the whole group showed no
marked differences. Included among the noncolorectal primaries were
adrenocortical carcinoma, adenocarcinoma of the kidney, spindle cell
sarcoma of the intestine, leiomyosarcoma of the stomach, glucagonoma,
neuroblastoma of the adrenal, ocular melanoma, sarcoma of the breast,
medullary carcinoma of the thyroid, squamous cell carcinoma of the
endocervix, and ovarian cancer. Fortner, et al. also published
favorable survival figures for noncolorectal hepatic metastases; but
this series possible included some liver resections for direct invasion rather than for truly metastatic tumor (11).

Palliative Hepatic Resection: Because of the broad range of
disease left behind after so called palliative resections and the
subjective nature of the assessment of palliation of pain and suffering, it is impossible to make definitive statements concerning
the efficacy of noncurative hepatic resections for malignant disease.
Nevertheless, some trends emerge.

There is agreement that resection of symptom producing functional
liver metastases of carcinoid tumors can offer excellent palliation
even if a small amount of tumor remains following surgical excision.

Foster and Berman reviewed a collected experience of 44 patients (9). Palliation of all but cardiac symptoms was achieved in 35 of the 36 patients in whom follow-up information was available, for a duration of a few weeks to more than six years. Six of seven of these patients who underwent repeat operation for recurrent symptoms achieved further significant palliation. Overall 11 patients were alive beyond three years, three patients died more than three years after resection, 13 patients were alive two to 24 months postresection, and 14 had died before three years. Foster and Berman (9) also cite two cases involving hepatic resections of metastatic insulinoma and gastrinoma respectively, with favorable outcomes.

There is little experience with palliative resection of liver metastases from other primary tumors. Foster and Berman mention two leiomyosarcomas and two melanomas metastataic to liver requiring emergent operation for rupture (9).

NIH Experience with Hepatic Resections for Hepatic Metastases from Colorectal Cancer: Seventy-seven patients with suspected liver metastases from colorectal cancers were seen by the Surgery Branch of the National Cancer Institute between January, 1980 and January, 1983 (22). After evaluation 47 patients were thought to be resectable for cure. Forty-six of these patients underwent exploratory laparotomy (one patient refused surgery) and 33 were resected of all gross disease. Reasons for unresectability included liver involvement judged too extensive to permit resection (six patients), a technically unresectable porta hepatis lesion (one patient), presence of metastatic pelvic peritoneal implant (one patient) and presence of metastases in lymph nodes draining the liver (five patients). The group included 23 men and 10 women ranging in age from 17 to 74 years (median 57 years). Median follow-up was 20 months (range 6 to 83 months) and was complete in all patients.

The operative procedures performed are summarized as follows: Twenty patients underwent wedge resections, 11 of which involved excisions in both lobes of the liver. Twelve lobectomies were performed (left - 3, right - 9), four of which also involved contralateral wedge resection. A single right trisegmentectomy with wedge excision from the left lateral segment was performed.

Twenty-one patients received intraperitoneal 5-FU as an adjuvant

following hepatic resection. Twelve patients did not receive chemotherapy.

Chemotherapy was initiated 10 to 74 days (median 34 days) after
resection and was given on days one through five of a 28 day cycle.
For the initial cycle 1040 mg of 5-FU was given in two liters of
Inpersol daily, and this daily dose was escalated by 65-130 mg in-
crements with subsequent cycles to a maximum of 1820 mg or until
limited by toxicity (usually fatigue or abdominal pain). Treatment
was continued for a total of 12 cycles unless toxicity or tumor recurrence indicated earlier cessation. The 21 patients received an
average of 9.4 cycles of chemotherapy (range 2-12), receiving a mean
of 6820 mg (range 4775-8255) of 5-FU per cycle.

Following resection patients were seen regularly in clinic.
Follow-up was complete in all patients. Time to recurrence and survival data were estimated and plotted using the Kaplan-Meier product
limit method. The Mantel-Haenszel test was used to compare outcome
between different groups of patients unless otherwise indicated. All
p-values cited are two-tailed.

Morbidity and Blood Loss: There were no intraoperative or in-hos-
pital deaths following either exploration or liver resection. Median
time to discharge following resection was 14 days (range 8-52 days).
Seven major and two minor postoperative complications occurred affecting nine of 33 patients (27%).

Intraoperative blood loss as estimated by the anesthesiologist
ranged from 350 cc to 16,000 cc (median 3000 cc). As shown in Figure
1 the occurrence of postoperative complications correlated with
intraoperative blood loss. Of 11 patients whose blood loss was
greater than 4000 cc, five (45%) experienced major complications.
Only two of 22 patients (9%) with blood loss less than 4000 cc
experienced a major postoperative complication. Estimated blood loss
in patients with complications averaged 4600 cc, versus 2600 cc in
patients without complications (p = 0.002, Wilcoxon Rank Order Test).

Survival: For all patients, median survival was 38 months with
estimated two year and four year survival of 72% and 53% respectively
(Figure 2A). The corresponding statistics for the 29 negative margin
patients were 40 month median survival with two and four year survival
of 80% and 55% respectively. Median disease-free survival for all

Figure 1.

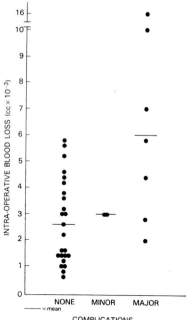

Figure 2A.

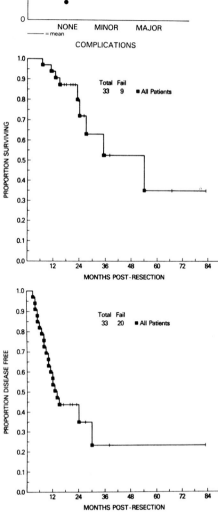

Figure 2B.

patients (Figure 2B) was 13 months, resulting in a 25 month interval between median time to recurrence and median time to death. Presently 13 patients are free of disease with follow-up ranging from six to 83 months. Of the 20 patients who have developed recurrent disease, the liver was the first site of recurrence in 11; five other patients developed hepatic recurrences subsequent to the discovery of other sites of recurrent disease. Thirteen of 20 recurrences (65%) were evident within one year of resection, and 19 of 20 (95%) occurred within 30 months.

The number of metastases resected and the distribution of metastases (unilobar versus bilobar) were predictive of survival. The status of the microscopic margins of the resected specimen was predictive of disease free survival. Median survival in patients with three or fewer metastases was significantly longer than in those with four or more metastases (44 months vs. 20 months, p = 0.028) (Figure 3). Only one of ten patients with more than three metastases resected is currently disease-free (at 19 months following right lobectomy for five metastases), whereas six of 12 patients with two or three metastases and six of 11 patients with solitary metastases resected are currently disease-free (minimum follow-up six months). Patients with three or fewer metastases resected had estimated two and four year survival of 86% and 59% respectively. There was no difference in survival between patients with solitary metastases and those with two or three metastases.

Patients with unilobar disease survived longer than those with bilobar disease (> 54 months vs. 23 months, p = 0.001) (Figure 4). This remained true when patients with solitary metastases were excluded from the analysis (p = 0.053).

All four patients with positive microscopic margins following resection developed recurrent disease within one year, but all survived beyond two years. Median disease-free survival in the positive margin patients was seven months versus 16 months in negative margin patients (p = 0.019).

The Dukes' stage of the primary lesion, the interval between bowel resection and detection of hepatic metastases, the method of detection of hepatic metastases (rising CEA versus other), the preoperative CEA level, and the type of operation performed (wedge resection versus

202

Figure 3.

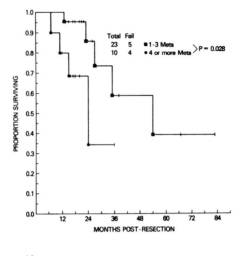

Figure 4.

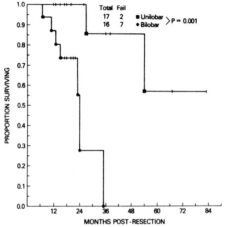

Figure 5.

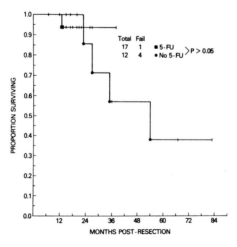

lobectomy) were not predictive of postresection survival.

Chemotherapy: As part of a pilot study, 21 of the patients under-going hepatic resection received intraperitoneal 5-FU via Tenckhoff catheter as a postresection adjuvant therapy. Seven patients were given a full 12 cycles of therapy, receiving an average of 7170 mg of 5-FU per cycle. Five patients received 9.2 - 11.8 cycles of intraperitoneal 5-FU (average 6344 mg/cycle), their therapy being terminated prior to completion of 12 cycles because of abdominal pain (two patients), disabling fatigue (one patient), nausea (one patient), or bacterial peritonitis (one patient). In nine patients chemotherapy was terminated because of documented tumor recurrence.

Overall, there was no difference in survival between patients who received intraperitoneal 5-FU and those who did not. However, pa-tients receiving chemotherapy had an average of 3.7 metastases re-sected whereas those not receiving chemotherapy had only 2.2 metas-tases removed; all four patients with greater than five metastases resected were in the chemotherapy group. When only patients with five or fewer metastases were compared, the patients receiving intraperitoneal 5-FU appeared to do better, but follow-up is limited (median 24 months for the no adjuvant group and 18 months in the 5-FU group) (Figure 5). Ten of the 12 patients (73%) who received adjuvant therapy and six of the eight patients (63%) who did not receive adju-vant therapy who developed recurrent disease had the liver as a site of tumor regrowth.

Hepatic resections for metastatic colorectal cancer is an estab-lished treatment regimen offering cure of this disease in 30-50% of carefully selected patients. In patients undergoing hepatic resection the incidence of complications correlated with intraoperative blood loss. Patients with three or fewer metastases resected or with uni-lobar disease had improved survival when compared with patients having more than three metastases or bilobar disease, respectively. Disease free survival was improved in patients with microscopically negative resection margins. Dukes' stage of the primary lesion, interval be-tween bowel resection and detection of hepatic metastases, preopera-tive CEA level, and type of operation performed were not predictive of postresection survival. Intraperitoneal 5-FU was well tolerated. There was a trend toward improve survival in patients receiving adjuvant chemotherapy, but this was not statistically significant. It is concluded that the number of metastases resected, the distribution of the metastases, and the technical adequacy of the excision are all predictive of outcome following hepatic resection of colorectal metastases. Encouraging results with the use of intraperitoneal 5-FU as a postresection adjuvant have led to the initiation of a prospective randomized trial investigating this modality at the NCI.

REFERENCES

1. Garre C. 1888. Beitraege zur Leber-Chirurgie. Bruns Beitr Klin Chir 4:181.
2. Keen WW. 1899. Report of a case of resection of the liver for the removal of a neoplasm, with a table of seventy-six cases of resection of the liver for hepatic tumors. Ann Surg 30:267.
3. Pringle JH. 1908. Notes on the arrest of hepatic hemorrhage due to trauma. Ann Surg 48:541.
4. Wendel W. 1911. Beitraege zur Chirurgie der Leber. Arch Klin Chir 95:887.
5. Lortat-Jacob JL, Robert HG. 1952. Hepatectomie droite réglée. Presse Med 60:549.
6. Lin TY, Hsu KY, Hsieh CM, Chen CS. 1958. Study on lobectomy of the liver: A new technical suggestion on hemihepatectomy and reports on three cases of primary hepatoma treated with left lobectomy of the liver. J Formosan Med Assoc 57:742.
7. Storm KF, Longmire WP, Jr. 1971. A simplified clamp for hepatic resection. Surg Gynecol Obstet 133:103.
8. Starzl TE, Bell RH, Beart RW, Putnam CW. 1975. Hepatic trisegmentectomy and other liver resections. Surg Gynecol Obstet 141: 429.
9. Foster JH, Berman MM. 1977. Solid liver tumors. In: Ebert P (ed), Major Problems in Clinical Surgery. Philadelphia, WB Saunders Co.
10. Hodgson WJB, Aufses A, Jr. 1979. Surgical ultrasonic dissection of the liver. Surg Rounds 2:68.
11. Fortner JG, MacLean BJ, Kim DK, Howland WS, Turnbull AD, Goldiner P, Carlon G, Beattie EJ, Jr. 1981. The seventies evolution in liver surgery for cancer. Cancer 47:2162.
12. Starzl TE, Iwatsuki S, Shaw BW, Jr, Waterman PM, VanThiel D, Diliz P HS, Dekker A, Bron KM. 1982. Left hepatic trisegmentectomy. Surg Gynecol Obstet 155:21.
13. Ottow RT, Barbieri BS, Sugarbaker PH, Wesley RA. Liver transection. A controlled study of four different techniques in pigs (submitted for publication).
14. Wilson SM, Adson MA. 1976. Surgical treatment of hepatic metastases from colorectal cancers. Arch Surg 111:330.
15. Adson MA, Van Heerden JA. 1980. Major hepatic resections for metastatic colorectal cancer. Ann Surg 191:576.
16. Attiyeh FA, Wanebo HJ, Stearns MW. 1978. Hepatic resection for metastasis from colorectal cancer. Dis Colon Rectum 21:160.
17. Bengmark S, Hafström L, Jeppsson B, Jönsson PE, Rydén S, Sundqvist K. 1982. Metastatic disease in the liver from colorectal cancer: An appraisal of liver surgery. World J Surg 6:61.

18. Thompson HH, Tompkins RK, Longmire WP, Jr. 1983. Major hepatic resection. A 25 year experience. Ann Surg 197:375.
19. Rajpal S, Dasmahapatra KS, Ledesma EJ, Mittelman A. 1982. Extensive resections of isolated metastasis from carcinoma of the colon and rectum. Surg Gynecol Obstet 155:813.
20. Iwatsuki S, Shaw BW, Jr, Starzl TE. 1983. Experience with 150 liver resections. Ann Surg 197:247.
21. Fortner JG, Silva JS, Golbey RB, Cox EB, MacLean BJ. 1984. Multivariate analysis of a personal series of 247 consecutive patients with liver metastases from colorectal cancer. I. Treatment by hepatic resection. Ann Surg 199:306.
22. August DA, Sugarbaker PH, Ottow RT, Gianola FJ, Schneider PD. Hepatic resection of colorectal metastases: Influence of clinical factors and adjuvant intraperitoneal 5-fluorouracil via Tenckhoff catheter on survival (submitted for publication).
23. Wood CB, Gillis CR, Blumgart LH. 1976. A retrospective study of the natural history of patients with liver metastases from colorectal cancer. Clin Oncol 2:285.
24. Blumgart LH, Allison DJ. 1982. Resection and embolization in the management of secondary hepatic tumors. World J Surg 6:32.
25. August DA, Sugarbaker PH, Schneider PD. Lymphatic dissemination of hepatic metastases: Implication for the follow-up and treatment of patients with colorectal cancer. Cancer (in press).
26. Foster JH. 1978. Survival after liver resection for secondary tumors. Am J Surg 135:389.
27. Martin JK, Moertel CG, Adson MA, Schutt AJ. 1983. Surgical treatment of functioning metastatic carcinoid tumors. Arch Surg 118:537.

RADIOTHERAPY IN THE TREATMENT OF LIVER METASTASES.

P. THOMAS.

The difference in number of articles on irradiation of liver metastases
in the United States and Europe probably reflects a difference in
interest in this subject.

Experience with the effects of irradiation on the liver is not new. Already in 1924 Case and Warthin reported on adverse effects of irradiation on the liver. In the period of 180 - 200 kV roentgen irradiation
the acute side effects were intensive, especially nausea and vomiting,
in a category of patients already prone to suffer from these symptoms.
The balance of therapy was mostly judged negative.

Moreover the liver is mostly only one of the many organs afflicted with
metastases. As long as there is no way to treatment of these metastases
it is hardly inspiring to treat liver metastases. Once systemic treatment of generalised metastases proved succesful, treatment of liver
metastases had to be reconsidered. This is the case with metastases of
mammary carcinoma, and may become feasible in metastases of small cell
bronchial carcinoma.

Tumours of the gastrointestinal tract are a common source of liver metastases, but are not a common indication for radiotherapy. We know that
the old axiom that gastrointestinal tumours, being adenocarcinomas, are
radioresistant is not true; nevertheless it is seldom possible to apply
a high dose without causing substantial damage to neighbouring organs.

Liver metastases of gastrointestinal tumours may well be radiosensitive,
this is only interesting when liver cells are less radiosensitive than
tumour cells.

This means there are the following questions to answer:

1. What is the radiation dose that can be applied to the liver without lasting injury?
2. Which tumours can be cured by this dose?
3. What are the indications for palliative irradiation of liver metastases?
4. When is elective liver irradiation indicated?
5. Which method of irradiation must be preferred?

1. Radiosensitivity of the liver.

Irradiation of para-aortic lymph nodes as in the treatment of Hodgkin's disease or seminoma implies irradiation of a substantial part of the left lobe of the liver. Irradiation of the right thoracic wall and of the right breast by tangential fields is impossible without irradiation of the ventrocranial portion of the right lobe of the liver. The only sign of effect of irradiation on the liver has been a band-like defect on the liver scintigram when colloidal ^{198}Au, which is absorbed by the liver reticulum cells, was used. This lead to the supposition that liver cells are relatively radioresistant. Once irradiation of the whole abdomen of big volumes including the whole liver came into use as in the treatment of ovarian carcinoma, or of nephroblastoma, it soon became clear that the radiosensitivity of the liver hardly differs from that of the kidney (Wharton, 1973; Tefft, 1969, 1970). Although Ingold (1965) stated that 3000 - 3500 rads in 3 - 4 weeks is a safe dose, Wharton (1973) described liver injury with doses of 2500 - 3000 rads. These differences may be due to differences in dose specification of irradiation methods. Anyhow, even if 35 Gy in 4 weeks is a safe dose, it is a relatively low dose to cure liver metastases.

Even with doses as low as 20 Gy midplane, daily fractions of 1 Gy, used in the abdominal-bath technic in the treatment of ovarian carcinoma changes in liver function can be found. In a group of 12 patients receiving this dose 3 weeks after a series of three to four CHAP 1 or V courses the SLDH (serum lactic dehydrogenase)-test was elevated in 10 patients. The 5-nucleotidase-test was elevated in five, the alkaline phosphatase in two patients. All these patients had no clinical signs of dysfunction of the liver. In contrast with Tefft's report none of our patients showed changes in the transaminase values. The liver function tests became normal within 4 months, mostly even within 4 weeks. In none of the patients in this series were there signs of late side effects.

It is of interest that Tefft e.a. have clearly shown the influence of regeneration of liver on radiosensitivity. After partial hepatectomy the risk of damage to the liver is greatly enhanced. Another observation of the same authors is that chemotherapeutic agents that depend on the liver for detoxification may give more serious toxic reactions, especially thrombocytopenia, when given during or shortly after liver irradiation. This observation has been confirmed by others (Haddad e.a., 1983). Anyhow, a relatively low dose of irradiation already gives a transient elevation of LDH in the majority of patients, a moderate dose of 35 Gy has been reported in the literature sometimes to result in an acute and eventually chronic hepatitis.

2. Curative irradiation.

A dose of 35 Gy given over a relatively long time is not one to cure many cancers. Theoretically it is a dose to cure leukemic liver involvement, probably most Hodgkin infiltrates too and certainly liver metastases of seminoma. Liver metastases of seminoma are nearly always part of a grossly disseminated seminoma, which can very well be cured by chemotherapy. Leukemia in the liver can be treated by chemotherapy as well. In Stanford, Kaplan (1968) has fostered the idea of elective treatment of the liver by irradiation, but this treatment modality has not played a significant role.

3. Is palliative irradiation of liver metastases indicated?

In 390 patients with untreated liver metastases Jaffe (1968) found a median survival of 75 days. Only 6,6% survived more than one year. Borgelt (1981) e.a. irradiated the whole liver to a dose of 2000 to 3000 rads/ 15 to 19 fractions in case of solitary metastases and if the tumour measured less than 1/3 of the liver volume he gave a boost of 2000 rads/10 fractions to the remaining tumour. In case of multiple hepatic metastases a dose of 2000 rads/10 fractions, 2100

rads/7 fractions, 2560 rads/16 fractions or 3000 rads/15 fractions
was given. One hundred and three of 109 patients could be analyzed.
The median survival was 11 weeks, hardly different from the Jaffe
material.

Most oncologists agree that in palliative medicine not the duration
of survival is a good criterium, but the improvement of the quality
of life.

In Borgelt's series only abdominal pain, nausea and vomiting, fever
and nightsweats improved in about 50% of the patients. Complete relief
of symptoms was seen in 34% of patients with nausea and vomiting, and
in 7% of those with fatigue and weakness. Pain relief occurred in
70% of the patients with severe pain.

With these results in mind one has to search for prognostic factors.
A patient who belongs to a category with a prognosis of one to two
months should not be irradiated for 2 - 3 weeks. Patients with extensive liver involvement as evidenced by abnormal chemistries, ascites
or jaundice have a median survival of less than one month (Jaffe).
Total bilirubin levels $>$ 1,5 mg% reduce the chance of favorable effect.
Turek-Maischeider (1975) restricts the indication to the young patient
who is not in a terminal condition.

Although irradiation of the liver is well tolerated if the dose does
not exceed 30 Gy, it should not be advocated with the expectation to
prolong life. Neither should it be given when medical treatment sufficiently alleviates symptoms. The best results will be obtained in
case of intensive pain, nausea and vomiting, and fever or nightsweats. Of course much depends on the wishes of the patient himself.

Not strictly belonging to my subject is
4. Elective irradiation of the liver.

Elective irradiation is the irradiation of organs or tissues in which
on statistical grounds the presence of micrometastases may be suspected but is not proven. It is a well known procedure especially with
cancers in the oropharynx and larynx. On theoretical grounds (L.
Cohen, 1968) and on the basis of the reduction of lymph node involvement at the time of the operation after preoperative irradiation of
rectal cancers (Roswit, 1975) one may conclude that relatively low

doses of 20 - 25 Gy may have some killing effect, resulting in an increase of disease free survival. Elective irradiation of the liver in the treatment of colorectal cancer has not yet been practised. In one arm of a not yet activated controlled clinical trial of the EORTC-Radiotherapy Cooperative Group on resectable rectal cancer postoperative radiotherapy includes pelvic irradiation and irradiation of the para-aortic nodes and liver up to 25 Gy in 19 fractions in four weeks. This trial may give us the answer to the question of the efficacy of low dose irradiation of occult liver metastases.

5. Methods of irradiation.

The most commonly employed method is external irradiation with photons. The method is simple and accurate, the dose distribution throughout the liver and its metastases is homogeneous and reproducible. Undesirable side effects on neighbouring organs are restricted and in the light of limited life expectancy acceptable.

Other methods of applying radiation to the liver are:
- injection of ^{198}Au
- injection of radioactive microspheres.

The problem of all intra-arterial or intravenous applications of radioactive material is and will remain the unpredictability of dose distribution. The blood supply of tumours and tumour metastases is erratic. Large parts of tumour nodules are necrotic and hypoxic.

Chamberlain e.a. (1983) have used ^{90}Yttrium microspheres with an average range of penetration of beta radiation in tissue of 0,25 cm. But in radiotherapy one is not interested in the average range, but in the volume that can obtain the prescribed dose. Moreover the problem is not to get a higher dose in the liver, but to get a high dose without radiation hepatitis as late effect. Much experimental work still has to be done before this method can be applied to patients unless under strict experimental conditions.

Are there ways to improve results?
1. Improvement will have to be looked for in the combination of

chemotherapy and radiotherapy.

2. The problem of chemotherapy is how to reach all tumour cells in badly vascularized metastases. Radiotherapy can be used to reduce the tumour volume as a first measure. The dose given should be small e.g. 10 - 12 Gy. After this short radiotherapy course chemotherapy should be given.

3. After chemotherapy a second course of radiotherapy may be given to a dose of 20 - 25 Gy. If it is possible to reduce the tumourload to a minimum, microspheres might be able to further improve the effects of therapy.

Patients with metastases of mammary carcinoma, who react favorably to medical treatment, are probably the best group to investigate the modalities of treatment of liver metastases.

But we must be aware of the fact that we mostly deal with patients with a very short future.

Conclusion.

The radiosensitivity of normal liver cells is such that the dose that can be given without a high probability of inducing radiation hepatitis, i.e. 35 Gy max., is too low for curative irradiation of most tumours.

Palliative irradiation does not influence the survival period. A substantial diminution of symptoms occurs in a minority of patients.

Severe pain is probably the best indication for palliative treatment.

The place of elective irradiation has still to be investigated.

As the dose is the limiting factor the combination with chemotherapeutic agents and irradiation may prove to be of value.

REFERENCES

1. Borgelt BB, Gelber R, Brady LW, Griffin T, Hendrickson FR. The palliation of hepatic metastases: results of the Radiation Therapy Oncology Group pilot study. Int. J. Radiation Oncology Biol. Phys., 1981, 7, 587-591.

2. Case JT, Warthin AS. Occurence of hepatic lesions in patients treated by intensive deep roentgen irradiation. Am. J. Roentgenol. and Rad. Therapy, 1924, 12, 27-46.

3. Chamberlain MN, Gray BN, Heggie JCP, Chmiel RL, Bennett RC. Hepatic metastases - a physiological approach to treatment. Br. J. Surg., 1983, 70, 596-598.

4. Cohen L. Theoretical iso-survival formulae for fractionated radiation therapy. Br. J. Radiol., 1968, 41, 522-528.

5. Haddad E, Le Bourgeois JF, Kuentz M, Lobo Ph. Livercomplications in lymphomas treated with a combination of chemotherapy and radiotherapy. Int. J. Radiation Oncology Biol. Phys., 1983, 9, 1313-1319.

6. Ingold JA, Reed GB, Kaplan HS, Bagshaw MA. Radiation hepatitis. Am. J. Roentgenol., 1965, 93, 200-208.

7. Jaffe BM, Donegan WL, Watson F, Spratt JS Jr. Factors influencing survival in patients with untreated hepatic metastases. Surg. Gynecol. Obstet., 1968, 127, 1-11.

8. Kaplan HS, Bagshaw MA. Radiation hepatitis: possible prevention by combined isotopic and external radiation therapy. Radiology, 1968, 91, 1214-1220.

9. Roswit B, Higgins GA, Keehn RJ. Preoperative irradiation for carcinoma of the rectum and rectosigmoid colon. Cancer, 1975, 35, 1597-1602.

10. Tefft M, Traggis D, Filler RM. Liver irradiation in children: acute changes with transient leukopenia and thrombocytopenia. Am. J. Roentgenol., Rad. Therapy, Nucl. Med., 1969, 106, 750-765.

11. Tefft M, Mitus A, Das L, Vawter GF, Filler RM. Irradiation of the liver in children: review of experience in the acute and chronic phases, and in the intact normal and partially resected. Am. J. Roentgenol., Rad. Therapy, Nucl. Med., 1970, 108, 365-385.

12. Turek-Maischeider M, Kazem I. Palliative irradiation for liver metastases. JAMA, 1975, 232, 625-628.

13. Wharton JT, Delclos L, Gallager S, Smith JP. Radiation hepatitis
    induced by abdominal irradiation with the cobalt 60 moving strip
    technique. Am. J. Roentgenol., Rad. Therapy, Nucl. Med., 1973, 117,
    73-80.

RADIOLOGICAL INTERVENTION TECHNIQUES IN THE PERCUTANEOUS TREATMENT OF
LIVER METASTASES

S. Wallace, C. Charnsangavej, C. H. Carrasco, W. Bechtel, K. Wright,
C. Gianturco

INTRODUCTION

Hepatic artery infusion (HAI) and hepatic artery embolization (HAE)
depend upon the concept that the treatment delivered to the hepatic
artery almost selectively affects the neoplasm. Hepatic metastases receive 90% of their blood supply from the hepatic artery, whereas normal
liver parenchyma has a dual supply from the hepatic artery (25%) and the
portal vein (75%); 50% of the oxygen supply comes from each source (1).

The transcatheter management of patients with inoperable hepatic
metastases by intra-arterial infusion and devascularization has been re-
surrected because of: (1) the greater technical expertise of the
angiographer in percutaneous selective catheterization of the vascular
supply to the neoplasm; (2) the surgeon armed with an implantable pump
which is associated with greater patient compliance; (3) the availability
of new chemotherapeutic agents and the use of combinations of cytotoxic
drugs; and (4) the appreciation of the value of peripheral embolization
which results in relative ischemia and in a decrease in the tumor cell
population.

Hepatic Artery Infusion (HAI)

Theoretically any drug delivered intravenously can be administered
intra-arterially as long as the concentration of the agent is tolerated
by the arterial endothelium. The rationale for intra-arterial infusion
is to expose the neoplasm to a higher concentration of the chemotherapeutic agent than is achieved by its intravenous delivery in order
to attain a greater therapeutic effect. The increase in local drug concentration also depends upon the rate of blood flow through the tumor
and the "first pass" effect. The cytotoxic effect is not only

1. Healey JE, Sheena KS: Vascular patterns in metastatic liver tumors.
   Surg Forum 14:121, 1963

concentration dependent but varies with the amount of uptake by the tumor, the metabolic activity of the tumor and of the drug; the sensitivity of the tumor to the drug, the local tumor environment (i.e., pH, pCO_2 and pO_2) as well as local and total body clearance of the drug. Ensminger et al. (2), Garmick et al. (3), and Kelsen et al. (4) demonstrated that after hepatic arterial infusion the hepatic extraction of floxuridine (FUDR),5-fluorouracil (5FU), Adriamycin, and cis-diamminedichloroplatinum (CDDP) was significantly greater than by the intravenous route. This increased hepatic extraction should be advantageous in the management of hepatic neoplasms.

Several modifications of the techniques for intra-arterial infusion of chemotherapeutic agents have been made to improve the effectiveness of this form of therapy including: a) higher concentrations of more effective chemotherapeutic agents or combinations of agents delivered over shorter infusion periods of up to 5 days depending upon the regimen; b) repeated cycles every 2 to 6 weeks as tolerated as long as there is evidence of a response; c) redistribution of flow through a single vessel to expose the entire neoplasm to the cytotoxic drugs; d) selective occlusion of vessels to increase concentration in the desired vessels and decrease complications in adjacent non-tumor bearing areas; and e) the use of a pulsatile flow pump to disrupt laminar flow in order to achieve a better distribution of the antineoplastic drugs.

ANATOMICAL CONSIDERATIONS

Familiarity with the variations of the hepatic arterial anatomy is essential for adequate transcatheter management of the neoplasms. The classic distribution of the celiac artery with its continuation into the common hepatic artery, which then gives off the right, middle, and left hepatic arteries only occurs in about 55% of people. An aberrant hepatic artery, originating from a source other than the celiac-hepatic artery was found in 41.5%. Thirty-one and one-half percent had only one aberrant hepatic artery while 10% had two or more. The right hepatic

2. Ensminger WD, Rosovsky A, Raso V, et al: A clinical-pharmacological evaluation of hepatic arterial infusions of 5-Fluoro-2-Deoxyuridine and 5-Fluorouracil. Cancer Res 38:3784-3792, 1978
3. Garmick MB, Ensminger WD, Israel M: A clinical-pharmacological evaluation of hepatic arterial infusion of adriamycin. Cancer Res 39:4105-4110, 1979
4. Kelsen DP, Hoffman J, Alcock N, et al: Pharmacokinetics of cisplatin regional hepatic infusions. Am J Clin Oncol (CCT) 5:173-178, 1982

artery is aberrant in 26%, usually arising from the superior mesenteric artery, and from the left hepatic artery in 27%, usually arising from the left gastric artery. Michels' study of 200 cadavers defined 10 anatomical variations of the hepatic artery (5). In our clinical experience, there are numerous variations of the variations described.

Michels also found 26 different extrahepatic collateral pathways in cadavers. Koehler et al. demonstrated angiographically extrahepatic and intrahepatic collateral channels after hepatic artery ligation (6). Collateral circulation through the internal mammary artery has been shown in monkeys by Doppman et al. following silicone embolization of the hepatic artery (7). The route through the vasa vasorum, arterioles of fine caliber in the wall of the hepatic arteries, hepatic veins, portal veins, biliary ducts, and the inferior vena cava was suggested by Michels (5), Bookstein et al. (8), and by Cho and Lunderquist (9). Charnsangavej et al. defined additional collateral vessels after hepatic artery occlusion secondary to peripheral and/or central embolization, surgical ligation, intra-arterial chemotherapy, or intimal injury from catheterization (10). Intrahepatic arterial collaterals developed in the portal triads and subcapsular areas between the lobes of the liver. Extrahepatic arterial collaterals were found in the ligaments which suspend the liver in the peritoneal cavity and through the structures that were closely attached to the liver.

TECHNICAL CONSIDERATIONS

Selective Catheterization: The delivery of chemotherapeutic or embolic agents requires more selective vascular catheterization. This is primarily

5. Michels NA: Blood Supply and Anatomy of the Upper Abdominal Organs. J.B. Lippincott, Philadelphia, 1965
6. Koehler RE, Korobkin M, Lewis F: Arteriographic demonstration of collateral arterial supply to the liver after hepatic artery ligation. Radiology 117:49-54, 1975
7. Doppman JL, Girton M, Kahn ER: Proximal versus peripheral hepatic artery embolization: Experimental study in monkeys. Radiology 128: 577-588, 1978
8. Bookstein J, Boijsen E, Olin T, et al: Angiography after end-to-side portocaval shunt: Clinical, laboratory, and pharmacoangiographic observations. Invest Radiol 6:101-109, 1971
9. Cho KJ, Lunderquist A: Peribiliary vascular plexus: The microvascular architecture of the bile duct in the rabbit and in clinical cases. Radiology 147:357, 1983
10. Charnsangavej C, Chuang VP, Wallace S, et al: Angiographic classification of hepatic arterial collaterals. Radiology 144:485-494, 1982

accomplished by tailoring the catheter configuration to that of the artery. For example, selective catheterization of the proper, right, left and middle hepatic arteries, which is absolutely essential for the optimal treatment of patients with secondary neoplasms of the liver is accomplished in 95% of our patients.

For the majority of vessels catheterized via the femoral route, 6.5Fr Torcon (Cook, Inc., Bloomington, Ind.) catheters are employed. The femoral approach is most frequently used because of the ease and famil-iarity with this route as well as the relatively short length of the infusion. In younger and smaller patients, especially females, studied by the femoral route, and all patients examined or treated from the brachial or axillary approach, a 5Fr polyethylene catheter which will accept a 0.035 in or 0.038 in guide wire is used. For children, 3.7Fr to 5Fr polyethylene catheters are preferred. The most common preformed catheter shapes found advantageous for our purposes are visceral, re-verse curve, right hepatic curve, cobra, etc. At times, the preshaped curves do not lay optimally in the anatomical contour of the hepatic artery. With the guide wire "anchored" in the vessel well beyond the catheter tip, the preformed catheter is exchanged for a polyethylene catheter shaped specifically for the vessel. Multiple exchanges of guide wires and catheters may be necessary to achieve the desired results. A coaxial system may also be employed, a 3Fr Teflon catheter will fit through a 6.5Fr catheter. Flow directed catheters or balloon catheters are necessary for certain circumstances.

Catheter Fixation: The catheter is positioned in the artery as close to the neoplasm as possible so that the infusion bathes the bulk of the tumor but spares the maximum of normal tissue. The catheter is fixed in position by taping it to the skin with plastic adhesive, covered with gauze squares and soft surgical tape, and connected to an infusion pump. At times, the catheter is fixed in place by suturing it to the skin.

Non-Thrombogenic Environment: A requirement for intra-arterial in-fusion is to create an intravascular non-thrombogenic environment. Systemic heparinization has been of considerable assistance in decreasing the complications resulting from the prolonged placement of the catheter. Any foreign body (needle, catheter or guide wire) placed into the blood stream will evoke clot formation within 10 minutes. A 3Fr catheter will result in less clot deposition than a larger bore catheter. The intra-arterial injection of 45 units/kg of aqueous heparin supplemented by intermittent catheter flushes (2-5 ml) of a solution of 1000 units of heparin in 500 ml of normal saline is adequate to maintain the activated clotting time (ACT) and partial thromboplastin time (PTT) at 1.5 to 2.0 times normal for approximately one hour during the catheterization (11).

With the incidence of vascular occlusion as high as 40% of patients with catheter placement of up to 9 months, a similar method of anticoagulation is used during the infusion (12). Systemic heparinization, i.e., maintaining the clotting parameters at 1.5 to 2.0 times normal, is accomplished by the continuous injection or infusion intravenously or intra-arterially of 10,000 to 25,000 units of aqueous heparin over each 24-hour period. Heparin and Adriamycin are incompatible and must be administered through different routes. Systemic heparinization is usually employed during the 5-day intra-arterial infusion of chemotherapy with the patient as an inpatient. At times, the catheter remains in place for months and Coumadin (5-10 mg/day) is more easily given to the outpatient to maintain the anticoagulation.

Catheter Position Monitoring: Following catheter placement, a radionuclide flow study is performed with 99m Technitium macroaggregated albumin as introduced by Kaplan et al. to monitor catheter position and flow characteristics (13). The infusion of chemotherapeutic agents at 50 ml/hour to 300 ml/hour is simulated and compared to the angiographic demonstration of the anatomical distribution of the contrast material which is usually injected at 2 ml to 12 ml/second.

For infusions longer than 24 hours, a conventional radiograph of the area of interest is obtained daily in the radiology department to check catheter position. During the period of infusion, the patient is usually at bed rest but may be allowed limited ambulation.

Choice and Frequency of Administration: In general those agents or combinations of agents most effective when delivered systemically

11. Wallace S, Medellin H, DeJongh DS, et al: Systemic heparinization for angiography. Amer J Roentgenol 116:204-209, 1972
12. Clouse ME, Ahmed R, Ryan RB, et al: Complications of long term transbrachial hepatic arterial infusion chemotherapy. Amer J Roentgenol 129:799-803, 1977
13. Kaplan WD, D'Orsi CJ, Ensminger WD, et al: Intra-arterial radionuclide infusion: A new technique to assess chemotherapy perfusion patterns. Cancer Treat Rep 62:699-703, 1978

should be the choices for intra-arterial therapy. Neoplasms refractory
to systemic chemotherapy may respond to arterial infusion of the same
agents at the same dose rate. In addition, those drugs compatible with
the intra-arterial route, as determined by the tolerance of the local
tissues, should be administered in that fashion while others can be delivered at the same time or sequentially, intravenously.

Because of the concentration of chemotherapeutic agents achieved
by the intra-arterial route, the response can frequently be assessed
after a single cycle by clinical, radiographic and biochemical parameters, including tumor markers. For the patient who is responding, the
intra-arterial route is continued at regular intervals - usually every
month as long as the treatment is tolerated. The surgically placed
catheter coupled with an implantable pump offers an excellent modality
for continuing intra-arterial therapy for the responding patient.
Therefore, the percutaneous placement assists in selecting the ideal
candidates for the more extensive and more expensive procedure, the instillation of the implantable pump. If the disease has not changed
after the first infusion, another cycle is administered. However, after
the second cycle with stable disease a new regimen should be instituted.
When there is obvious progression of the disease after the first infusion, a change in protocol should be initiated at the time of the
second catheterization. With failure after a maximum of 3 cycles of
intra-arterial chemotherapy, embolization or chemoembolization is available and at times may be the initial preferred approach.

Redistribution of Vascular Supply: An aberrant hepatic artery
which occurs frequently is a significant obstacle to hepatic artery infusion. The use of multiple catheters increases the time of the
procedure, the risks to the patient, the radiation exposure, and the
patients' discomfort. Transcatheter occlusion of the aberrant artery
is performed to redistribute the hepatic arterial flow to a single
vessel (14). This is accomplished by the placement of a stainless steel
coil and/or a Gelfoam segment at the origin of the replaced hepatic
artery.

Selective Occlusion for Infusion: Temporary or permanent occlusion
of branch vessels can minimize the exposure of normal tissues and

14. Chuang VP, Wallace S: Hepatic arterial redistribution for intra-
     arterial infusion of hepatic neoplasms. Radiology 135:295-299, 1980

maximize the infusion of the tumor to the chemotherapeutic agents. The gastroduodenal artery is frequently obstructed at its junction with the common hepatic artery to lessen gastroduodenal complications and to increase the concentration of the cytotoxic agents to the liver (15). This allows the placement of the catheter in the common hepatic artery in the event of a trifurcation of its branches into the right hepatic, left hepatic and gastroduodenal arteries. Selective occlusion as described is not associated with ischemia because of adequate collateral circulation.

Pulsatile vs. NonPulsatile Flow: The flow rate for intra-arterial infusion is slow, 50 ml/hour to 300 ml/hour, at a constant pump pressure. Even at seemingly optimal catheter position, there may be laminar flow at this slow rate which results in unequal distribution of the chemotherapeutic agent. A pulsatile pump at 1 to 3 pulses per second was devised by Gianturco (Cook, Inc., Bloomington, Ind.). This pump interrupts laminar flow and creates turbulence which results in greater dispersion which significantly improves the distribution in 20% of patients treated by hepatic arterial infusion.

COMPLICATIONS OF HAI

Vascular trauma is associated with superselective catheterization, higher concentrations of drugs, shorter infusion times or a combination of these factors (15). This trauma results in a 17% incidence of occlusion or stenosis and aneurysm, 6%. Gastrointestinal complications predominate. Unavoidable infusion of the gastroduodenal, and gastric and cystic arteries has resulted in dyspepsia, gastritis, duodenitis, and ulcers in 11.6%, and has on occasion resulted in cholecystitis and pancreatitis (16,17). Placement of the infusion catheter beyond the gastroduodenal will decrease the unintentional infusion. Frequently, the gastroduodenal artery has hepatopedal flow allowing safe placement in the common hepatic artery. Otherwise, occlusion of the gastroduodenal artery with a steel coil is performed in selected patients

17. Carrasco CH, Freeny PC, Chuang VP, et al: Chemical cholecystitis associated with hepatic artery infusion chemotherapy. Amer J Roentgenol 141:703-706, 1983
18. Soo CS, Wallace S, Chuang VP, et al: Injury to the intima of the hepatic artery. Radiology 143:373-378, 1982
19. Chuang VP, Wallace S, Stroehlein J, et al: Hepatic artery infusion chemotherapy: Gastroduodenal complications. Amer J Roentgenol 137:347-350, 1981

who develop serious gastrointestinal complaints. These problems are more prevalent with chemotherapeutic agents as vinblastine, Mitomycin C, and Adriamycin.

CRITERIA FOR RESPONSE

The parameters utilized to define response include liver function studies, radionuclide scintigraphy, ultrasonography, computed tomography, magnetic resonant imaging, angiography, carcinogenic embryonic antigen, alpha fetaprotein, and other markers that may be specific for the particular neoplasm. Those that define the hepatic involvement are employed on a sequential basis.

Tumor response is classified as CR (complete response), i.e., the resolution of the neoplastic process in the liver; PR (partial response) is a decrease of at least 50% in the product of the two largest perpendicular diameters of the lesions measured.

Arbitrarily, HAI is limited to a course of 3 cycles at monthly intervals and for responders, continued treatment as long as there is response. Usually a response can be detected after the first cycle if the neoplasm is sensitive to the treatment. If the disease remains stable after the first cycle, a second cycle of HAI is given. Failure to respond after the first or second cycle has precipitated the investigation of other interventional alternatives, including a change in the agents for HAI, hepatic artery embolization, or chemoembolization.

Hepatic Artery Embolization (HAE)

The concept of treating hepatic neoplasms by hepatic artery ligation was suggested by Markowitz in 1952 (17). Physiologic blood flow studies in patients using radioactive xenon demonstrated a 90% decrease in tumor blood flow after hepatic artery ligation, as compared to 35 to 40% decrease to normal liver parenchyma (18). Mori et al. reported selective destruction of the tumor without damage to the normal liver after ligation of the hepatic artery for metastatic gastric carcinoma (19). The response to surgical ligation is temporary, in part due to the formation of collateral circulation which may occur instantaneously.

17. Markowitz J: The hepatic artery. Surg Gynecol Obstet 95:644-646, 1952
18. Gelin LE, Lewis DH, Nilsson L: Liver blood flow in man during abdominal surgery. Acta Hepatosplenol 15:21, 1968
19. Mori W, Masada M, Miyanaga T: Hepatic artery ligation and tumor necrosis in the liver. Surgery 59:359, 1966

TECHNICAL CONSIDERATIONS

More lasting devascularization of an hepatic neoplasm can be achieved by peripheral embolization with particulate material such as polyvinyl alcohol foam (Ivalon); Gelfoam; Gelfoam plus a sclerosing agent; or a combination of peripheral embolization and central occlusion with stainless steel coils (20). Peripheral sequential unilobar embolization using Ivalon particles is our preferred approach. Following peripheral embolization of one lobe (100-200 mg), the patient returns in 1 month for the embolization of the remaining lobe. Significant intrahepatic collaterals usually develop in the previously embolized lobe and repeat embolization is performed.   During the third angiographic study, any collaterals to the liver, either intra or extrahepatic are completely occluded. The patient is usually followed clinically for 3 to 6 months prior to another angiographic study and HAE is repeated if necessary. If there are metastases outside the liver, systemic chemotherapy is administered in conjunction with or following HAE. At times when one lobe of the liver is embolized, the catheter is left in the artery to the other lobe for concomitant chemotherapy. After embolization, a normal distribution through intrahepatic collaterals occurs in 24 to 48 hours which allows for infusion after occlusion into the same artery. Thus far over 300 patients have been treated by HAE.

INDICATIONS

The indications for embolization are: (1) preoperatively to facilitate surgery for a resectable neoplasm; (2) failure to respond to systemic or intrahepatic arterial chemotherapy; (3) multiple hepatic arteries; (4) failure of surgery; (5) as primary treatment; and (6) to control pain and/or hemorrhage.

CONTRAINDICATIONS

The contraindications to hepatic artery embolization are still being formulated. Cirrhosis, portal vein and biliary tract obstruction, and extensive metastatic disease are only relative restrictions. In patients with neoplasms coexisting with cirrhosis, the hepatic artery flow assumes a greater proportion of the oxygen transport and nutritive function. This is a relative problem and decisions are made on the basis of therapeutic options.

20. Gianturco C, Anderson JH, Wallace S: Mechanical devices for arterial occlusion. Amer J Roentgenol 124:428-435, 1975

Portal vein involvement by tumor is more frequently thought of in association with primary hepatic neoplasms, but can also occur in metastatic disease. Patients with intrinsic or extrinsic obstruction of the portal vein without reversal of flow or demonstration of extra-hepatic venous collaterals, have tolerated hepatic devascularization. At the other end of the spectrum, in the face of tumor thrombosis obstructing the portal vein with an extensive collateral network, we have been reluctant to embolize. Those situations in between vary considerably and are managed individually depending upon the patient's general medical status, the presence of intrahepatic portal vein collaterals, minimal extrahepatic venous collaterals, and the availability of therapeutic alternatives.

We have treated some patients with hepatic neoplasms and jaundice by hepatic artery embolization. In these patients with signs of biliary obstruction, confirmed by laboratory studies, HAE has been performed gradually and sequentially over a 3-month period with surprisingly good results. However, with hepatocellular damage as the cause of jaundice, if this can be established, embolization has not as yet been employed.

The estimation of tumor replacement of 70% or greater has been considered, by some, a contraindication to hepatic artery devascularization. Because it is difficult to accurately determine the extent of involvement, we have treated a few patients by HAE under these circumstances with relatively few consequences. In the absence of therapeutic alternatives, this was done by sequential partial embolization over a period of several months. Careful monitoring of fluids and electrolytes has been critical in minimizing hepatorenal complications.

RESULTS

The survival statistics must be compared to those presented by Jaffe et al. who reported a median survival of 75 days with untreated metastases from various primary tumors and a mortality of 26% within 30 days of the time of diagnosis (21). The surgical mortality within 30 days of a major lobectomy (extended right lobectomy) ranged from 30 to 35% (22).

21. Jaffe BM, Donegan WL, Watson F, et al: Factors influencing survival in patients with untreated hepatic metastases. Surg Gyn Obstet 127:1-11, 1968
22. McBride CM, Wallace S: Cancer of the right lobe of the liver. Arch Surg 105:289-296, 1972

The median survival from the time of the hepatic artery embolization in our first 43 patients with long term followup was 11.5 months. Most of these patients had already failed systemic chemotherapy, hepatic artery infusion, and surgery (23).

COMPLICATIONS

The posthepatic embolization syndrome consists of pain, fever, nausea, and vomiting, which usually lasts from 3 to 5 days. Abnormal liver function studies become even more abnormal for 5 to 7 days but sometimes for as long as 3 weeks before returning to pre-embolization levels. Nonspecific gas formation following tumor embolization occurs in almost all patients. This is due to air introduced during the embolization and to gas released by necrosis of the neoplasm.

Of the first 100 patients treated by HAE, there were 7 deaths which occurred within 1 month of the procedure. Three deaths were most probably related to the embolizations, the result of hepatic failure and hepatic encephalopathy, and/or the "hepatorenal" syndrome, while 4 patients probably died of extensive metastases. The "hepatorenal" syndrome was observed in 4 patients, one of whom failed to respond to therapy consisting of hydration, electrolytes, and corticosteroids.

PORTAL VEIN INFUSION AFTER HEPATIC ARTERY OCCLUSION

The contributions of the portal vein to the vascular supply to hepatic neoplasms have been reviewed and shown by Lin et al. to be significantly more than 10% (24). Arterioportal communication exists at the peribiliary arterial plexus, the vasa vasorum of the portal vein and direct anastomoses in the sinusoids. Ekelund et al. in rats, and Taylor et al. in patients demonstrated that following hepatic artery occlusion, portal vein perfusion to the metastases was significantly increased (25,26).

Nine patients at M. D. Anderson Hospital have been treated by portal vein infusion. In 4 patients whose celiac or common hepatic artery was occluded centrally as the result of HAI, the portal vein

23. Chuang VP, Wallace S: Hepatic artery embolization in the treatment of hepatic neoplasms. Radiology 140:51-58, 1981
24. Lin G, Hagerstrand I, Lunderquist A: Portal blood supply of liver metastases. Amer J Roentgenol (In Press)
25. Ekelund L, Lin G, Bengmark S: The blood supply of experimental liver tumors following intra-arterial embolization with Gelfoam powder and absolute ethanol (In Press)
26. Taylor I, Bennett R, Sheriff S: The blood supply of colorectal liver metastasis. Br J Cancer 38:749, 1978

was infused through a surgically placed catheter in a branch of the middle colic vein. Five patients received 9 courses of chemotherapy through percutaneous transhepatic placement of a catheter into the portal vein after purposeful peripheral and central occlusion of the hepatic artery. It is still too early to evaluate the effect of this form of treatment.

Colon Carcinoma

ADJUVANT TREATMENT

More than 60% of Dukes' C colorectal carcinoma patients are destined to have a recurrence of their disease (27). Most of these relapses take place in the liver. In an attempt to reduce the frequency of hepatic metastases, adjuvant hepatic arterial infusion was initiated in 25 patients with floxuridine (FUDR) and Mitomycin C every 5 to 6 weeks for 3 cycles. The estimated time to relapse of 25% of these patients is 20 months. This compares well to 16 months for 121 patients given BCG by scarification and 11 months for 75 patients treated by surgery for the primary colonic lesion alone. The preliminary results must be followed for at least 5 years for statistically significant data (27).

RESECTABLE LIVER METASTASES

Ten patients with resectable or potentially resectable liver metastases were given 2 hepatic arterial infusions of FUDR and Mitomycin C. This was done to facilitate surgery by reducing the size of the tumors. Lobectomy or wedge resection was then performed followed by 2 or more cycles of HAI. The median survival of this group is 15.5 months. Some of these patients have been followed for close to 4 years (27).

NONRESECTABLE LIVER METASTASES

Fifty-five patients with metastases, colorectal carcinoma confined to the liver were treated with HAI of FUDR and Mitomycin C. Thirty-one patients had HAI alone, while 14 had HAI as well as arterial occlusion for either redistribution of the hepatic arterial blood flow; intentional occlusion, both peripheral and central, for treatment; or inadvertent occlusion, usually central, as a complication of HAI. Twenty-two of these patients had failed systemic chemotherapy with intravenous fluoropyrimidines.

27. Patt YZ: Hepatic arterial infusion of floxuridine, Adriamycin, and mitomycin C for primary liver neoplasms. Cancer Bulletin 36:29-31, 1984

A complete remission was observed in 5.5% (3 patients) and a partial remission in 47.5% (26 patients) for a total response rate of 53%. The median survival of those treated with infusion plus occlusion was 15 months compared to 8 months for infusion alone. Of the 22 patients who failed previous intravenous 5FU, 10 patients (45.4%) responded to HAI of FUDR and Mitomycin C. The median survival rate of the 10 responders was 14 months as opposed to 6 months for nonresponders. A significant decrease in CEA levels was observed only among responding patients (28).

The treatment cycle consisted of Mitomycin C at 10 mg/m^2 as a single dose and FUDR, 100 mg/m^2 per day for 5 days. This was repeated at monthly intervals as long as the patient continued to respond.

Breast Carcinoma

Systemic chemotherapy with various regimens has resulted in substantial palliation to the patient with liver metastases from breast carcinoma, but long term remissions are rare. The treatment of refractory metastatic liver involvement has been disappointing.

HEPATIC ARTERY INFUSION (HAI)

A variety of agents has been investigated for the intra-arterial management of liver metastases. Once again, it should be stressed that the preferred intravenous combinations should be explored for its intra-arterial effectiveness. If these fail to result in a reasonable response, alternative agents, vinblastine (Velban), cis-diamminedichloroplatinum (CDDP), or a combination of both, have been encouraging (29,30,31).

Ten of 20 evaluable patients treated by HAI of CDDP, 100 to 120 mg/m^2 over 2 hours achieved an objective decrease in the size of their hepatic metastases - 1 complete response and 4 partial responses for a response rate of 25%. Five patients had a minor response, 5 patients experienced stabilization of disease and 6 progressed. The median time

28. Patt YZ, Wallace S, Freireich EJ, et al: The palliative role of hepatic arterial infusion and arterial occlusion in colorectal carcinoma metastatic to the liver. Lancet 1:349-351, 1981
29. Yap HY, Salem P, Hortobagyi GN, et al: Phase II study of cis-dichloro-diammineplatinum (II) in advanced breast cancer. Cancer Treat Rep 62:405-408, 1978
30. Fleishman G, Yap HY, Chuang VP, et al: Percutaneous hepatic arterial infusion of cis-diamminedichloroplatinum (II) for metastatic breast cancer in the liver. J Clin Oncol (In Press)
31. Yap HY, Fleischman G, Fraschini G: Intra-arterial infusion for liver metastases from breast cancer. Cancer Bulletin 36:27-29, 1984

to progression was 18 weeks (range 8-26 weeks) for responding patients, 12 weeks for stable disease, and 6 weeks for progressive disease. The median duration of survival from the onset of HAI was 8.5 months for the responders compared to 3 months for the nonresponders.

Eleven of 15 patients who were treated with continuous HAI of Velban, 1.6 to 2.0 mg/m^2 per day for 5 days at 4-week intervals, are evaluable for response. There were 4 partial responders (36%), 4 patients experienced a minor response, 2 patients had stable disease and one progressed. The median survival time was 8.5 months from onset of HAI for the responding patients.

Ten of 14 patients are presently evaluable for response to a HAI combination of CDDP (100 mg/m^2) followed by Velban (1.6 mg/m^2 a day for 5 days). A partial response was achieved in 8 of 10 patients (80%). The median survival time as yet has not been reached and all but one responder has remained alive and in remission from 1 to 8 months.

The toxicities were worse than with either drug alone and included nausea, vomiting, renal failure, hepatitis and fever with severe neutropenia and thrombocytopenia. Arteritis and arterial occlusion was more frequent probably as a result of Velban and the presence of the catheter. Otherwise, catheter related complications included displacement, local bleeding, sepsis, and gastric ulceration. The high response rate is encouraging but a slight dose reduction is in order.

HEPATIC ARTERY EMBOLIZATION (HAE)

For those patients that fail HAI or for further palliation after successful intravenous or intra-arterial therapy, a few patients have been subjected to HAE. HAE probably has a place in the therapeutic management of liver metastases which is still to be established.

Metastatic Hormone Producing Tumors

Eighteen patients with various APUDOMAS (hormone-producing tumors) metastatic to the liver underwent hepatic artery embolization. In one group of 14 patients, hepatic artery embolization was the only antineoplastic therapy employed. A partial remission of the hepatic metastases occurred in 8 of the 11 living patients. Three deaths occurred in this group. In addition to hepatic artery embolization, a second group of 4 patients received concurrent hepatic artery infusions of chemotherapeutic agents. A partial remission occurred in 3 of these patients (32).

Seven of these 18 patients had carcinoid with hepatic metastases. Six of these 7 patients were treated by hepatic artery embolization; 5 of the 6 had a partial response with symptomatic improvement of their diarrhea and flushing. One of these patients died 5 days after HAE from hepatic failure. The seventh patient was lost to followup after receiving one course of HAE and HAI of CDDP.

Hepatic artery embolization offers significant palliation for patients with APUDOMAS metastatic to the liver by reducing the tumor bulk and thus decreasing the production of pharmacologically active substances secreted by functioning tumors. The impact of this treatment on the survival of patients with APUDOMAS is impossible to evaluate because of their usual prolonged course.

Chemoembolization

Chemoembolization is the combination of intra-arterial infusion of a chemotherapeutic agent and arterial embolization of the vascular supply as proposed by Kato et al. (33). In addition to the direct effect of ischemia on the neoplasm by occlusion, the emboli increase the transit time through the tumor vascular bed, theoretically the contact time of the chemotherapeutic agent with the neoplastic cells, increase the local drug concentration, and possibly increase tissue permeability to the drug because of anoxia. The cytotoxic effect is not only to the neoplasm but to the vessel embolized and infused, producing vasculitis and occlusion. The systemic toxic effect may be reduced by metabolism of the drug on its first passage through the infused organ, thereby confining the higher concentration of the chemotherapeutic agent to the target organ.

Kato, et al. (1980) (33) combined peripheral arterial embolization with intra-arterial infusion by creating microencapsulated Mitomycin C. The microcapsules consisted of 80% Mitomycin C as the core and 20% ethylcellulose as the shell with a mean particle size of 225 um. The ethylcellulose micorcapsules protect the Mitomycin C from enzymatic inactivation, slowly releasing concentrated Mitomycin C into the surrounding tissues, thereby preventing its rapid clearance from the

32. Carrasco CH, Chuang VP, Wallace S: Apudomas metastatic to the liver; Treatment by hepatic artery embolization. Radiology 149:79-83, 1983
33. Kato T, Nemoto R, Mori H, et al: Arterial chemoembolization with microencapsulated anticancer drug. JAMA 245:1123-1127, 1981

target organ. The mechanical occlusion of the small vessels results in multiple focal areas of ischemia. The potential effects of intra-arterial chemoembolization with the injection into an artery over minutes is probably a function of prolonged drug action and ischemia.

A similar concept has been applied by using different materials to decrease blood flow. Aronsen et al. (34) and Dakhil et al. (35) used biodegradable starch microspheres injected into the catheter prior to infusion chemotherapy. Biodegradable starch microspheres (Spherex), specially formulated cross-linked starch spheres of 40 microns in dia-meter, cause an occlusion of small arterioles and are degradable by serum amylase with the half life of 15 to 30 minutes. The occlusion enhances the contact time between the chemotherapeutic agent and the tumor.

At M. D. Anderson Hospital and Tumor Institute, cis-diammine-dichloroplatinum (CDDP) in concentrated form (10 mg/ml) or Mitomycin C mixed with Ivalon or Gelfoam particles, is used for peripheral emboli-zation; it is hoped that this combination will enhance both the embolization and the chemotherapeutic effects.

34. Aronsen KF, Hellekant C, Holmberg J, et al: Controlled bleeding of hepatic artery flow with enzymatically degradable microspheres combined with oncolytic drugs. Eur Surg Pes 11:99, 1979
35. Dakhil S, Ensminger W, Cho K, et al: Improved regional selectivity of hepatic arterial bischlorethylnitrousourea with degradable microspheres. Cancer 50:631-635, 1982

INTRA-ARTERIAL INFUSION OF CYTOTOXIC DRUGS FOR THE TREATMENT OF
LIVERMETASTASES

T.J.A. Kuijpers, A.T. van Oosterom, E.H. Overbosch, E.A. de Bruijn, M.
Oudkerk

Regional infusion chemotherapy has been used now over more than two
decades. Today its application is limited mainly to primary and
secondary liver malignancies, although it has been used in other types
of cancer as well. This survey concerns hepatic arterial infusion (HAI)
in metastatic liver disease, and its current investigational methods of
application.

HISTORY

The first report about intra-arterial chemotherapy was presented by
Bleichroder (1) who in 1912 attempted a therapy for puerperal sepsis by
infusion of Collargol at the aortic bifurcation. In 1950 Bierman et al
(2) and Klopp et al (3) almost simultaneously originated the arterial
infusion technique by administering nitrogen mustard for a variety of
neoplasms. Almost a decade later, Sullivan et al (4) administered an
a.timetabolite, 5-fluorouracil (5-FU) by arterial infusion. Since that
time, HAI has been in use in palliation of hepatic malignancy. The
original method for HAI was proximal ligation and subsequently distal
infusion of cytotoxic agents beyond the ligation via a catheter placed
at surgery (5).

The majority of groups now, prefer infusion therapy through whether
percutaneously or surgically placed hepatic artery catheters, which has
been used regularly for the past 10 years. The combination of infusion
and embolization techniques are applied more frequently too. Some
authors believe that we are: "Only at the threshold of a new
therapeutic approach, in which the radiologist is the prime
catalyst".(6) Probably this statement is too optimistic since the
development of monoclonal antibodies, microspheres and other devices,

which have the possibility to carry cytotoxic drugs to tumors.

INTRODUCTION

The liver as one of the major organs of the body is most frequently
involved by metastases. Almost 70% of all patients who died of cancer
show liver metastases (7).

The most important primary cancers, prone to develop liver metastases
are carcinomas of the gastrointestinal tract, pancreas, lung, breast
and melanoma. In a large series of autopsies of cancer patients 2,5%
had metastases only to the liver (8). Especially those types of cancers
that spread primarily to the liver are considered for regional
chemotherapy. Such a pattern is frequently seen in colon and rectum
malignancies, however other types like breast carcinoma may also
present with secondary liver disease only. Colorectal carcinoma may
metastasizes to the liver up to 70% (9), however in approximately half
of this group, the liver is the only detectable site of clinical
metastases. This is the major reason why this group of cancers are the
prime candidates for intra-arterial infusion therapy.

The natural history of patients with liver metastases is poor. However
it must be stated, that there is a wide variation in survival in this
group of patients, when asymptomatic liver metastases are distinquished
from clinically symptomatic lesions (10). Asymptomatic liver
metastases, or synchronous lesions are discovered either at surgery,
during staging or as the result of routine follow up after curative
cancer resections. Symptomatic patients (metachronous liver
metastases), will complain of upper abdominal pressure, fatique, pain,
jaundice and or ascites. The difference in survival between synchronous
and metachronous lesions is reported by Cady et al (11). They showed a
mean survival of 13 month (mo) and a median survival of 7 mo in
patients undergoing colonic resections with synchronous metastases.
Other authors reported similar data (12,13). Shorter survival rates
were presented by Jaffe et al (14), without categorizing the clinical
status of the patients. In their group of patients with untreated liver
metastases, the median survival after diagnosis is 75 days and only 7%
survived 1 year.

Generally the outcome of patients with diffuse metastases is dismal,
however it is important to remember that if multiple organs are

involved the length of the survival generally depends on the extent of the hepatic metastases (14). Other prognostic factors in survival are the degree of differentiation, and the site and histologic type of the primary tumor.

The histology of many tumors, indicating a low radiosensitivity is often a contraindication for radiotherapy. The optimal therapy for metastatic liver disease is surgical resection, but this can only be performed if the lesion is located in a resectable segment or lobe and if the remaining liver tissue is normal (15). Unfortunately, this situation occurs only in about 6% of patients with liver metastases (8).

The effects of intravenous or systemic chemotherapy in patients with gastrointestinal metastatic carcinoma has been well established. In a recent review of clinical trials, the mean response rate of liver metastases in colorectal carcinoma, has been 23% (16). This is slightly higher than earlier similar reports, in which the response rate has been about 10-14% (17-21). The poor response rate following intravenous chemotherapy in the past has led to the application of regional intrahepatic delivery of drugs by intra-arterial administration.

RATIONALE FOR INTRA-ARTERIAL INFUSION

Secondary hepatic neoplasms receive their blood supply almost completely (95%) from the hepatic artery, whereas normal liver tissue has a dual supply from the portal vein (75%) and from the hepatic artery (25%). Because of the altered perfusion the hepatic artery is an ideal route for selective delivery of chemotherapeutic agents. The administration of drugs which are metabolized by normal liver tissue, will result in both relatively high intracellular concentrations of the applied drug in tumor cells and low systemic concentrations, with reduced side effects (22). HAI with several drugs produces higher intrahepatic and lower systemic concentrations, than are achieved using corresponding systemic intravenous administrations (22,23,25). This results in an increase in therapeutic index and virtual elimination of systemic toxicity, which has been demonstrated by several authors (22-25). Therefore in patients, with metastatic disease confined to the liver, without any other signs of tumor spread, treatment with transcatheter intraarterial infusion seems a promising step.

VARIATIONS IN VASCULAR ANATOMY

Adequate catheter position is essential in HAI technique.
For that reason familiarity with the variations of the hepatic arterial
anatomy is mandatory. The classic distribution of the celiac trunc with
its branches is found in about 55% of the cases (fig. 1). In the
remaining 45% there is an aberrant arterial anatomy (26,27). Both right
and left hepatic arteries are aberrant in about a quarter of the cases,
in which the right hepatic artery usually arises from the superior
mesenteric artery and the left hepatic artery from the left gastric
artery. In about half the patients the gastroduodenal artery originates
midway between the origin of the common hepatic artery from the celiac
trunc and the division point of the common hepatic artery (27).
Placement of the catheter beyond the gastroduodenal into the proper
hepatic artery is the optimal position for HAI. The right gastric
artery is usually small and originates from the left hepatic artery
(42%), or the proper hepatic artery (40%) (27). Infusion of this vessel
with chemotherapeutic agents is considered to significantly contribute
to dyspepsia, gastritis and ulceration.
The cystic artery originates as a single trunc (75%) or as a double
trunc (25%). Multiple variants of the cystic artery have been described
(27). Infusion proximal to the origin of the cystic artery may be
associated with cholecystitis. In conclusion in 20% of patients with
liver metastases, HAI is not applicable because of anomalous hepatic
arteries or inaccessible arterial supply to the liver (28). In our
series of patients this percentage is about 10. Therefore exact
knowledge of the vascular anatomy is of major importance.

HEPATIC ARTERIAL INFUSION METHODS

Generally there are two methods to place the catheter in the hepatic
artery: the surgical and the percutaneous method.

SURGICAL APPROACH

For each patient the hepatic arterial blood supply is defined by a
preoperative selective celiac and superior mesenteric angiogram. At
normal anatomy, the gastroduodenal artery is selected for catheter
placement. The artery is ligated distally and a small arteriotomy is

234

fig. 1
Normal anatomy of the celiac trunc

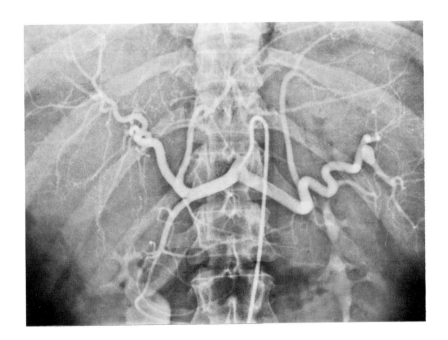

performed. A silastic catheter is then introduced into the vessel and carefully positioned, so the end of the catheter is just at the origin of the gastroduodenal artery. It is important not to extend the catheter in the proper or common hepatic arteries since this may lead to trombosis. In order to insure total liver perfusion the catheter has to be placed in positions other than the gastroduodenal artery according to the vascular anatomy (15). Ligation of an accessory vessel is routinely performed. Ligation of aberrant vessels can result in development of intrahepatic collaterals. Therefore, these vessels remain in situ and to achieve total infusion, two catheters are placed. In a series of 110 patients single catheter placement in the gastroduodenal artery was feasible in 55%. Two catheters were placed in 16% (15). Alterations in blood flow secondary to anatomic variations or to celiac atheromatous disease has led to the placement of the catheter through the splenic artery in 31% of these series. Elective cholecystectomy proved not to be necessary, however, care has to be taken to eliminate indirect perfusion of the stomach (29). Catheter positioning can be controlled, postoperatively, by using transcatheter technetium-aggregates. Continuous infusion will be obtained by an implantable pump placed in a subcutaneous pocket.

Another advantage of this method is the careful assessment of the extent of the disease at laparotomy and the appropiate obtainment of biopsies. However it is well known that surgery of a patient with advanced liver metastases result in a mortality rate, up to 30% (5). This is an important consideration for treatment selection of patients, with a predictable short survival. Mortality rate varies from 2 to 4%, depending on the patient selection (15,30,31).

Thrombosis of the hepatic artery, using an implantable pump system, occurs in less than 5% (32). Patients with extrahepatic metastases as well as liver involvement have a poor prognosis. The presence of extrahepatic disease, therefore, must be considered as an absolute contraindication for the surgical placement of an hepatic artery catheter.

PERCUTANEOUS APPROACH

Superselective placement of the catheter by the radiologist has expanded the role of the angiography to include infusion chemotherapy,

embolization and pharmacologic manupulation of the vascular system
(33). Superselective catheterization is accomplished in 85-95% of the
patients, dependent on the experience of the angiographer (34).
Selective celiac and superior mesenteric angiograms are performed in
each new patient to obtain an anatomic road map of the visceral
arteries and portal system (34). Angiographic catheterization is done
by the Seldinger technique, through the femoral artery with
subsequently selective catheterization of respectively celiac trunc and
hepatic arteries. If the femoral route fails and or long term infusion
is required, left brachial or axillary approach offers an alternative
route for the introduction of the catheter. In our experience the
latter offers the best catheter stability during bolus injection of the
drug.

Multiple catheter sizes are available varying in diameter from 7 to 5
French (2,3 to 1,7 mm). Generally, the first size is used in the
selective series. The 5 French catheter is selected for smaller
patients or for smaller arteries such as brachial catheterization and
for infusions lasting longer than one week. Brachial artery trombosis
cannot be adequately prevented by heparinization of the catheter or by
systemic heparinization (35,36). The catheter size is therefore an
important factor to prevent arterial trombosis. Many different catheter
curves have been described (34), and various exciting names have been
applied to catheters with similar curves. It is essential that the
catheter configuration matches the arterial anatomy as closely as
possible to decrease intima dissection rate and increase catheter
stability. Chuang et al(34) introduced the "tailor made catheter"
principle, corresponding to the vascular anatomy. Optimally, a
three-dimensional concept of the arterial anatomy is neccessary in
using the right catheter.

Additional digital subtraction angiography series can be very helpfull
in order to accomplish the "tailor made catheter" principle.
Digital subtraction angiography is a fast and easy method, in
intra-arterial use, to locate the superselective catheter position and
to exclude back flow during bolus injection of the drug. The catheter
is placed as close as possible to the target area, generally distal to
the origin of the gastroduodenal artery or in the left or right hepatic
artery. If the catheter tip cannot be placed distal to the origin of

the gastroduodenal artery, the angiographer must determine the flow
direction in this vessel, to avoid drug infusion to stomach or
duodenum. Some authors prefer embolization of the gastroduodenal
artery before infusion starts, minimizing gastro-intestinal symptoms,
which is the most frequent complication of HAI chemotherapy (37-40).
Once the catheter is in a satisfactory position it is connected to an
infusion-pump for long term infusion or to a syringe to inject the drug
directly (bolus infusion). The catheter position should be checked
daily, when long term infusion is performed, since displacement of the
catheter is a frequently observed complication (15-40%) (41,42).
Conventional radiographs of the abdomen or isotopic flow studies can be
obtained to ascertain the position of the catheter (43). Manupulation
of a catheter for repositioning, in patients with long term infusion,
increases the risk of infection, so broad spectrum antibodies may be
required. The main risk of the superselective catheterization itself is
injury and dissection of the intima of the arterial wall, which may
cause acute obstruction of the vessel. The incidence, including
complete and partial thrombosis ranges from 15 to 50% (35,42,44).
Generally, this complication does not cause serious problems since
collateral vessels as well as intrahepatic anastomoses will be
sufficient (45-47). Thrombosis of both, the hepatic artery and the
portal vein lead to acute liver insufficiency and mortality. This is the
reason to visualize the patency of the portal vein before the
superselective catheterization can be started. However, thrombosis of
the portal vein is a relative contraindication because of the poor
prognosis of the patient (48). The arterial branch supplying the
gal bladder is often included within the infusion territory. First,
because of the multiple anatomic variants of the cystic artery and
secondly, this artery is too small for preventive embolization.
Nevertheless, arterial infusion chemotherapy is generally well
tolerated by the gal bladder.Symptomatic cholecystitis occurred only in
4 out of 700 HAI with chemotherapeutic agents (49).

Recently, we reviewed our series of HAI over the last 3 years.
The series include 35 patients with symptomatic liver metastases
without demonstrable extrahepatic involvement. In 23 patients the
primary was colorectal cancer, in 6 patients breast cancer. In nearly

all patients the only treatment applied was an intra-arterial hepatic bolusinfusion with Mitomycin-C (MMC), which was performed in 73 courses. In 23 patients 2 to 4 infusions were administered with a four to six weeks interval. The technique of the HAI was performed as described above, and in 34% succeeded by axillary or brachial approach. At each course, if adequate catheter positioning was obtained, 20-30 mg MMC was injected over a ten minutes period. Thereafter the catheter has been removed and the patient remained hospitalized for one day only. The most frequent anatomic variation was a partial or complete origin of the proper hepatic artery from the superior mesenteric artery (fig. 2). Unsuccesfull catheterization of the proper hepatic artery was present in 15%, mainly as a result of complications during angiography. Intima dissection of the hepatic artery as a complication of the technical procedure was encountered in 11%.

A subsequent occlusion of the hepatic artery was seen in 4%. Mortality occurred in two patients. One died of liverinsufficiency due to thrombosis following partial dissection of the common hepatic artery, the portal vein being occluded by a tumor localization. In the other patient a dispositioning of the catheter occured during the second HAI leading to infusion of MMC in the gastric artery and subsequent severe toxic gastritis. A subsequent pulmonary complication lead to the death of the patient.

Our experience led us to the following selection criteria for percutaneous intermittent hepatic arterial infusion:

CRITERIA FOR PATIENT SELECTION

1. Metastatic liver cancer without any other demonstrable extra-hepatic signs of tumor spread or local recurrence.
2. Severe liver dysfunction due to involvement of the liver not exceeding 75% of its volume.
3. An adequate portal vein, demonstrated by selective angiography prior to HAI. However, a thrombosis of the portal vein is not an absolute contraindication for HAI.
4. Colorectal and breast cancer as primary tumors.
5. Good general condition of the patient (WHO performance < 3).
6. Consent of the patient.

CHEMOTHERAPEUTIC AGENTS

Generally the chemotherapeutic agents applied for the treatment of
liver metastases can be divided in two groups according to their
mechanism of action.

1. The cell-cycle specific drugs, like 5-FU and 5-fluoro-
    2-deoxyuridine (5-FUDR) (antimetabolites).
2. The cell-cycle non-specific drugs like MMC, Cisplatin
    and Adriamycin (intercalating and alkylating agents).

The Pyrimidine antimetabolites act in a specific part of the
cell-cycle, inhibiting RNA and DNA synthesis. Therefore prolonged
exposure of the tumor to the antimetabolite affects most of the
vulnerable cells of the tumor population as they enter the RNA
synthesis phase. The intercalating agents act on cells in all phases of
the cell-cycle. The intercalating agents, like most cytotoxic agents,
have a steep dose response curve. So, bolus injection with peak
exposure may produce maximal damage to the nucleic acids of the cells.
Schedule dependency is based on this concept. The pharmacokinetic
principles defining the advantages of intra-arterial drug infusions has
been described by Eckman et al (49) and Chen and Gross (51). Eckman et
al showed that the advantage of increased drug delivery in HAI is
determined by factors that influence the time interval for drug delivery
and the arterial drug levels obtained (concentration x time) . Marked differences are seen in drug levels by comparing arterial versus venous infusion.
Chen and Gross demonstrated that this advantage was dependent on the rate of
drug elimination in the rest of the body and the blood perfusion rate
into the target organ. So, rapid elimination of the drug elsewhere in
the body and lowered blood flow rate into the target lesion will
increase the regional advantage of HAI. These main pharmocokinetic
principles are applied to hepatic arterial chemotherapy. There are
five drugs which are regularly used in HAI, either as single agents or
in combination therapy. The average daily dose of these drugs delivered
by arterial infusion are summarized in table I.

fig. 2
Anatomic variation in which the hepatic artery originates from the
superior mesenteric artery

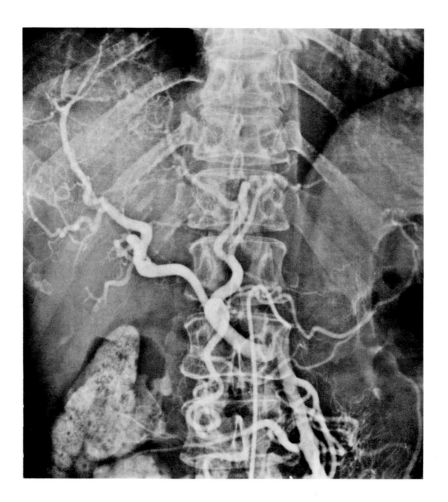

CANCER CHEMOTHERAPEUTIC AGENTS APPLIED
IN ARTERIAL LIVER INFUSION

Drug	Daily dose	Days
5-FU	10 - 25 mg/kg	5-21
5-FUDR	0,1 - 0,3 mg/kg	5-21
MMC	12 - 18 mg/m2	1
Adriamycin	10 - 30 mg/m2	1-3
Cisplatin	10 - 40 mg/m2	1-3

Drug selection for use in HAI include agents with short half-lives,
which indicate that they have a high total body clearance. 5-FU and
5-FUDR have half-lives of about 10 minutes. Adriamycin, MMC and
Cisplatin respectively about 60, 40 and 30 minutes (22,52).
5-FU, 5-FUDR and MMC are the most commonly used drugs today, especially
in metastatic colorectal cancer (22,28). In relation to the time
schedule, drugs can be delivered in a number of ways. Long-term
infusion, up to three weeks with 5-FU or 5-FUDR as single agents is
most frequently applied in HAI. In a series of 419 patients reported by
Ansfield et al (53). 5-FU was used in 15-20 mg/kg/day for 21 days. They
showed a response rate of 55%. Continuous infusion with 5-FUDR as a
single agent reveal response rates from 35 to 76% (54,55).
Combinations of drugs are used to improve their therapeutic index in
the treatment of liver metastases. Oberfield et al (56) administered
5-FU for ten days, followed by continuous infusion of 5-FUDR via a
portable pump system. They reported a response rate of 54%. Virtually
all combinations of drugs have been applied. The disadvantage of the
fluorinated pyrimidines is that these drugs have to be administered
over at least a five-day period, which necessitates the application of
an infusion pump or hospitalization during that period. MMC can be
administered in high dose bolus injection and may yield a 30-50%
response rate (57-59). Only one day of hospitalization is required
without serious discomfort of the patient. The treatment is free of
other cytotoxic side effects as nausea, vomiting and myelotoxicity
(58). Trombocytopenia is the most frequently observed side-effect of

MMC (28,58). In a series of 30 patients treated with bolus injection of MMC, trombocytopenia was the major complication, which occured at a median dose of 45 mg/m2 in 11 patients (59).

Adriamycin showed antitumor activity against hepatoma (60). This drug is also used in short-term infusions up to 3 days, single or in combination with MMC and 5-FUDR, for the treatment of metastases from unknown primary sites. Cisplatin, used in combination with other chemotherapeutics is particular effective in metastases originated from melanoma (61).

INFUSION EQUIPMENT

The first ambulatory infusion pump was the Watkins, chronometric infusion device in 1963 (62). Battery driven infusion pumps have been designed and employed for precise drug delivery (Auto syringe R, Cornud R). This development made chemotherapy available to ambulatory patients, minimizing costs and discomfort to the patient. Infusion systems employing pressure-energy sources have been designed for external (Alza-pump) and internal or implantable designs (Infusaid R, and Port-A-Cath R). Recently, Lokich reviewed the external and internal infusion pumps (Infusaid R) (63). External pumps show high risk of hepatic arterial trombosis, catheter occlusion and displacement. However, unsuccesful therapy can easily be stopped. The implanted pumps require surgical placement of both catheter and pump. The latter is a comfortable system without compromising activities but with relative high costs. The implanted system is preferred, generally, in patients having primary hepatic cancer who are likely to undergo surgery, particularly since the high response rate. The external pump with the percutaneously placed catheter is regularly used in patients with extra-hepatic tumor. The accuracy of the present infusion systems proved to be excellent and in the future, modifications will be directed to decrease the weight and the size of the mechanical system, while the reservoir system can be expanded.

CONCLUSIONS

Until now there is no optimal chemotherapeutic treatment schedule which increases survival significantly in patients with metastatic colorectal cancer (64-69). The difficulties in comparing the results of HAI with

intravenous chemotherapy are based on the differences between the
treatment techniques (selection of drugs and duration of
administration) and the patient selections. The major variations in HAI
technique include the application of a single drug versus a combination
of drugs, the use of short versus long-term therapy, and percutaneous
versus surgical catheter placement. There is no study which compares
the efficacy of surgically placed catheters with percutaneous placed
catheters and the superiority of long-term infusions over short-term
infusions has also not been demonstrated. The patient selection may
differ in terms of referral patterns. For example, patients who are
selected in HAI series have liver-only or liver-limiting disease, while
those in systemic series have more often also extrahepatic disease.
The heterogeneity of the patient population represents also prior
therapy and presence or absence of symptoms (synchronous versus
metachronous lesions). Recently, Huberman reviewed the current status
between HAI and systemic chemotherapy (28). He concluded that:

1. Reported response rates are significantly higher with HAI, than
   with systemic therapy.
2. Many patients receive significant benefit with HAI.
3. Placement of the catheter percutaneously is associated with a
   lower complication rate than at surgery, but there are more
   difficulties in catheter displacement.
4. There is, however, no survival advantage with HAI over systemic
   chemotherapy. His major conclusion was that there are no data
   available who clearly support the superiority of HAI over
   systemic therapy.

There is only one randomized trial comparing HAI of 5-FU with
intravenous 5-FU in patients with liver metastases of colorectal
carcinoma (72). In 12 patients the catheter was placed at surgery since
liver metastases were found at laparotomy. The other 19 patients
received a percutaneous placed catheter. The response rate was higher
with HAI than with systemic 5-FU, an observation also known from
non-randomized studies. The difference, however (34% versus 23%) was
not statistically significant. The median survival appeared to be the
same in both groups (about 13 to 10 mo). Nevertheless, the experimental
design can be criticized. As pointed out by the authors of the study,
the median survival in the systemic groups is similar to that reported

in non-randomized trials of HAI using 5-FUDR or longer treatment
schedules. Indeed, all patients did receive maintenance intravenous
5-FU after the arterial infusion. In two ongoing studies preliminary
data do not show any superiority of HAI over prolonged systemic
infusion. What is shown however is that the type of progression is
widely different and that local toxicity of HAI in both series is much
higher than previously reported (70,71).

There are two other problems, not mentioned before, which concern the
quality of life and the costs of the total treatment. It is known that
the response rate in HAI is nearly equal for all different techniques.
Therefore social reasons should play a major role in the choice of the
appropriate treatment.

Patients with complaints and large liver metastases (metachronous
lesions) could therefore be treated with percutaneous short-term
infusion in a procedure with an only one day hospitalization. Patients
without complaints who appear to have liver metastases at surgery
(synchronous lesions) may be treated better by long-term chemotherapy
using an implantable pump system. However it must be stated that until
now, it is unknown whether palliation in patients with metachronous
lesions cannot be equally obtained with symptomatic therapy only. It is
possible that the quality of life is better when symptomatic treatment
is started when complaints arise. Again, no such comparative study is
available. The costs of the total treatment of HAI, varies mainly with
the technique of catheter placement (radiographic vs surgical) and the
infusion method (bolus injection vs pump). The costs of
hospitalization, radiographic control studies and the constant need for
medical supervision, particularly in long-term infusion must also be
taken in consideration.

The most important benefit of HAI is the possible increase in response
rate, not uniformely resulting in a prolonged survival. The question is
whether the higher response rate justifies the routine use of HAI,
including the high costs and discomfort of the patient. Therefore until
the claimed superiority of this treatment has undoubtful been
demonstrated in randomized studies this treatment procedure remains
experimental.

REFERENCES
1. Bleichroder F.: Intraarterielle Therapie. Berl Klin Wschr 1912 49: 1503.
2. Bierman H.R., Byron R.L., Miller F.R., et al: Effects of intra-arterial administration of nitrogen mustard. Am. J. Med 1950, 8: 535.
3. Klopp C.T., Crandall A., Bateman J. et al: Fractionated intra-arterial cancer chemotherapy with methyl bis amine hydrochloride: A preliminary report. An Surg 1950, 132: 811.
4. Sullivan R.D., Miller E., Sikes M.P.: Antimetabolite-metabolite combination cancer chemotherapy: Effects of intra-arterial methotrexate-intramuscular citrovorum factor therapy in human cancer. Cancer 1959, 12: 1248.
5. Sullivan R.D., Norcross J.W., Watkin's E. Jr: Chemotherapy of metastatic liver cancer by prolonged hepatic artery infusion. New Eng. J. Med 1964, 220: 321.
6. Chuang V.P., Wallace S.: Interventional Approaches to Hepatic Tumor Treatment. Seminars in Roentgenology 1983 Vol 18, 2: 127.
7. Ariel I.M., Pack G.T.: Intra-arterial chemotherapy for cancer metastatic to liver: Arch Surg 1965, 91: 851.
8. Pikren J.W., Tsukada Y., Lane W.W.: Livermetastases: Analysis of autopsy data, in Weis L, Gilber H.A. (eds): Liver metastases. Boston, G.K. Hall.
9. Kemeny N., Yagoda A., Braun D. et al: Therapy for metastatic colorectal carcinoma, with a combination of methyl-CCNU, 5-fluorocoracil, vincristine and streptozotozin. Cancer 1980, 45: 876.
10. Cady B.: Natural History of Primary and Secondary Tumors of the Liver. Seminars in Oncology 1983 Vol 10, 2: 127.
11. Cady B., Monson D.O., Swinton N.W. Sr: Survival of patients after colonic resection for carcinoma with simultaneous liver-metastases. Surg. Gyneol. Obstet 1970, 131: 697.
12. Modlin J., Walker H.S.J.: Palliative resections in cancer of the colon and rectum. Cancer 1949, 22: 767.
13. Ransom H.K.: Carcinoma of the colon: A study of end-results of surgical treatment. Arch. Surg. 1952, 64: 707.
14. Jaffe B.M., Donegan W.L., Watson F. et al: Factors influencing untreated hepatic metastases. Surg. Gyneol. Obstet 1968, 127: 1.
15. Niederhuber J.E., Ensminger W.D. Surgical considerations in the management of hepatic neoplasia. Sem, in Onc. 1983 Vol 10, 2: 135.
16. Kemeny N.: The systemic Chemotherapy of Hepatic Metastases. Sem in Onc. 1983 Vol. 10, 2: 148.
17. Leane L.: The chemotherapy of colorectal cancer. Cancer 1974, 34: 972.
18. Ariel I.M.: Systemic 5-FU in hepatic metastases from primary colon or rectal cancer. NY state J. Med., 1972, 772: 1041.
19. Rapaport A.H., Burleson R.C.: Survival of patients treated with systemic flurouracil for hepatic metastases. Surg. Gyneol. Obstet. 1970, 130: 773.
20. Priestman T.J., Hanham I.W.F.: Results of 27 cases with hepatic metastases treated by combination chemotherapy. Brit. J. Cancer 1973, 26: 466.
21. Young C.W., Golbey R.B.: Evaluation of therapeutic response of large bowel cancer to fluorinated pyrimidines in relation to

clinical patterns. Proc Am Assoc Cancer Res 1960, 3: 293.

22. Ensminger W.D., Rosowsky A., Raso V. et al: A clinical pharmacological evaluation of hepatic arterial infusion of 5-FUDR and 5-FU. Cancer Res 1978, 38: 3784.

23. Sullivan R.D., Young C.W., Miller E. et al: The clinical effects of the continuous administration of fluorinated pyrimidines. Cancer Chemother Rep 1960, 8: 77.

24. Sullivan R.D., Miller E., Chryssochoos T. et al: Clinical effects of the continuous intravenous and intra-arterial infusion of cancer chemotherapeutic compounds. Cancer Chemother. Rep 1962, 16: 499.

25. Khazei A.M., Patel D.D., Morgenthaler F.R. et al: Chronic infusion of 5-FUDR into the hepatic artery of the dog. J.Surg Res 1970, 10: 343.

26. Chuang V.P., Wallace S.: Hepatic arterial redistribution for intra-arterial infusion of hepatic neoplasms. Radiology 1980, 135: 295.

27. Michels N.A.: Blood Supply and Anatomy of the Upper abdominal organs. Philadelphia, Lippincott Co, 1955.

28. Huberman M.S. Comparison of systemic chemotherapy with hepatic arterial infusion in metastatic colorectal carcinoma. Sem. in Onc. 1983. Vol 10, 2: 238.

29. Norsete T., Ansfield F., Wirtanen G. et al: Gastric ulceration in patients receiving intrahepatic infusion of 5-fluorouracil. An Surg 1977, 186: 734.

30. Cady B. An Surg 1973, 178: 156.

31. Labelle J.J., Lucas R.J., Eisenstein B. et al. Arch Surg 1968, 96: 683.

32. Lokich J., Ensminger W.: Abulatory pump infusion devices for hepatic artery infusion. Sem in Onc 1983 Vol 10, 2: 183.

33. Clouse M.E., Roentgenographic techniques for the diagnosis and management of liver tumors. Sem in Onc 1983 Vol 10, 2:159.

34. Chuang V.P., Soo C.S., Carrasio C.H., Wallace S.: Superselective catheterization technique in hepatic angiography AJR 1983, 141: 803.

35. Goldman M.L., Bilbao M.K., Rosch J. et al: Complications of indwelling chemotherapy catheters. Cancer 1975, 36: 1983.

36. Tyler U, Forsberg L., Owman T.: Heparinized catheters for long-term intra-arterial infusion of 5-fluorouracil in liver metastases. Cardiovasc. Radiol. 1979, 2: 111.

37. Chuang V.P., Wallace S., Stroehlein J. et al: Hepatic artery infusion chemotherapy gastroduodenal complications. AJR 1981, 137: 347.

38. Granmayeh M., Wallace S., Schwarten D.: Trans catheter occlusion of the gastroduodenal artery. Radiology 1979, 131: 59.

39. Hall D.A., Clouse M.E., Gramm H.F.: Gastroduodenal ulceration after hepatic arterial infusion chemotherapy. AJR 1981 136: 1216.

40. Kuribayashi S., Phillips D.A., Harrington D.P. et al: Therapeutic embolization of the gastroduodenal artery in hepatic artery infusion chemotherapy AJR 1981, 137: 1169.

41. Burrows J.H., Talley R.W., Drake E.L. et al: Infusion of fluorinated pyrimidines into hepatic artery for treatment of metastatic carcinoma of the liver. Cancer 1967, 20: 1886.

42. Clouse M.E., Ahmed R., Ryan R. et al: Complications of long-term

transbrachial hepatic arterial infusion chemotherapy. AJR 1977, 129: 799.

43. Bledin A.G., Kantarijian H.M., Kim E.E. et al: 99m Tc-labeled macroaggregated albumin in intrahepatic arterial chemotherapy. AJR 1982, 139: 711.

44. Lucas R.J., Tumacder O., Wilson G.S.: Hepatic artery occlusion following hepatic artery catheterization. Ann Surg 1971, 173: 238.

45. Michels N.A.: Collateral arterial pathways to the liver after ligation of the hepatic artery and removal of the celiac axis. Cancer 1953, 6: 708.

46. Michels N.A.: Newer anatomy of the liver: Variant blood supply and collateral circulation. JAMA 1960, 172: 125.

47. Plengvanit U, Vhearanai O., Sindhvananda K. et al: Collateral arterial blood supply of the liver after hepatic artery ligation. An Surg 1972, 175: 105

48. Greenfield A.J.: Regional chemotherapy. Chapter 16 Anantanasoulis. Interventional Radiology 1982.

49. Carrasio C.H., Freeny P.C., Cherqug V.P. et al: Chemical cholecystitis associated with hepatic artery infusion chemotherapy AJR 1983, 141: 703.

50. Eckman W.W., Patlak C.S., Fenstermacher J.D.: A critical evaluation of principles governing the advantages of intra-arterial infusions. J. Pharmacokinet. Biopharm 1974, 2: 257.

51. Chen H.S.G., Gross J.F.: Intra-arterial infusion of anticancer drugs: Theoretic aspects of drug delivery and review of responses. Cancer Treat Rep 1980, 64: 31.

52. van Oosterom A.T., de Bruijn E.A., den Hartogh J. et al: Pharmatokinetik intravenoser, intrahepatischer und intra-vesikaler. Gabe von Mitomycin. Mitomycin C. Profil eines Zytostatikums. Aktuelle Onkologie 1984, 10: 1.

53. Ansfield F.J., Ramikez G., Davis H.L. Jr et al: Further clinical studies with intrahepatic arterial infusion with 5-fluorouracil. Cancer 1975, 36: 2413.

54. Reed M.L., Vaitkevicus V.K., Al-Sarkaf M. et al: The practicality of chronic hepatic artery infusion therapy of primary and metastatic hepatic malignancies. Cancer 1981, 47: 402.

55. Buroker T., Samson M., Correa J. et al: Hepatic artery infusion of 5-FUDR after prior systemic 5-FU. Cancer 1976, 60: 1277.

56. Oberfield R.A., Mc Caffrey J.A., Polio J. et al: Prolonged and continuous percutaneous intra-arterial infusion chemotherapy in advanced metastatic liver adenocarcinoma from colorectal primary. Cancer 1979, 44: 414.

57. Kinami Y., Miyazaki I.: The superselective and the selective one shot method for treating inoperable cancer of the liver. Cancer 1978, 41: 1720.

58. van Oosterom A.T., de Bruijn E.A., Langenberg J.P. et al: Intra-arterial hepatic infusion of Mitomycin-C: Clinical data and pharmacokinetic profiles in Mitovaqun-C ed. Ogawa VI,eral Excerpta Medica, Amsterdam 1982, 30 ...

59. Mattsson W., Jonsson K., Hellekant C. et al: Short-term intra-arterial Mitomycin-C in hepatic metastases. Acta. Rad 1980, 19: 321.

60. Bern M.M., Mc Dermott Jr W., Cady B. et al: Intra-arterial hepatic infusion and intravenous Adriamycin for treatment of

hepato cellular carcinoma. Cancer 1978, 42: 399.

61. Calvo D.B., Patt Y.Z., Wallace S. et al: Phase I-II trial of percutaneous intra-arterial cis-diamminechloroplatinum for regionally confined malignancy. Cancer 1980, 45: 1278.

62. Watkins E. Jr: Chronometric infusor. New Eng J. Med 1963, 269: 850.

63. Lokich J., Ensminger W.: Ambulatory Pump Infusion Devicer for hepatic artery infusion. Sem in Onc. 1983 Vol 10,2: 1983.

64. Moertel C.G.: Clinical management of advanced gastrointestinal cancer. Cancer 1975, 36: 675.

65. Moertel C.G.: Chemotherapy of gastrointestinal cancer. Clin. Gastr. Enterol. 1976, 5: 777.

66. Moertel C.G.: Chemotherapy of gastrointestinal cancer. New Eng. J. Med. 1978, 299: 1049.

67. Schein P.S., Kisner D., Mac. Donald J.S.: Chemotherapy of large intestinal carcinoma. Cancer 1975, 36: 2418.

68. Carter S.K.: Large bowel cancer: The current state of treatment. JNCI 1976, 56: 3.

69. Heal J.M., Schein P.S.: Management of gastrointestinal cancer. Med. Clin. North Am 1977, 61: 991

70. Kemeny N., Daly J., Oderman P., Chu H., et al: Randomized study of intrahepatic vs systemic infusion of fluorodeoxyuridine in patients with liver metastases from colorectal carcinoma ASCO proceedings 3 no 551, p 141, 1984

71. Stagg R., Friedman M., Lewis B., Ignoffor et al: Current status of the NCOG randomized trial of continuous intra-arterial versus intravenous floxuridine in patients with colorectal carcinoma metastatic to the liver. ASCO proceedings 3 no 577, P 148, 1984.

NEW TREATMENT MODALITIES

INTRAPERITONEAL CHEMOTHERAPY -- A POSSIBLE ROLE IN THE TREATMENT OF HEPATIC
METASTASES

J.L. SPEYER

INTRODUCTION

In recent years there have been a number of clinical investigations
utilizing intraperitoneal (ip) chemotherapy for the treatment of intra-
cavitary and intrahepatic disease. The aim of this locoregional therapy
is to provide high intratumor concentrations of antineoplastic agents
while reducing the systemic exposure to these toxic drugs.

In gastrointestinal malignancies particularly those of the colon and
rectum the intraperitoneal space is a major site of recurrence. Local or
diffuse seeding of the peritoneal cavity can frequently be seen (1, 2, 3).
In rectal tumors local recurrences are quite common (4). It is, however,
well known the primary site of metastases for these malignancies is the
liver (1, 2, 3, 4). It is important to note that the putative route of
tumor seeding of the liver is through the portal venous system (3, 4, 5, 6).
While there are numerous studies to indicate that the primary blood supply
of hepatic metastases is arterial, this applies to larger tumor nodules
that have parasitized the hepatic blood supply (5, 6). Moreover, in studies
by Taylor (6, 7) it has been shown that even complete ligation of the
arterial vessels leading to tumor often results in a residual rim of viable
tumor that is being supplied by the portal system. Clearly then, both
the arterial and portal blood supplies to the liver must be considered
when delivering local chemotherapy. In order to plan hepatic locoregional therapy, consideration must be given to tumor size and blood
supply, hepatic extraction of the drug, systemic elimination of the drug
and of course the intrinsic antitumor activity of the drug for the tumor
in question. For microscopic disease the portal circulation may indeed be
the predominant route of concern.

Some additional theoretical support for portal vein infusions has
been well explicated by Collins (8) who points out that for small

intrahepatic metastases mixing of arterial with portal blood supply yields relatively equivalent drug exposure whether the drug is delivered via the hepatic arterial or portal system. Depending on the drug and its hepatic extraction, either hepatic arterial or portal venous infusions are attractive for the treatment of hepatic metastases since these routes may yield higher intrahepatic drug levels with possibly lower systemic concentrations than might be obtained by peripheral infusion. In fact if there is significant extraction by the liver then the systemic exposure may be even lower than it would be if the drug were infused through the peripheral venous system. For large tumor nodules which have developed their own arterial blood supply hepatic arterial infusions become attractive since drug should reach the majority of the tumor without being degraded by hepatic enzymes and since the tumor exposure is equivalent to hepatic arterial concentration without dilution from the portal system (8, 9).

There are numerous trials in the literature to support the possible role of the intraarterial infusion of hepatic metastases particularly with fluoropyrimidine drugs (9, 10, 11, 12, 13). The high systemic clearance (9, 14) as well as significant hepatic extraction (9, 14) make these excellent candidates for intrahepatic infusion. These are also the single most active class of compounds for the treatment of most GI malignancies. Portal venous infusions of fluoropyrimidines also have been tried either by cannulating the portal vein through the remnant of the umbilical vein or by direct placement of a catheter into the portal vein at surgery. Taylor (15) has recorded a number of trials using this approach in Great Britain with good results. Other investigators have had similar results (16). Nevertheless, there are a number of problems associated with either the direct portal or arterial infusions. Firstly, these require placement of semi-permanent catheters. While this can be done by the percutaneous route for the arterial catheters the current recommendation is, if possible, to place them surgically at the time of laparotomy, so that the catheter can be best positioned and careful observation be made at the time of surgery of the distribution of catheter flow (10, 18). This can either be done by an intraoperative macroagregated albumin (MAA) scan (17) or with a fluorescein injection and Woods Lamp inspection (18). The general aim of these techniques is to prevent high concentration drug flow to organs other than the liver such as the stomach, small bowel, and biliary tree where excessive toxicity may occur. Another problem encountered in the past has been non-uniform distribution of the infused drugs because of catheter positioning or streaming of the drug in the vessel (19). Some of the newer techniques of checking the drug flow with MAA scan have also helped to reduce this problem but it still persists. Non-uniform distribution of drug means that part of the liver is not being perfused by the drug and any tumor in those areas will therefore only be exposed to drug concentrations equivalent to those recirculating in the systemic circulation, thereby eliminating the possible benefit derived from direct infusion. There are additional hazards associated with catheters, including bleeding and infection (20, 21). The introduction of the implantable pump systems and infusion ports (22) has simplified these problems to some degree but considerable expense associated with the need for intraoperative placement of catheter, expensive pumps and repeat scans to check catheter placement still limit the general applicability of these techniques and are only justified if there is clearcut therapeutic advantage.

In patients with small volume hepatic metastases, intraperitoneal therapy has possible merit as a route of drug delivery. First of all, it is a treatment which results in high local drug concentrations at the peritoneal surfaces. This would clearly be an advantage over routine systemic or direct arterial or portal venous infusions. Many patients do recur locally and the argument has been proposed that for some drugs the peritoneal surfaces do not receive optimal drug concentrations during systemic therapy (23). Secondly, if the drug is cleared substantially into the portal system, then intraperitoneal therapy could provide a means for delivering high concentrations of drug to the liver. A high local intraperitoneal concentration can clearly be achieved (23). Ideally then, the liver and intrahepatic tumor would be perfused by a high concentration portal infusion. Since the drug would enter the portal system via capillary, diffusion homogeneous mixing would occur and the drug distribution to the liver and the tumor would be limited only by the anatomy of the portal system. Finally, intrahepatic drug metabolism would remove a portion of the total drug and the systemic circulation would be exposed to lower drug concentrations and less toxicity than if the drug were given intravenously.

The concept of intraperitoneal chemotherapy is not at all new and has been utilized as long as chemotherapy has been available (23). Unfortunately, early trials did not have available the drugs we now have and were flawed by a variety of methodological problems. These include only treating patients with ascites, delivering drug in very small volumes of fluid usually for only one or two treatments and not using conventional response criteria. Therefore the effect of this therapy until more recent years was at best uncertain and it was, for the most, part abandoned. Dedrick (24) and his colleagues at the National Cancer Institute reconsidered this route of drug administration in a theoretical paper and provided a strong rationale for again investigating this form of locoregional therapy. Drawing on toxicologic data by Torres (25) as well as their own pharmacokinetic modeling, they proposed guidelines for intraperitoneal chemotherapy. It should be given in large volumes of fluid. Specifically, this should be as much fluid as the patient can tolerate to assure adequate distribution of drug. They also indicated that the ideal drugs for administration by this route were those that egressed slowly from the peritoneal cavity and which had a rapid systemic clearance. Intraperitoneal instillation would therefore result in a high concentration difference between the intraperitoneal fluid and the systemic circulation, thus yielding high drug concentrations where the tumor might be and exposing the normal tissue in the rest of the body to lower drug concentrations. They further reasoned that since the potential advantage of direct surface exposure of tumor with drug over the intravascular route is highest at the tumor surface and limited by the depth of diffusion, such therapy would ideally be directed at small tumor volumes (minimal residual disease). Large tumor masses would receive most of their drug exposure via their own vascular supply and little additional advantage would be gained by surface exposure.

Initial trials of intraperitoneal chemotherapy at the National Cancer Institute were done by a team of researchers using first methotrexate (26), 5 Fluorouracil (5 FU) (27), and adriamycin (28). In the NCI 5FU trial the drug was delivered in a 2 liter volume of 1.5% dextrose dialysate through a semi-permanent implanted Tenckhoff catheter. This is the same technique which has been used by a number of centers for chronic ambulatory peritoneal dialysis. Other researchers have now examined a number of other agents including cisplatinum (29, 30), melphalan (30), cytosine arabinoside (30), bleomycin (31), BCG (32), and interferon (33). In the initial Phase I studies it was found that patients could tolerate this treatment quite well and that chemotherapy could safely be delivered by this method. Patients receiving 5FU (27) received approximately 8 consecutive 2 liter infusions with 1040 mg of 5FU/2L with a 4 hour dwell time (resulting in a total of 8 grams of drug during the infusion period). This was repeated every 2 - 4 weeks. The limiting toxicities were the systemic effects mainly myelosuppression. Patients experienced some nausea and vomiting and mild chemical peritonitis was noted in some patients. In the initial study of 5FU the intraperitoneal drug concentrations were approximately 300 times higher than the simultaneously measured systemic drug concentrations thus proving that the predicted intraperitoneal pharmacokinetic advantage could be obtained by drug administration by this route for treatment of small volume intraperitoneal disease. The question remained though as to whether delivering 5FU by the intraperitoneal route could result in high portal concentrations of drug delivered to the liver. A study was designed to investigate this problem by researchers at the National Cancer Institute.

METHODS

A group of 4 patients with known hepatic metastases from carcinoma of the colon had a Tenckhoff catheter placed at the time of laparotomy for investigation of their tumor. In addition, prior to surgery, a hepatic venous catheter, a peripheral artery catheter, and a peripheral venous catheter were placed. Also a catheter was placed in the portal vein by cannulating the **remnant** of the umbilical vein (see Fig I). These permitted direct measurement of intraperitoneal drug concentration (through the Tenckhoff catheter) as well as measurement of drug concentration systemically as it enters the liver through the portal and hepatic arterial system and leaves the liver via the hepatic vein. The concentration of drug in the peripheral artery was used as a measure of the concentration in the hepatic artery. The peripheral artery was more convenient and less hazardous to cannulate, and assuming little or no metabolism of drug in blood or vessel walls, the concentrations of drug in both vessels would be identical when drug is administered ip since they both would carry recirculating drug, i.e. drug absorbed into the portal system or systemic venous circulation, entering the heart and then the arterial circulation with equal concentration in all arteries.

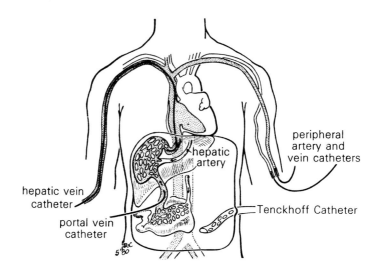

Figure I. Tenckhoff catheter and vascular catheters for drug delivery and blood sampling. The administered drug was intraperitoneal 5-Fluorouracil.

Within 4 hours after surgery, patients were treated with a standard 2 liter dialysate containing 1040 mg of 5FU in 1.5% dextrose dialysate (Inpersol, Abbott Laboratories) containing 1000 units of heparin and 8 meq KCl. The fluid was permitted to remain in the abdomen for 4 hours and then was drained in the usual fashion which is described elsewhere (27, 34). At baseline and during this time blood samples of hepatic venous, portal venous, hepatic arterial, and peripheral venous blood were obtained. Eight consecutive 4 hour exchanges were performed.

5FU concentrations were measured by an HPLC assay as described elsewhere (27).

RESULTS

All patients tolerated the treatments well. The toxicities observed included nausea and the systemic side effects of 5 Fluorouracil, mainly myelosuppression. These have been described elsewhere in detail (34).

Table I. 5FU concentrations during intraperitoneal 5FU therapy

	Exchange 1	Exchange 7
Area Under The Curve (mm x min)		
Intraperitoneal [a]	330 ± 73	275 ± 52
Portal Vein	3.8 ± 0.65	6.3 1 1.4
Peripheral Artery (Hepatic)	1.1 ± 0.26	2.7 ± 0.85
Hepatic Vein	0.97 ± 0.44	2.5 ± 1.3
Peripheral Vein	0.90 ± 0.32	2.3 ± 1.1

a = ± S.E.

The drug concentrations measured for the four patients are detailed in Table I. Measurements were made during the first and seventh exchanges. These are also depicted for a single patient in Figure II. Over the four hour dwell time, the intraperitoneal drug exposure area under the curve (AUC) of concentration x time was high and greatly exceeded all of the intravascular drug concentrations. The ratio of AUC between the peritoneal fluid and systemic drug concentration was 318 which was similar to that reported earlier (27). The portal drug concentrations measured was higher than those in the hepatic venous systemic, arterial and systemic venous circulations, throughout the treatment period. Peak portal concentrations were rapidly achieved and ranged from 22-120 uM. Likewise the portal venous drug exposure exceeded that in the other vessels (Fig III). In exchange 1 the portal 5FU exposure (measured as AUC) was 4.0 times the hepatic venous exposure, 4.2 times the peripheral venous exposure and 3.6 times the peripheral arterial (or hepatic arterial exposure). These values differed in exchange 7 but the qualitative relationships remained. The AUC ratios were 2.5, 2.8 and 2.5 for the hepatic vein, peripheral vein and hepatic artery respectively.

Intraperitoneal instillation of 5FU results in high portal venous concentrations of the drug. These are clearly higher than those achieved in either the systemic venous or hepatic arterial systems. When given by this route these portal drug levels compare favorably with 5FU levels achievable by other routes of delivery.

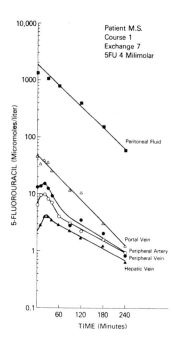

Figure II. Plasma levels and intraperitoneal fluid levels for a patient receiving 1040 mg of 5 Fluorouracil in 2 liters of dialysate.

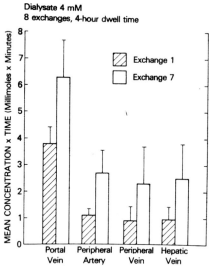

Figure III. Drug exposure (area with curve of concentration x time) for patients receiving 1040 mg of 5 Fluorouracil in 2 liters of dialysate. Data for first and seventh exchanges are given.

A standard intravenous bolus of 5FU results in peak systemic levels
in excess of 100 uM but these fall off rapidly with a T ½ of 10-20 minutes
(14, 35). Portal exposure by this route should be equivalent to that in
the system circulation less any extrahepatic metabolism within the GI tract
or within blood vessels, since a drug administered into the peripheral
circulation must first pass through the abdominal viscera before entering
the portal system. The enzyme dihydrouracil reductase is
ubiquitous and may remove some portion of peripherally infused drug or
for that matter of recirculating drug if the drug is infused directly into
the hepatic artery or portal vein. Because of the short exposure half
life and the desire for higher local concentration other routes and
schedule have been tried. Continuous peripheral venous infusion 5FU
(30 mg/kg/24 hrs for 5 days) results in prolonged drug exposure, but
steady state levels which can be safely achieved remain in the range 1-3
uM with significant systemic toxicity. Moreover,clinical trials of this
route have not generally achieved improved results of therapy (37).

Intraarterial 5FU yields prolonged drug exposure with an estimated
drug concentration of 12 uM (34) and a calculated portal or systemic
concentration of 1 uM. This method is of course not limited to 24 hours
of exposure. The studies of Ensminger et al (9, 11) with implanted pumps
and FudR have demonstrated that prolonged infusions are technically feasible
and reasonably safe. They take advantage of high hepatic drug extraction
(9) and the high local drug concentrations result in reduced systemic
toxicity and increased antitumor efficacy (11). Other investigators have
reported lower response rates with FudR (12, 13). All have reported
serious toxicity with drug induced hepatitis, gastritis and sclerosing
cholangitis (11, 12, 13). Some of these problems can be lessened by
careful intraoperative or post-operative study to determine that high
local drug concentrations are confined to the liver (11). MAA scans done
intraoperatively can also help insure uniform drug distribution (19).
This technique can also be applied to portal infusions where streaming or
shifting of catheter position can also lead to non-uniform hepatic drug
exposure.

Direct portal infusions can result in local drug concentrations and
hepatic exposure similar to those achievable by arterial infusions. Just
as for arterial infusions, they can be directed if desired to selectively
infuse one lobe of the liver. The new technology of implantable pumps or

infusion ports and safer portable delivery systems can also be applied to portal infusions.

The portal drug levels achievable by intraperitoneal 5FU instillation are as good or better than those achievable by other routes of administration. Peak portal concentrations ranged from 22 to 120 uM and remained in excess of 10 uM for most of the treatment period. Earlier work with ip 5FU (27) demonstrated that eight 4 hour exchanges given every 2-3 weeks resulted in limiting systemic toxicity. The potential duration of portal venous exposure of 5-FU using the intraperitoneal route is thus limited to about 36 hours when consecutive instillations are employed. Other schedules such as a single daily instillation x5 repeated monthly are being tested by other investigators (38). At present, the optimal balance between duration of locoregional infusion and maximal achievable concentrations is not known. While portal levels achieved using the ip route exceed those that can be safely maintained by systemic infusion (37) and exceed those usually reached during arterial infusions (9, 14), these infusions are generally given for a longer duration of time than possible by the ip route in this concentration range. Shorter and higher concentration arterial infusion can also be achieved.

Another way to assess the possible role of this route is to ask how much drug is delivered via the portal system during ip administration. One must recall that the liver has a dual blood supply receiving contributions from the portal vein and hepatic artery. Moreover for ip drug instillation the drug delivered through the portal vein is a function of both the drug delivered directly from the ip drug pool as well as the amount of drug that is not metabolized in a first pass through the liver and is recirculating into the portal vein from the system circulation. Furthermore one must account for any metabolism in blood vessels or the GI tract that would decrease the amount of recirculating drug. The fraction of ip drug that appears in the portal vein (F) can be calculated using the equation F = drug appearing in portal veins/ip dose. The drug appearing in the portal vein is determined by measured drug concentration (AUC portal), blood flow and possible GI tract metabolism, (Range 0-100%). For ethical and technical reasons we did not make direct flow measurements in our patients but used estimates obtained from the literature (27). Using estimates for portal vein flow ranging from 1-1.5 L/min we calculated F at from 29% to 100% (mean value 0.56). Using this mean value for F and

assuming that a mean of 83% (27) (measured in earlier work) of ip 5FU is
absorbed in 4 hours, then about 430 mg of ip 5FU reaches the liver via
the portal vein during each exchange (37 mg/kg/24 hours). This is in
addition to the higher concentration direct drug exposure of the peritoneal
surfaces provided by this route and compares favorably to total doses that
can be delivered by other infusion routes. It is certainly more 5FU than
can be delivered safely by IV bolus.

Another possible advantage of the ip route of 5FU is homogeneous
exposure of the liver to drug since the drug enters the portal system by
diffusion at many levels. Intraperitoneal 5FU seems most likely to be
useful in the adjuvant setting or in early disease when tumor cells have
seeded the liver via the portal route and have not yet gained their own
arterial blood supply. It eliminates the need for expensive laparotomies
and pumps since the dialysis catheter can be placed even in an out-patient
setting. The potential infections of indwelling dialysis catheters must,
however, be considered though this can be kept to a low level by careful
asceptic technique (39).

Intraperitoneal chemotherapy directed at hepatic metastases may be
applicable to other drugs with similar considerations as for 5FU. The drug
employed must not be locally sclerotic to peritoneal surfaces. It should
have a slow clearance from the abdomen and rapid systemic clearance.
Preferably there should be some first pass drug removal by the liver.
Drugs with short half lives (rapid clearance) maximize the pharmacokinetic
advantage since with long half lives the recirculating drug fraction becomes
increasingly important and the relative advantage of a local infusion is
diminished. Of course the two most important elements are 1) that the drug
have activity against the tumor and 2) that higher concentrations than can
be safely delivered by systemic infusions will result in higher response
rates. Finding drugs that fit all these criteria is unfortunately difficult
particularly when we consider the low response rates for many drugs against
hepatic metastases of GI tract origin. Nevertheless, there is room to
reconsider the role of drugs such as cytosine arabinoside and cisplatinum
when high locoregional concentrations can be achieved. Moreover, the ip
route may be considered as new drugs come to clinical trials.

The value of local infusions of 5FU has not been fully established.
If further consideration of locoregional 5FU is still a viable issue, then
further exploration of the intraperitoneal route for patients with

microscopic or small bulk intrahepatic disease appears warranted.

REFERENCES

1. Cass AW, Million RR, and Pfaff WW. 1976. Patterns of recurrence
    following surgery alone for adenocarcinoma of the colon and rectum.
    Cancer. 37:2861-2865.
2. Dionne L. 1965. The pattern of blood-borne metastasis from carcinoma
    of rectum. Cancer. 18:775-781.
3. Taylor FW. 1962. Cancer of the colon and rectum: A study of routes
    and metastases and death. Surgery. 52:305-308.
4. Gunderson LL, and Sosin H. 1974. Areas of failure found at reoperation
    (second or symptomatic look) following "curative surgery" for
    adenocarcinoma of the rectum. Cancer. 34:1278-1292.
5. Ackerman NB, Lien WM, Kondi ES, Silverman NA. 1969. The blood supply
    of experimental liver metastases. 1. The distribution of hepatic
    artery and portal vein blood to "small" and "large" tumors. Surgery.
    66:1067-1072.
6. Taylor I, Bennett R, and Sherriff S. 1979. The blood supply of
    colorectal liver metastases. Br J Cancer. 39:749-756.
7. Taylor I. 1978. Cytotoxic perfusion for colorectal liver metastases.
    Br J Surg. 65:109-114.
8. Collins JM. 1984. Pharmacokinetic rationale for intraarterial
    therapy. Proceedings of Conference on Intra-arterial and
    Intracavitary chemotherapy.
9. Ensminger WD, Rosowsky A, Raso V, Levin DC, Glode M, Come S, Steele G,
    and Frei E, III. 1978. A clinical-pharmacological evaluation of
    hepatic arterial infusions of 5-Fluoro-2'-deoxyuridine and 5-fluorouracil
    Cancer Res. 3784-3792.
10. Barone RM, Byfield JE, Goldfarb PB, Frankel S, Ginn C, and Greer S.
    1982. Intra-arterial chemotherapy using an implantable infusion
    pump and liver irradiation for the treatment of hepatic metastases.
    Cancer. 50:850-862, 1982.
11. Niederhuber JE, Ensminger W, Gyves J, Thrall J, Walker S, and Cozzi E.
    1984. Regional chemotherapy of colorectal cancer metastatic to the
    liver. Cancer. 53:1336-1343.
12. Lewis BJ. 1984. Intraarterial versus intravenous FudR for
    colorectal cancer metastatic to the liver: A Northern California
    Oncology Group Study. Proceedings of Conference on Intraarterial
    and Intracavity Chemotherapy - University of California at San Diego.
13. Kemeny N. 1984. Randomized study of intraarterial vs. systemic
    infusion of flurodeoxyuridine in patients with liver metastases from
    colorectal carcinoma. Proceedings of Conference on Intraarterial and
    Intracavity Chemotherapy - University of California at San Diego.
14. Collins JM, Dedrick RL, King FG, Speyer JL, and Myers CE. 1980.
    Non-linear pharmacokinetic models for 5-fluorouracil in man:
    Intravenous and intraperitoneal routes. Clinical Pharmacology and
    Therapeutics. 25:235-246.
15. Taylor I, Brooman P, Rowling JT. 1977. Adjuvant liver perfusion in
    colorectal cancer: Initial results of a clinical trial. British
    Medical Journal. 2:1320-1322.
16. Almersjo O, Gustavsson B, and Hafstrom L. 1976. Results of regional
    portal infusion of 5-Fluorouracil in patients with primary and
    secondary liver cancer. Annales Chirurgiae et Gynaecologiea.
    65:27-32.

17. Kaplan WE, Ensminger WD, Come SE, Smith EH, D'Orsl CJ, Levin DC, Takvorian RW, and Steele GD. 1980. Radionuclide angiography to predict patient response to hepatic artery chemotherapy. Cancer Treat Rep. 64:1217-1222.

18. Barone RM. 1984. Technical aspects of arterial access and contrast infusion. Proceedings of Conference on Intraarterial and Intracavity Chemotherapy - University of California at San Diego.

19. Kaplan WD, O'Orsl CJ, Ensminger WD, et al. 1978. Intraarterial radionuclide infusion: A new technique to assess chemotherapy perfusion patterns. Cancer Treat Rep. 62:669.

20. Goldman ML, Bilbao MK, Rosch J, and Dotter CT. 1975. Complications of indwelling chemotherapy catheters. Cancer. 36:1983-1990.

21. Fortner JG, and Pahnke LD. 1976. A new method for long term intrahepatic chemotherapy. Surgery, Gynecology & Obstetrics. 143:979-980.

22. Ensminger W, Niederhuber J, Dakhil S, Thrall J, and Wheeler R. 1981. Totally implanted drug delivery system for hepatic arterial chemotherapy. Cancer Treat Rep. 65:393-400.

23. Speyer JL, and Myers CE. 1982. Intraperitoneal chemotherapy of ovarian cancer. In: William CJ, Whitehouse JMA, (Eds). Recent Advances in Clinical Oncology. Churchill Linvingstone. Edinburgh, 181-195.

24. Dedrick RL, Myers CE, Bungay PM, and DeVita VT, Jr. 1978. Pharmacokinetic rationale for peritoneal drug administration in the treatment of ovarian cancer. Cancer Treat Rep. 62:1-11.

25. Torres IG, Litterst CL, Guarino AM. 1978. Transport of model compounds across the peritoneal membrane in the rat. Pharmacology. 17:330-340.

26. Jones RB, Collins JM, Myers CE, et al. 1981. High-volume intraperitoneal chemotherapy with methotrexate in patients with cancer. Cancer Res. 41:55-59.

27. Speyer JL, Collins JM, Dedrick RL, Brennan MF, Londer H, DeVita VT, and Myers CE. 1980. Phase I and pharmacologic studies of intraperitoneal 5-Fluorouracil. Cancer Res. 40:567-572.

28. Ozols RF, Young RC, Speyer JL, Sugarbaker PH, Green R, Jenkins J, and Myers CE. 1982. Phase I and pharmacologic studies of adriamycin administered intraperitoneally to patients with ovarian cancer. Cancer Res. 42:4265-4269.

29. Howell SB, Pfeifle CL, Wung WE, et al. 1982. Intraperitoneal cisplatin with systemic thiosulfate protection. Ann Int Med. 77:845-851.

30. Howell SB. Phase I trials and pharmacokinetics of intraperitoneal cisplatinum, melphalan and cytarabine. Proceedings of Conference on Intraarterial and Intracavity Chemotherapy - University of California at San Diego. 1984.

31. Markman M. Bleomycin. Personal communication.

32. Bast RC, Berek SS, Obrist R, et al. 1983. Intraperitoneal immunotherapy of human ovarian carcinoma with corynebacterium Parvum. Cancer Res. 43:1395-1401.

33. Spiegel R. Personal communication.

34. Speyer JL, Sugarbaker PH, Collins JM, Dedrick RL, Klecker RW, Jr, and Myers CE. 1982. Portal levels and hepatic clearance of 5-Fluorouracil after intraperitoneal administration in man. Cancer Res. 41:1916-1922.

262

35. Christophidis N, Vajda JFE, Lucas I, Drummer O, Moon WJ, and Louis WJ. 1978. Fluorouracil therapy in patients with carcinoma of the large bowel: A pharmacokinetic comparison of various rates and routes of administration. Clinical Pharmacokinetics. 3:330-335.
36. MacMillan WE, Wolberg WH, and Welling PG. 1978. Pharmacokinetics of fluorouracil in humans. Cancer Res. 38:3479-3482.
37. Hillcoat BL, McCulloch PB, Figueroedo AT, Ehsan MH, and Rosenfeld JM. 1978. Clinical response and plasma levels of 5-Fluorouracil in patients with colonic cancer treated by drug infusion. Br J Cancer. 38:719-724.
38. Sugarbaker P. Personal communication.
39. Jenkins JF, Sugarbaker DH, Gianoa FJ, Myers CE. 1982. Technical consideration in the use of intraperitoneal chemotherapy administered by Tenckhoff catheter. Surg Gynecol Obstet. 154:858-864.

ACKNOWLEDGEMENTS

The author gratefully acknowledges the assistance of Peggy Nixdorf in the preparation of the manuscript and the assistance of many colleagues of the NIH (USA) particularly Drs. Jerry Collins, Charles Myers, and Paul Sugarbaker.

THE INFUSAID PUMP AND HEPATIC REGIONAL CHEMOTHERAPY

P.D. SCHNEIDER, P.H. SUGARBAKER, F.J. GIANOLA

INTRODUCTION

The Infusaid pump is a totally implanted device for continuous drug infusion. It is automatically recharged with each refill of the device. This pump remains the single such device with United States Food and Drug Administration approval for physician use in regional drug delivery. The first clinical use of the device was to deliver anticoagulation therapy in the form of heparin (7,28,29) followed by the first use of the device to deliver intrahepatic FUDR (5-fluoro-2-deoxyuridine) (6). More recently, the device has been used for delivery of intrathecal morphine, for regional head and neck chemotherapy, and for insulin delivery (30). Significantly, this pump may represent the most sophisticated biomedical device that the average U.S. physician has ever had to directly manage on a regular basis.

The potential value of the device for regional drug therapy and the management of metastatic malignancy to the liver was obvious despite a Central Oncology Group study, published in 1979, which suggested no advanvantage of regional delivery of 5-FU compared with systemic 5-FU (17,18). This multi-institutional trial, utilizing a variety of arterial catherization techniques and a short term infusion of three weeks, was well founded and a significant model study, but the availability of FUDR, a newer and possibly better regional agent (11,13), and the Infusaid pump provided theoretical and practical improvements in drug and delivery systems which apparently covered all the objections to regional therapy and the COG data in particular. Although the Infusaid pump appears to be a substantial advance, it is important to distinguish the device itself, its reliability, and the role it plays in regional chemotherapy, from the efficacy of the regional approach to metastatic colorectal cancer in the liver.

The first data suggesting an advantage of FUDR and the Infusaid device over standard 5-FU regimens and previous intrahepatic chemotherapy drugs and devices appeared only recently, in 1981 (12). However, although the initial data with the use of this device continues to be encouraging, there is sufficient available information both from trials and from general, non-trial experience to suggest that the strategy of intrahepatic chemotherapy with the current best technology suffers from substantial limitations vis-a-vis attempted palliation for the colorectal cancer patient. Too, once again, randomized prospective trials demonstrate the danger of comparing patients undergoing new treatments to historical controls. This paper will discuss these points and demonstrate that the Infusaid pump is a tool for regional or systemic drug treatment and not an answer to the problem of metastatic disease in the liver of the colorectal cancer patient.

This paper will point out the formidable problems of regional drug toxicity, and the appearance of metastatic disease at extrahepatic sites -- a continuing challenge to the oncologist. Also, as is apparent from on-going trials, modern staging -- guided by CEA levels and abdominal and lung computed tomography -- can detect metastatic disease at an earlier stage. Thus, patients who are treated in current trials are likely to do well from the standpoint of survival and, certainly, are likely to do much better than patients available for historical controls (15). This points again to the continued need to support ongoing clinical trials in this area as the only means to accurately judge the usefulness of this new therapy.

CURRENT TRIALS

With the initial reports of the possible efficacy of the Infusaid pump and FUDR for liver metastatic colorectal cancer (1,3,8,9,12), the only available completed study in the literature was and remains that of the Central Oncology Group (17,18). It was immediately perceived to be important to compare purported current best regional therapy for metastatic liver disease to the best available systemic therapy. Thus, the goals were not only to investigate the device as a means to prolong the lives of colorectal cancer patients, but also to attempt to disclose a "standard therapy" for liver metastatic colorectal cancer in

view of the general dissatisfaction with systemic 5-FU and its low
(20%) disease response rate. Although many modern oncologists feel
that 5-FU alone is not adequate therapy for metastatic disease apparently confined to the liver, there is agreement that some standard
against which to compare any emerging therapies is required. Thus, in
addition to finding possibly effective new therapies there exists a
need to "standardize" therapy in order to evaluate new modalities.
At the present time, there are six National Cancer Institute supported
trials of regional versus systemic therapy of colorectal hepatic metastases. Their selection for funding was designed to address these
goals. One of these trials, an intramural N.C.I. trial, will be
discussed in greater detail in a later section. However, a brief
overview of the current trials and their aims is informative.

There are five extramural N.C.I. cooperative groups conducting
trials. Table 1 lists the groups, the methods of staging, the eligibility, the treatment arms, the provision for crossing over from systemic failure to intrahepatic therapy, and the end points of each
trial. Each of the trials addresses, in individual fashion, certain
concerns such as: (1) whether to perform surgical staging on all
patients, (2) whether to include patients with limited extrahepatic
disease, (3) whether patients who fail systemic drug therapy should be
crossed over to receive intrahepatic therapy, and (4) whether the
response rate or survival is the better end point. All the trials
compare hepatic infusion to variations of "standard treatment" and to
new variations of "standard treatment". There are theoretical and
practical reasons for the differences in the various studies. Thus,
as will be discussed, with the completion of all of these trials, all
the nuances of regional therapy with the Infusaid pump and continuous
intrahepatic FUDR infusion will have been addressed.

One concern is the issue of laparotomy for staging -- a central
problem in the strategic approach to hepatic metastatic disease. If
all patients undergo a laparotomy to enter a trial and only patients
with disease confined to the liver are included, there will be a substantial number of patients excluded from the trial who would have
been included had radiologic criteria alone been used. Thus, if systemic therapy is effective, utilizing the available radiologic screen-

Table 1. U.S. National Cancer Institute Supported Trials of Regional
          versus Systemic Chemotherapy for Colorectal Cancer Liver
          Metastases

GROUP	LAPAROTOMY FOR STAGING *	ELIGIBILITY
I ENSMINGER CONSORTIUM	All Patients	1. Liver Mets Only - Laparotomy 2. Measurable Disease
II NORTH CENTRAL ONCOLOGY GROUP	HAI Patients Only	1. Liver Mets Only - Preop Radiological Exam 2. Measurable or Non-Measurable Disease in Liver
III NORTHERN CALIFORNIA ONCOLOGY GROUP	HAI Patients Only	1. Liver Mets Only - Preop Radiological Exam 2. Measurable Disease
IV MEMORIAL SLOAN-KETTERING CANCER CENTER	All Patients	1. Liver Mets Only - Laparotomy 2. Measurable Disease
V PIEDMONT ONCOLOGY GROUP	HAI Patients Only	1. Liver Mets Predominate No Extra Hepatic Mass >3 cm - Radiological Exam or Laparotomy
VI NATIONAL CANCER INSTITUTE SURGERY BRANCH	HAI Patients Only	1. Liver Mets Only - Radiological Exam 2. Measurable or Non Measurable Disease in Liver 3. No Peritoneal Carcinomatosis

*All groups pursue extensive radiological evaluation.
 H.A.I. - Hepatic artery infusion.

Table 1. U.S. National Cancer Institute Supported Trials of Regional
(cont.)   versus Systemic Chemotherapy for Colorectal Cancer Liver
          Metastases

GROUP	TREATMENT ARMS*	SYSTEMIC FAILURES CROSSOVER?	END RESULTS
I ENSMINGER CONSORTIUM	A. FUDR HAI	YES	1. Tumor Response
	B. FUDR HAI + Syst 5-FU, MITO		2. Survival
	C. Syst 5-FU: 5 Day Infusion q 4 Wks.		
II NORTH CENTRAL ONCOLOGY GROUP	A. FUDR HAI	NO	1. Survival
	B. Syst 5-FU: 5 Day Infusion q 5 Wks.		2. Time to Progression
			3. Tumor Response
III NORTHERN CALIFORNIA ONCOLOGY GROUP	A. FUDR HAI	YES	1. Tumor Response
	B. Syst FUDR: Cont. Inf.		2. Time to Progression
			3. Survival
IV MEMORIAL SLOAN-KETTERING CANCER CENTER	A. FUDR HAI	YES	1. Tumor Response
	B. Syst FUDR: Cont. Inf.		2. Survival
V PIEDMONT ONCOLOGY GROUP	A. FUDR HAI	YES	1. Tumor Response
	B. Syst 5-FU: Weekly Bolus		2. Survival
VI NATIONAL CANCER INSTITUTE SURGERY BRANCH	A. FUDR HAI	NO	1. Survival
	B. Syst FUDR: Cont. Inf.		2. Time to Progression
			3. Tumor Response

*HAI - Hepatic Artery Infusion - Alternate 2 weeks on/off.
 Systemic Continuous Infusion - Alternate 2 weeks on/off.
 FUDR - 5-fluoro-2-deoxyuridine.
 Mito - Mitomycin C.

ing modalities, one could arrive at a reasonable assessment of a given
patient's extent of disease, and begin systemic therapy without having
the patient assume the risk of laparotomy and the potential risk of
catheter and pump complications which might necessitate subsequent
surgery. However, equally important is the concept of securing accurate
information about response rates and survival from patients with exactly
comparable disease. Thus, the strategy of laparotomy after radiologic
evaluation ensures comparability of the arms of the study but will
exclude patients who have assumed a strategic risk and become ineligible
because of operative findings, thus "failing" the operative approach.

When considering eligibility, an additional issue of importance has been considered. This is the belief that liver disease is
the major cause of death in the colorectal cancer patient (4,17). A
higher response rate by disease in the liver to a given treatment
should, in theory, result in prolongation of survival assuming, of course,
that extrahepatic metastatic disease does not become a clinical problem.
Of the six trials listed, all but one compare systemic therapies to
hepatic arterial infusion. The exception is an important trial --
that of Ensminger and colleagues. The existence of a third treatment
arm in the Ensminger study is revealing in and of itself. Ensminger,
having had the largest early experience with the Infusaid device, reported
high response rates to regional arterial chemotherapy. However, increases
in deaths due to extrahepatic metastases prompted the addition of a
third arm to their proposed trial to address the issue of controlling
liver disease as well as extrahepatic metastatic sites (2,27). This
addition, a combined regional and systemic treatment arm, from a group
with the most experience to date with the Infusaid pump, points to a
possible underlying weakness of all regional therapy strategies.

A final issue addressed by these assorted trials is the question
of "crossing over" -- allowing failures in one arm to receive the
alternate treatment. One must assume that the major goal of palliative
therapies is to prolong survival. If response rates do in fact correlate
with survival, "crossing over" is not an important problem. This
information, however, is not yet available for the Infusaid pump and
FUDR and the major question in any trial of regional therapy
versus systemic therapy remains, "Will the therapy prolong survival?"

Only two trials appear to directly address this question: those of the North Central Oncology Group and the National Cancer Institute, Surgery Branch. It is probable that all trials will, in fact, provide an indication of survival and additional information can be gained from crossover trials, aside from information about time to progression and tumor response. Such information might supply answers to such crucial questions as whether treating a patient with systemic FUDR will prejudice the chances of his responding to intrahepatic therapy. Anecdotal comments seem to indicate this to be a reality. Thus, the various trials will address, when all are completed, the full spectrum of problems and techniques in the therapy of hepatic metastatic disease by continuous FUDR infusion .

NCI Surgery Branch Trial

The National Cancer Institute, Surgery Branch trial was initiated in August, 1982. As an example of the general arrangement of the trials discussed above, this will be described in some detail. The organization of this trial was based on the data gleaned from the Central Oncology Group trial published in 1979 (17,18). From the outset, our trial was planned as a controlled randomized trial of FUDR infusion via the hepatic artery compared to systemic FUDR infusion for the palliation of colorectal metastases to the liver. The goals were to examine, as a primary objective, survival; to examine objective response; and to establish a standard treatment modality against which to compare possibly effective new modalities such as monoclonal anti-bodies, liver irradiation (3,22,3), and new chemotherapeutic agents or schedules (4,10,14,31).

Each patient is evaluated with standard blood tests, including a complete blood count, platelet count, prothrombin time, partial throm-boplastin time, thrombin time, electrolytes, liver function tests, creatinine, a carcinoembryonic antigen determination, a hepatitis associated antigen level; an electrocardiogram; and a chest x-ray. Patients receive full lung tomography, a liver scan, a liver CT, and an enhanced liver CT with an ethiodized oil emulsion (EOE-13). In addition, patients receive a barium enema and celiac and superior mesenteric artery angiography.

   Patients are eligible for participation who have hepatic metastatic
disease only by this preoperative evaluation. In addition, at our institution, where an aggressive approach to surgical resection
is undertaken, patients must be unresectable by virtue of having a
number of metastases (generally greater than four) or a location of
metastases which precludes hepatic resection. Patients who are poor
risks for liver resection are eligible for the trial as are those
who refuse liver resection.

   Patients are excluded who have non-colon primaries, preoperative
evidence of extrahepatic metastatic disease, a less than 2 month life
expectancy, an unresectable local recurrence of a primary noted at
laparotomy, and peritoneal carcinomatosis determined at laparotomy.
Obviously, those who decline to participate are excluded. Patients
with node metastases determined only at surgery, and not radiologically,
are eligible.

   Preoperatively, patients are randomized to receive intrahepatic or
systemic FUDR if they have a proven diagnosis and are unresectable by
radiologic evaluation. Patients may be randomized intraoperatively if
the diagnosis is proven and they have been determined to have unresectable
hepatic metastatic disease. There is no pre-randomization stratification.
Thus, patients who are explored with a view toward possible resection
are asked to participate in this trial preoperatively so that randomization
can be carried out, if appropriate. After randomization, patients
who receive intrahepatic therapy receive the Infusaid model 400 pump
with single or dual catheters (20,26). Patients are begun, two to
three weeks postoperatively on 0.3 mg of FUDR/kg/day, on a two week on -
two week off cycle. Systemic patients receive the Infusaid model 400
pump in the infraclavicular position with the catheter placed in the
superior vena cava. Patients are begun on 0.125 mg of FUDR/kg/day.
These patients are maintained on a two week on - two week off schedule.
All intrahepatic patients have required dose reductions and increasing
intervals between the cycles of drug therapy. Systemic patients have
not tolerated their initial dose without need for reduction when,
early on in the trial, a dose of 0.15 mg/kg/day was utilized. The
reduced dose is mildly toxic in most patients.

Follow-up evaluation includes a CBC, a SMAC, and a CEA at two week intervals; and a chest x-ray, and an MAA liver scan at one month intervals for those patients with intrahepatic pumps (21). At three month intervals, patients receive a liver CT and a liver EOE CT.

Response is defined as disappearance of 50% of visible lesions; or a 50% decrease in the size of any well described lesion; or disappearance of lesions 2 cm in size or greater. Progression is defined as doubling in the size of any lesion or the appearance of any new lesion. All these criteria are based on liver CT or liver EOE CT determinations of maximal perpendicular lesion diameters.

As with the majority of other trials, selection criteria have been formalized on an objective basis. That is, some criteria previously used for defining response, such as changes in liver function tests have not been included. No crossover of systemic failures is planned in order to evaluate survival.

NCI Trial Results to Date. Since the trial was approved in August, 1982, 21 patients have been randomized into the study with a median follow-up of 13 months. Table 2 lists the numbers per group and those responding at 3, 6, 9, and 12 months from the inception of treatment. A single death has occurred and that in the systemic treatment arm. The patient died one year after therapy was initiated.

Table II. Responses to Therapy (Those responding versus those eligible for evaluation for intervals after therapy was initiated).

	NUMBER PTS.	RESPONSE			
		3 MO	6 MO	9 MO	12 MO
SYSTEMIC FUDR	8	3/8	3/8	0/3	0/3
INTRAHEPATIC FUDR	12	8/11	4/10	4/5	3/3

Between 3 and 6 months, of the 4 failing patients, two developed lung metastases and two had progression in the liver.

Toxicity. Chemical hepatitis occurs in 100 percent of patients receiving intrahepatic FUDR, requiring dose reductions and increasing intervals between drug cycles -- often 4-8 weeks. A peculiar, idiosyncratic response has occured in approximately every 2 in 5 patients. This entity has been well characterized by Stagg, Hohn et al. in presentations at the meetings of the American Society of Clinical Oncology and the American Association for the Study of Liver Disease (19,25). Seven of 16 hepatic infusion arm patients developed, without forewarning, liver function abnormalities including marked elevation of bilirubin and a persistent elevation of alkaline phosphatase two to three times above previously normal levels. Three patients in our series meet the criteria for this extreme sensitivity to FUDR. Endoscopic cholangiopancreatography in the San Francisco patients has demonstrated an appearance of biliary sclerosis not unlike sclerosing cholangitis. Percutaneous cholangiography has shown this in two of three such NCI patients. Liver biopsies have evidence of periportal round cell infiltration and bile stasis. This toxicity requires a marked reduction in or discontinuance of FUDR.

Major toxicities in the systemic group have been nausea, vomiting, and diarrhea generally occuring during the first toxic cycle, which is usually the first cycle. The original dose of 0.15 mg/kg/day (24) has been reduced to a starting dose of 0.125 mg/kg/day without further major toxic complications.

Table III lists our complications including hospitalizations and technical complications.

Table III. Complications of Therapy - Systemic (S)/Hepatic (H)

6 Hospitalizations Drug Toxicity 3S/3H
6 Technical Complications in 5 Pts (1S/5H)
  -RHA Occlusion at 4 months
  -Connector Disruption
  -Post-op Bleeding
  -LHA Occlusion at 6 months
  -Angiography Catheter Dissection found at operation
  -Catheter in Neck (S)
1 Perforated ulcer, bile duct necrosis (H)
1 Duodenal ulcer, uncomplicated (H)

A single non-responder in the hepatic artery infusion group was randomized to have a catheter placed but could not have this accomplished
secondary to dense post-inflammatory scarring in the periportal region
which precluded hepatic arterial placement of the catheter. Too few
patients are available for survival analysis. Limited information
about median time to recurrence is available: for hepatic artery
infusion six months median time to recurrence has been noted versus 3
months for systemic therapy patients.

Data From Other Ongoing Trials

Data from the previously mentioned trials is available only in
abstract form. Information from those abstracts (American Society of
Clinical Oncology and Society for Surgical Oncology, 1984) and information
from pre-trial experience suggests, however, that the initial non-trial
results are not being fully reproduced. Although the Infusaid pump is
reliable with a less than 1% failure rate, the technical difficulties
of vessel occlusion and GI ulceration related to catheter infusion
remain -- although reduced in incidence. Patients followed with MAA
scans at one month intervals may demonstrate good catheter perfusion
for prolonged periods followed by occasional unanticipated sudden
occlusion of major or segmental branches of hepatic arterial anatomy.
Thus, although therapy delivered directly to the liver may afford a
high initial response rate, this response may not be durable, because
1) late segmental arterial occlusion may occur impairing drug delivery,
or, 2) chemical hepatitis or biliary sclerosis may occur leading to a
dose reduction or cessation of therapy. In our trial, both of these
problems have occurred, leading to progression of the liver disease.

The pump is well tolerated and, once the dose is standardized, continuous chemotherapy can usually be achieved without difficulty and
with mild toxicity, whether FUDR is delivered systemically or intra-
hepatically. Infusion toxicities compared with bolus schedule toxicities
of 5-FU or FUDR have pointed out that, esentially, new classes of
drugs have been created by using old drugs and new infusion schedules
(16,31). This is born out by the fact that some patients in each of
our arms who have received previous 5-FU therapy and have been classified
as non-responders are now responding to FUDR. Too, no hair loss, marrow

toxicity, or renal deterioration has occurred in patients receiving systemic, continuous FUDR as opposed to the occurrence of such toxicity in patients receiving 5-FU.

A major flaw in the strategy of regional chemotherapy may be indicated by the appearance, in all series, of extrahepatic metastatic disease in the face of responding liver disease (2,19). Ensminger, et al., with the earliest experience, realized this and, as previously discussed, added a third arm to their trial. With the availability of the two catheter pump, both regional and systemic chemotherapy may be possible, allowing a simple combination approach. Another significant problem with regional therapy remains unpredictable liver toxicity. Chemical hepatitis and biliary sclerosis, both acute and chronic, remain problems; and newer methodologies for evaluating hepatic toxcity may better guide therapy (5). Too, if new data regarding blood supply to metastases (23) and anecdotal clinical response (14) is accurate, the portal infusion route may avoid direct toxicity to the end arterioles nourishing the bile ducts and may thus avoid biliary sclerosis.

CONCLUSION

Current trials must be completed. However, there is evidence that this will not be simple. Dissemination of this new technology has slowed accrual into several of the trials previously mentioned. Complication rates, the response rates, and the durability of response, as well as that crucial parameter, survival, must be assessed. Yet, even at this point, current data point to the continued need for innovation in the treatment of hepatic metastatic colorectal cancer. The delivery of FUDR by infusion pump has improved our understanding of the therapeutic problems of such an approach but need for alternative approaches is already apparent. Such approaches might well include regional drug delivery (3,4,10,14,22,27,33). If so, the Infusaid pump may be viewed as the current best means of achieving reliable regional infusion. Those conducting trials addressing regional drug delivery will find the pump to be reliable and acceptable to patients. It is important to realize, however, that the pump is not an answer to the problem of liver metastatic cancer; it is merely a device for the delivery of agents which, for the present time, are unequal to the task.

ACKNOWLEDGEMENTS

Dr. John Y. Killen of the Cancer Therapy Evaluation Branch, Division of Cancer Treatment kindly provided the data on NCI extramural trials. Ms. Rosalind Blackwood and Ms. Mary Ann Bodnar prepared the manuscript.

REFERENCES

1. Balch, C.M., Urist, M.M., and McGregor, M.L.: Continuous regional chemotherapy for metastatic colorectal cancer using a totally implantable infusion pump. Amer. J. Surg. 145:285-290, 1983.
2. Balch, C.M., Urist, M.M., Soong, S-J., amd McGregor, M.L.: A prospective Phase II clinical trial of continuous FUDR regional chemotherapy for colorectal metastases to the liver using a totally implantable drug infusion pump. Ann. Surg. 198:567-573, 1983.
3. Barone, R.M., Byfield, J.E., Goldfarb, P.B., et al.: Intraarterial chemotherapy using an implantable infusion pump and liver irradiation for the treatment of hepatic metastases. Cancer. 50:850-862, 1982.
4. Bengmark, S., Fredlund, P., Hafstrom, L.O., and Vang, J.: Present experiences with hepatic dearterialization in liver neoplasm. Progr. Surg. 13:141-166, 1974.
5. Bircher, J.: Quantitative assessment of deranged hepatic function: A missed opportunity? Sem. Liver Ds. 3:275-284, 1983.
6. Buchwald, H., Grage, T.B., Vassilopoulos, P.P., et al.: Intraarterial infusion chemotherapy for hepatic carcinoma using a totally implantable infusion pump. Cancer. 45:866-869, 1980.
7. Buchwald, H., Rohde, T.D., Varco, R.L., et al.: Long-term continuous intravenous heparin administration by an implantable infusion pump in ambulatory patients with recurrent venous thrombosis. Surgery. 88:507-516, 1980.
8. Cohen, A.M., Kaufman, S.D., Wood, W.C., and Greenfield, A.J.: Regional hepatic chemotherapy using an implantable drug infusion pump. Am. J. Surg. 145:529-533, 1983.
9. Cohen, A.M., Wood, S.D., Greenfield, A.J., et al.: Transbrachial hepatic arterial chemotherapy using an implanted infusion pump. Ds. Colon Rectum. 23:223-227, 1980.
10. Dahl, E.P., Fredlund, P.E., Tylen, V., Bengmark, S.: Transient hepatic dearterialization followed by regional intraarterial 5'-fluorouracil infusion as treatment for liver tumors. Ann. Surg. 193:82-88, 1981.
11. Ensminger, W.D., Gyves, J.W.: The clinical pharmacology of hepatic artery chemotherapy. Sem. Oncol. 10:176-182, 1983.
12. Ensminger, W.D., Niederhuber, J., Dakhil, S., et al.: Totally implanted drug delivery system for hepatic arterial chemotherapy. Cancer Treatment Rep. 65:393-400, 1981.
13. Ensminger, W.D., Roskowsky, A., Raso, V., et al.: A clinical pharmacology evaluation of hepatic arterial infusions of 5-fluoro-2-deoxyuridine and 5-fluorouracil. Cancer Res. 38:3784-3792, 1978.
14. Fortner, J.G., Silva, L.S., Cox, E.B., et al.: Multivariate analysis of a personal series of 247 patients with liver metastases from colorectal cancer. II. Treatments by intrahepatic chemotherapy. Ann. Surg. 199:317-324, 1984.

276

15. Goslin, R., Steele, G., Zamcheck, N., et al.: Factors influencing survival in patients with hepatic metastases from adenocarcinoma of the colon and rectum. Ds. Colon Rectum. 25:749-754, 1982.
16. Goldman, P.: Rate controlled drug delivery. NEJM. 307:286-290, 1982.
17. Grage, T.B., Shingleton, W.W., Jubert, A.V., et al.: Results of a prospective randomized study of hepatic artery infusion with 5-fluorouracil vs. intravenous 5-fluorouracil in patients with hepatic metastases from colorectal cancer. Front. Gastrointest. Res. 5:116-129, 1979.
18. Grage, T.B., Vassilopoulos, P.P., Shingleton, W.W., et al.: Results of a prospective randomized study of hepatic artery infusion with 5-fluorouracil in patients with hepatic metastases from colorectal cancer: A Central Oncology Group Study. Surg. 86:550-555, 1979.
19. Hohn, D., Stagg, R., Ignofo, R., et al.: Incidence and prevention of complications of cyclic hepatic artery infusions of Floxuridine: Severe biliary sclerosis, gastritis and ulcer. Abstract - Amer. Soc. Clin. Oncol. Toronto, 1984.
20. Hughes, K.S., Villela, E.R.: An improved technique for regional perfusion chemotherapy in the presence of a replaced right hepatic artery using a single implantable pump. Surg. 95:355-357, 1984.
21. Kaplan, W.D., Ensminger, W.D., Come, S.E., et al.: Radionuclide angiography to predict patient response to hepatic artery chemotherapy. Cancer Treatment Rep. 64:1217-1222, 1980.
22. Kinsella, T.J.: The role of radiation therapy alone and combined with infusion chemotherapy for treating liver metastases. Sem. Oncol. 10:215-222, 1983.
23. Lin, G., Lunderquist, A., Hagerstrand, I., and Boitsen, E.: Post Mortem examination of the blood supply and vascular pattern of small liver metastases in man. Surg. In press.
24. Lokich, J.J., Sonneborn, H., Paul, S., Zipoli, T.: Phase I study of continuous venous infusion of 5-fluoro-2-deoxyuridine chemotherapy. To be published.
25. Melnick, J., Hohn, D., Stagg, R., et al.: Cholestasis and biliary sclerosis in patients receiving hepatic arterial infusion of floxuridine (FUDR). Abstract - Amer. Assoc. Study Liver Ds. Chicago, 1983, pg. 47.
26. Niederhuber, J.E., and Ensminger, W.D.: Surgical considerations in the management of hepatic neoplasia. Sem. Oncol. 10:135-147, 1983.
27. Niederhuber, J.E., Ensminger, W., Gyres, J., et al.: Regional chemotherapy of colorectal cancer metastatic to the liver. Cancer. 53:1336-1343, 1984.
28. Rohde, T.D., Blackshear, P.J., Varco, R.L., and Buchwald, H.: One year of heparin anticoagulation: An ambulatory subject using a totally implantable infusion pump. Minnesota Med. 60:719-722, 1977.
29. Rohde, T.D., Blackshear, P.J., Varco. R.L., and Buchwald, H.: Protracted parenteral drug infusion in ambulatory subjects using an implantable infusion pump. Trans. Am. Soc. Artif. Intern. Organs. 23:13-16, 1977.
30. Rupp, W.M., Barbosa, J.J., Blackshear, P.J., et al.: The use of an implantable insulin pump in the treatment of type II Diabetes. NEJM. 307:265-270, 1982.

31. Speyer, J.L., Sugarbaker, P.H., Collins, J.M., et al.: Portal levels and hepatic clearance of 5-fluorouracil after intraperitoneal administration in humans. Cancer Res. 41:1916-1922, 1981.
32. Stagg, R., Friedman, M., Lewis, B., et al.: Current status of the NCOG randomized trial of continuous intra-arterial versus intravenous floxuridine in patients with colorectal carcinoma metastatic to the liver. Abstract - Amer. Soc. Clin. Oncology - Toronto, May 1984.
33. Webber, B.M., Soderberg, C.H., Leone, L.A., et al.: A combined treatment approach to management of hepatic metastases. Cancer. 42:1087-1095, 1978.

RECEPTOR-MEDIATED ENDOCYTOSIS BY NORMAL AND PROLIFERATING HEPATOCYTES
AND LIPOSOMAL DRUG DELIVERY

ALLAN W. WOLKOFF, M.D., RICHARD J. STOCKERT, Ph.D. AND PHILIP S.
SCHEIN, M.D.

Receptor-mediated endocytosis is a process common to many species
and cell types. One of the best characterized systems in which this
process occurs is that of the hepatocyte receptor for
asialoglycoproteins (1). This receptor was first described by Ashwell
and Morell in studies of plasma disappearance of ceruloplasmin (2). In
these studies performed in rats, they determined that native
ceruloplasmin had a circulating half-life of 55 hours. Like virtually
all mammalian plasma proteins, with the exception of albumin,
ceruloplasmin is a glycoprotein consisting of a protein core with
complex carbohydrate side-chains attached via aspartate residues. The
terminal carbohydrate in these chains is sialic acid; the penultimate
is galactose. Removal of sialic acid, exposing galactosyl residues,
resulted in a reduction in circulating half-life to minutes rather
than hours. Plasma clearance of asialoceruloplasmin as well as most
other asialoglycoproteins represents uptake into hepatocytes. This
uptake is mediated by a specific liver cell membrane receptor, hepatic
binding protein (HBP) (3).

HBP is a membrane glycoprotein which has been solubilized in
detergent and purified from rat, rabbit and human liver. As
demonstrated in studies performed in isolated perfused rat liver, HBP
is necessary for uptake of asialoglycoproteins by hepatocytes (4). In
these studies, rat liver was first perfused with 100 mg of non-immune
goat IgG (Figure 1). Following IgG infusion, a mixture of ^{125}I-
Asialoorosomucoid (ASOR), ^{3}H-Bilirubin and ^{131}I-Albumin was injected
as a small bolus into the portal vein. Albumin was used as a non-
transported reference. Its extracellular space of distribution is
that of bilirubin, which circulates bound to it, and is similar to

that of ASOR, a protein of comparable molecular weight. Following injection, all effluent coming from the hepatic vein was collected in aliquots every 1-2 seconds without recirculation. In this way, uptake of bilirubin and ASOR during a single pass through the liver could be quantitated. Following this study, anti-HBP IgG was infused and the study repeated (Figure 2). Analysis revealed that uptake of ASOR was reduced by over 80% following anti-HBP infusion, while bilirubin uptake did not differ from control. These studies also revealed that uptake of bilirubin which occurs by facilitated diffusion rather than by endocytosis is independent of uptake of ASOR.

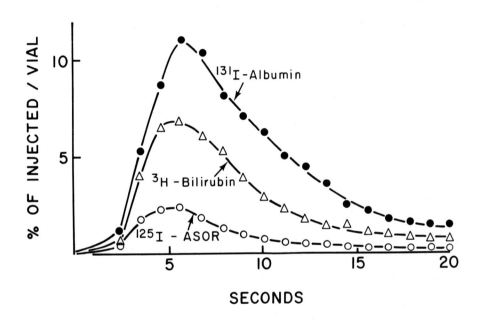

Figure 1: Hepatic venous outflow patterns of ^{131}I-Albumin, ^{3}H-Bilirubin, and ^{125}I-Asialoorosomucoid (ASOR) following simultaneous injection into the portal vein of an isolated perfused rat liver following pre-infusion of non-immune goat IgG. (Reprinted from reference 4 with permission).

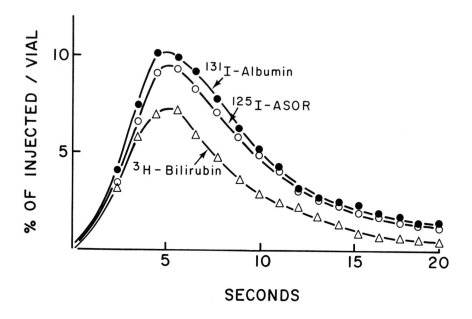

Figure 2: The same liver as in Figure 1 was then infused with anti-HBP IgG and the transport study was repeated. There was a marked reduction in uptake of ^{125}I-ASOR as indicated by increased recovery, while uptake of ^{3}H-Bilirubin was unchanged. (Reprinted from reference 4 with permission).

Newer studies have revealed that endocytosis of ASOR following binding to HBP is a complex event (5). Following binding of ligand to cell surface HBP, the ligand-receptor complex is internalized into a prelysosomal compartment that has been termed the endosome. The endosome interior becomes acidified resulting in dissociation of ligand and receptor (6). The ligand and receptor segregate from each other; receptor eventually recycles to the cell surface, while ligand enters lysosomes where degradation takes place. Recent studies have identified specific inhibitors of these steps (Figure 3) .

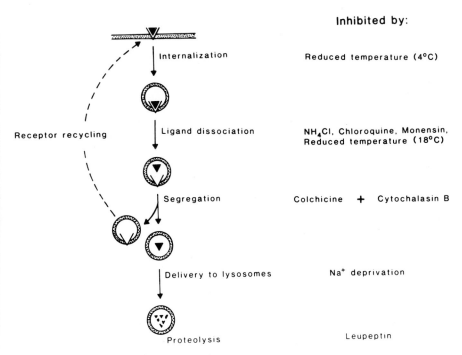

Figure 3: Schematic diagram of receptor-mediated endocytosis of asialoglycoproteins and its inhibitors. Based on these and other studies, five discrete steps in uptake and catabolism can be quantitated. Inhibitors of each of these steps have been identified. Inhibitors are assigned on the basis of their most proximal site of action as a wave of prebound ligand moves through the pathway. (Reprinted from reference 5 with permission).

The liver cell plasma membrane plays an important role in receptor-mediated endocytosis. Because the liver cell surface may undergo marked changes during proliferation, we studied transport of ASOR and bilirubin by regenerating rat liver (7). The rat hepatocyte divides approximately once per year, and mitosis in hepatocytes is infrequently seen in normal liver (8). Following two-thirds hepatectomy, rapid cellular proliferation occurs throughout the remaining liver remnant, and is associated with expression of oncofetal antigens (9-11). Studies performed with hepatocytes in culture suggest that hepatocyte replication is associated with modulated expression of several intracellular and secreted proteins including ligandin, pyruvate kinase, and α-1-fetoprotein (12). Altered liver cell plasma membrane function during regeneration has also been suggested. Studies of the interaction of plasma membrane,

prepared from regenerating liver, with insulin and glucagon revealed
an increased number of insulin receptors and reduced number of
glucagon receptors (13). Amino acid uptake by hepatocytes was found to
be increased several-fold during liver regeneration (14). This
finding which may be due to an altered plasma membrane transport
mechanism, is blocked by pretreatment with colchicine, a microtubule
disrupter. Changes in other liver cell plasma membrane enzymes occur
in regeneration, including a doubling of (Na^+-K^+)-ATPase activity and
a reduction in glucagon-stimulated adenyl cyclase activity (15).

As a measure of specific hepatocyte function, transport of ^{3}H-
Bilirubin and ^{125}I-ASOR was determined using the single-pass indicator
dilution method in the isolated perfused regenerating liver (7). This
method permits quantitation of uptake rates independent of hepatic
mass. Results were compared to those obtained in sham-operated rats.
As seen in Figure 4, liver weight increased progressively with time
after two-thirds hepatectomy, and returned to normal by six days.
Uptake of ^{3}H-Bilirubin and ^{125}I-ASOR fell by over 50% and 80%,
respectively, reaching a nadir at the time of greatest cell
proliferation (Figure 5). Uptake returned to normal by six days.
These studies of transport of anions and asialoglycoproteins during
liver regeneration revealed functional maturation similar to that seen
during development.

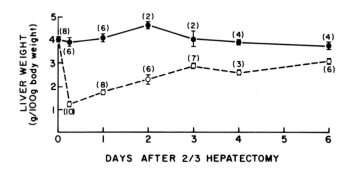

Figure 4: Liver weight in sham-operated rats (●) and two-thirds
hepatectomized rats (O) at various times after surgery. (Reprinted
from reference 7 with permission).

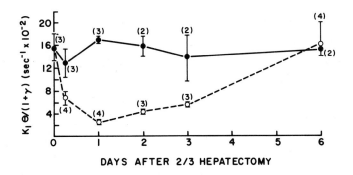

Figure 5: Influx rate of ^{125}I-ASOR ($k_1\theta/(1 +\gamma)$) in perfused liver from sham-operated (●) and partially hepatectomized rats (o). Rate constants were calculated from indicator dilution curves. Similar results were obtained in studies of ^{3}H-Bilirubin transport. (Reprinted from reference 7 with permission).

That hepatocellular proliferation alone is not responsible for the transport alterations seen during liver regeneration was demonstrated in perfused liver from rats pretreated with nafenopin (16). Nafenopin (2-methyl-2p-(1,2,3,4,-tetrahydro-1-naphthyl) phenoxy propionic acid) is a hypolipidemic drug which induces rapid liver growth characterized by hepatocellular hypertrophy and hyperplasia similar to that seen during regeneration (17-20). After nafenopin treatment, the liver has morphologic features of regeneration including proliferation of smooth endoplasmic reticulum, enlargement of peroxisomes and Golgi, and dilated and tortuous bile canaliculi (21,22). Despite a 40% increase in liver weight 24 hours after two days of nafenopin, there was no change in transport of bilirubin or ASOR, unlike results seen in regeneration (Figure 6). However, uptake of the water soluble organic anions, BSP and conjugated bilirubin was reduced by 50% (Figure 6). These studies suggest that hepatocellular proliferation alone is not responsible for the transport alterations seen during liver regeneration. Nafenopin effectively unmasks differences in uptake of bilirubin and other more water soluble organic anions such as sulfobromophthalein and conjugated bilirubin, suggesting that their uptake mechanisms are partially independent. As discussed below, reduced uptake of ASOR during liver regeneration is a consequence of reduced numbers of cell surface receptors for this ligand. Whether there are analagous alterations in organic anion interaction with liver cell surface membranes during regeneration or after nafenopin-treatment remains to be determined.

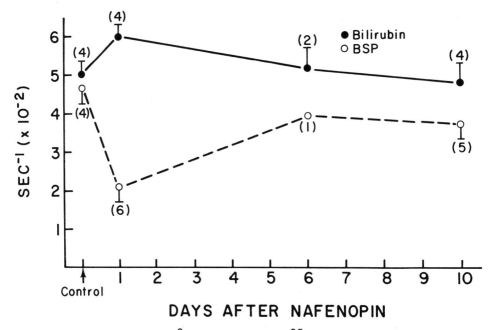

Figure 6: Influx of ^{3}H-Bilirubin and ^{35}S-BSP in isolated perfused liver of rats pretreated with nafenopin. There was no change in influx of either compound in corn oil fed controls. Despite the marked proliferative response similar to that seen in regeneration, influx of bilirubin remained constant, as did influx of ASOR. In contrast, BSP influx was significantly reduced.

Reduced uptake of ASOR during liver regeneration could be due to a number of factors. That it is due to reduced levels of HBP on the liver cell surface, however, has been demonstrated (23). In these studies, isolated hepatocytes were prepared from livers at various times after two-thirds hepatectomy. Binding of ^{125}I-ASOR to the cell surface or to solubilized cell homogenates was determined as was uptake and degradation of this ligand (Figures 7 and 8). Results were compared with identical studies performed in cells obtained from sham-operated rats. Similar to results in perfused liver, there was reduced uptake of ASOR by hepatocytes obtained during the period of active cell proliferation. This was accompanied by an 80% loss of receptor from the cell surface. Total cell receptor, as determined in the solubilized homogenates, was normal (Figure 8).

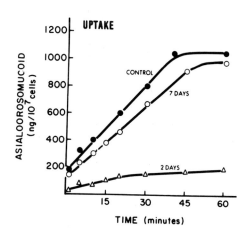

Figure 7: Uptake of ASOR by isolated hepatocytes obtained from sham-operated rats or rats 2 days (Δ) or 7 days after two-thirds hepatectomy. Similar to results in perfused liver, uptake is reduced during the proliferative phase of regeneration. (Reprinted from reference 23 with permission).

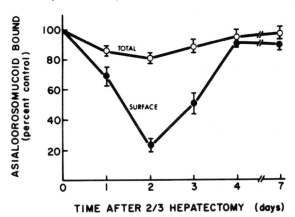

Figure 8: Binding of ASOR by intact hepatocytes (●) and cell homogenates (o) at various times after two thirds hepatectomy. During the time of active cell proliferation, there was an 80% loss of receptor from the cell surface. (Reprinted from reference 23 with permission).

286

The modulation of liver cell HBP content seen during regeneration
is similar to that which has been observed in the mouse during
development (24). As seen in Figure 9, fetal mice have no detectable
receptor until the nineteenth day of gestation, and develop normal
adult levels by 5 days postpartum. Maternal liver has a tripling of
HBP activity in the last trimester, with a fall to normal levels
shortly after birth.

These studies suggested that hepatocytes during regeneration
entered a state of "dedifferentiation". Other studies have revealed
altered liver cell membrane enzyme activities during
hepatocarcinogenesis (25). Based on these data, Stockert and Becker
(26) studied HBP content of rat liver following exposure to the
chemical carcinogen AAF (N-2-acetylaminofluorene). As has been
described, this drug induces formation of neoplastic nodules and
hepatocellular carcinoma in rat liver (27). These nodules can be
dissected free of other liver tissue and studied biochemically. HBP,
as assayed by specific binding of ^{125}I-ASOR, was reduced by almost 70%
in neoplastic nodules and by 95% in areas of hepatocellular carcinoma.

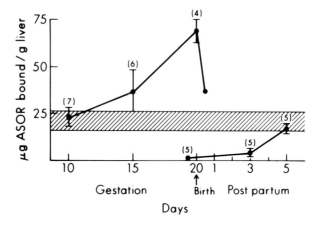

Figure 9: Asialoglycoprotein receptor binding activity in pregnancy,
fetal and neonatal development. The hatched area indicates control
male and virgin female mouse liver activity. Pregnant mice (●) have
supranormal receptor activity while developing mice (●) do not have
detectable receptor activity until the nineteenth day of gestation.
(Reprinted from reference 24 with permission).

These studies have suggested potential new directions in treatment of hepatocellular carcinoma. Exciting studies along these lines have recently been performed by Wu and colleagues (28) in studies of methotrexate. The lack of specificity for neoplastic tissue which results in injury to normal as well as malignant cells, has limited the clinical usefulness of this drug. In addition, hepatotoxicity frequently complicates treatment with high levels of methotrexate. These investigators synthesized a covalent conjugate of folinic acid with asialofetuin with the goal of directing this methotrexate antagonist to receptor-bearing cells, sparing them from methotrexate toxicity. Less differentiated cells not containing HBP, would be killed by methotrexate.

Two cultured cell lines were used for these studies. One was a relatively undifferentiated human hepatocellular carcinoma line, PLC/PRF/5, which lacks HBP. The other was a more differentiated human hepatocellular carcinoma line, HepG2. This is the only cultured cell line which has been found to express HBP. As seen in Figure 10, PLC/PRF/5 receptor negative cells were killed by methotrexate both in the presence and absence of the asialofetuin-folinic acid conjugate. Methotrexate also killed HepG2 cells, but this effect was eliminated by adding the folinic acid conjugate to the medium. Thus, these studies reveal specific rescue of differentiated cells based upon the presence of a specific receptor on the cell surface. They may have important implications in the design of clinical chemotherapeutic protocols.

A similar line of investigation has been conducted on liposome delivery of drugs. Rahman and colleagues (29,30) incorporated adriamycin into liposomes composed of phosphatidylcholine and cholesterol mixed with stearyl amine (positively charged) or phosphatidylserine (negatively charged). Lipsosomal incorporation may result in internalization of drug into cells by endocytosis. Use of adriamycin has been limited by its cardiac toxicity. Electron microscopic studies have demonstrated degeneration of myofirils and mitochondrial distortion, as well as a reduction in cardiac myocytes.

288

Pharmacokinetic studies have revealed avid uptake into heart muscle. Incorporation of adriamycin into positively charged liposomes effectively retarded the in vivo uptake of drug in cardiac tisssue when compared to free drug or drug incorporated into negatively charged lipsosmes (Figure 11). In this situation, adriamycin was preferentially concentrated in liver, spleen and lungs. Electron microscopic studies revealed that the myocytes and myofibrillar structure of cardiac muscle were well preserved. Importantly,, anti-tumor activity against murine ascitic P388 leukemia and Lewis lung carcinoma was identical whether adriamycin was administered alone or entrapped in positively charged liposomes (Figure 12). These studies and the studies presented above, suggest that liposomes may be developed to deliver their contents to specific cell types by targeting them to particular cell surface receptors.

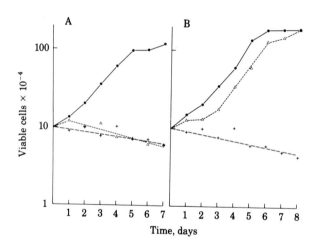

Figure 10: Specific rescue of methotrexate (MTX)-treated HBP containing cells by an asialofetuin-folinic acid conjugate. (A) PLC/PRF/5 receptor-negative cells grown in the absence of MTX (●) in 0.5 uM MTX (+), or in 0.5 uM MTX/15 uM asialofetuin-folinic acid conjugate (Δ). (B) HepG2 receptor-positive cells grown under the same conditions. (Reprinted from reference 28 with permission).

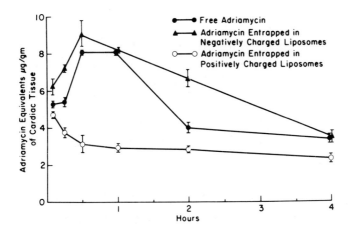

Figure 11: Adriamycin disposition in mouse heart following i.v. administration of free and liposome-entrapped drugs. (Reprinted from reference 29 with permission).

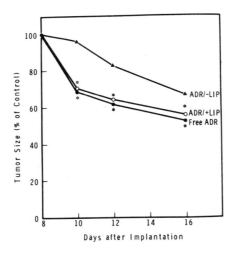

Figure 12: Treatment of mice given implants of Lewis lung carcinoma. Adriamycin (4 mg/kg) was administered i.v. to mice on days 8, 10 and 12 after tumor implantation, as free drug (Free ADR) or drug entrapped in positive (ADR/+ LIP) or negative (ADR/-LIP) liposomes. The percentage of reduction of tumor mass was assessed by measuring the largest perpendicular diameter of the primary tumor. The asterisk indicates statistical difference from control (P < 0.05). (Reprinted from reference 29 with permission).

REFERENCES

1. Stockert RJ, Morell AG. 1982. Endocytosis of Glycoproteins. In The Liver: Biology and Pathobiology. ed. IM Arias, H Popper, D. Schachter and DA Shafritz. Raven Press, New York, pp. 205-217.
2. Morell AG, Gregoriadis G, Scheinberg IH, Hickman J, Ashwell G. 1971. J Biol Chem 246:1461-1467.
3. Hudgin RL, Pricer WE Jr, Ashwell G, Stockert RJ, Morell AG. 1974. J Biol Chem 249:5536-5543.
4. Stockert RJ, Gartner U, Morell AG, Wolkoff AW. 1980. J Biol Chem 255:3830-3831.
5. Wolkoff AW, Klausner RD, Ashwell G, Harford J. 1984. J Cell Biol 98:375-381.
6. Harford J, Wolkoff AW, Ashwell G, Klausner RD. 1983. J Cell Biol 96:1824-1828.
7. Gartner U, Stockert RJ, Morell AG, Wolkoff AW. 1981. Hepatology 1:99-106.
8. Steiner JW, Perz ZM, Taichman LB. 1966. Exp Mol Pathol 5:146-181.
9. Bonney RJ, Walker PR, Potter VR. 1973. Biochem J 136:947-954.
10. Sell S, Nichols M, Becker FF, et al. 1974. Cancer Res. 34:864-871.
11. Naughton BA, Kaplan SM, Roy M, et al. 1977. Science 196:301-302.
12. Leffert H, Mora T, Sell S, et al. 1978. Proc Natl Acad Sci USA 75:1834-1838.
13. Leffert HL, Koch KS, Moran T, et al. 1979. Gastroenterology 76:1470-1482.
14. Walker PR, Whitefield JE. 1978. Proc Natl Acad Sci USA 75:1394-1398.
15. Bruscalupi G, Curatola G, Lenaz G, et al. 1980. Biochim Biophys Acta 597:264-273.
16. Gartner U, Stockert RJ, Levine WG, Wolkoff AW. 1982. Gastroenterology 83:1163-1169.
17. Hess R, Maier R, Staubil W. 1969. Adv Exp Med Biol 4:483-489.
18. Best MM, Duncan CH. 1970. Atherosclerosis 12:185-192.
19. Beckitt R, Weiss R, Stitzel R, et al. 1972. Toxicol Appl Pharmacol 23:43.
20. Moody DE, Rao MS, Reddy JK. 1977. Virchows Arch B Cell Pathol 23:291-296.
21. Novikoff AB, Novikoff PM, Mori M, et al. 1975. J Histochem Cytochem 23:314.
22. Leighton F, Coloma L, Koenig C. 1975. J Cell Biol 67:281-309.
23. Howard DJ, Stockert RJ, Morell AG. 1982. J Biol Chem 257:2856-2858.
24. Collins JC, Stockert RJ, Morell AG. 1984. Hepatology 4:80-83.
25. Gravela E, Feo F, Canuto RA, Garcea R, Gabriel L. 1975. Cancer Res 35:3041-3047.
26. Stockert RJ, Becker FF. 1980. Cancer Res 40:3632-3634.
27. Stout DL, Becker FF. 1978. Cancer Res. 38:2274-2278.
28. Wu GY, Wu CH, Stockert RJ. 1983. Proc Natl Acad Sci USA 80:3078-3080.
29. Rahman A, Kessler A, More N, Sikic B, Rowden G, Woolley P, Schein PS. 1980. Cancer Res 40:1532-1537.
30. Rahman A, More N, Schein PS. 1982. Cancer Res 42:1817-1825.

ACKNOWLEDGEMENT: This work was supported by NIH grants AM-23026, AM-17702, AM-32419 and AM-32972.

ISOLATED REGIONAL LIVER PERFUSION IN THE TREATMENT OF HEPATIC
METASTASES

C.J.H. van de Velde, U.R. Tjaden, B.J.L. Kothuis

THE BASIS FOR REGIONAL ISOLATED LIVER PERFUSION

Regional cancer chemotherapy is a means of exploiting dose-
response effects by delivering more drug to regionally confined
tumors. It is based on the separation of the target organ from
the rest of the body since many chemotherapeutic agents display
a steep dose-response for toxicity and for therapeutic effect[1].

Dose-response effects

The principles of cancer chemotherapy as elucidated by
Skipper and co-workers[2] were the basis of the design of many
clinical protocols. These principles include:

1. The killing effect of drugs is a logarithmic function
   (fractional cell kill). That is, a given dose kills a constant fraction of cells, regardless of the number present
   at the start.
2. The most effective dose of most drugs is the maximum tolerated dose.

An example of an experimental tumor system demonstrating
this is given in Fig. 1. The doubling or tripling of the 1/4
dose regimen did not produce a shrinkage of measurable tumor
growth. Only the maximum tolerated dose produced a 50% reduction in volume. Such a situation in the clinic would be interpreted as 'no response' at the first three dose levels. The
slope of the dose-response is related to the sensitivity of
the tumor to a given drug. In the marginally sensitive gastrointestinal tumors a twofold difference in the dose may result
in less impressive evidence for the superiority of the high
dose. However, a prospective randomized clinical trial testing
four different systemic dosage regimens of 5-FU showed that

the most toxic regimen (an intravenous loading course of 12 mg/ kg/day) significantly improved responses and duration of responses in colon-rectum cancer patients[3].

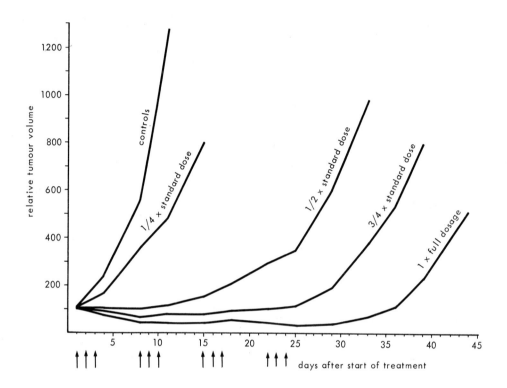

FIGURE 1. 2661 carcinoma in CBA/Rij mice.

Growth delay of flank tumors dependent upon chemotherapy dose; 5-8 animals per group, each carrying two tumors.

Hepatic arterial infusion

A major impetus for hepatic arterial chemotherapy was the demonstration that 95% of tumor blood supply of established metastases came from the hepatic artery and only 5% from the portal vein[4]. From a physiologically based pharmacokinetic model, it was calculated that only 5-Fluorouracil (5-FU) shows a significant increase in response rate in the treatment of metastatic hepatic cancer when infused intra-arterially compared to systemic routes of administration[5]. The benefit of

such treatments is suggested by clinical reports of objective
response rates of 35-83% in uncontrolled series[6],[7],[8].

In experimental tumor models, trials can easily be designed
in a reproducible manner. Figure 2 shows the results of continuous 5-FU treatment for 7 days on induced liver metastases in
a rat model. The intra-arterial treatment gave significantly
better results than other routes of administration. This was
however not translated in a significantly improved survival[9].

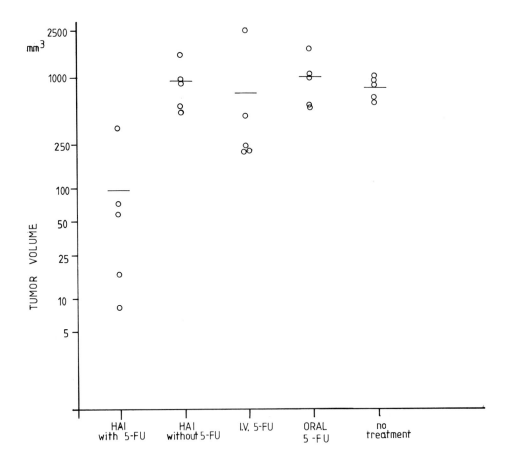

FIGURE 2. Tumor growth, according to treatment.

On the horizontal axis, 5 groups of 5 rats each, killed on
the 11th day after inoculation of 2×10^6 Walker 256 cells
into the median lobe of the liver. On the vertical axis, the
volume of the tumor plotted in natural logarithms. The intra-
arterial treatment with 5-FU gave significantly better results
than the other methods (P < 0.05).

The sole exception to successful clinical series of therapy
in selected patients with hepatic cancer was a randomized trial
of hepatic arterial versus intravenous chemotherapy for metastatic colorectal carcinoma. A modest improvement in objective
response (34 versus 23% for the systemically treated group)
was not translated into improved survival[10]. However, if survival alone is used as an endpoint, the evaluation of quality
of life may be overlooked. In the absence of adequate reproducible guidelines for evaluating the quality of life, response to infused drugs is assessed from two parameters:
1) the percentage of patients showing a major response and
2) the median survival. In table I a number of reports on
hepatic arterial infusion therapy is summarized.
Generally, responses (± 59%) and median survival data (± 12
months) are somewhat better than those in the Grage study and
far better than reported response rates (15-20%) after systemic 5-FU administration[11]. Especially when compared to series
of patients with untreated hepatic metastases which reveal a
median survival of 5-6 months[20,22], hepatic arterial chemotherapy *seems* to be effective. The published reports however,
generally provide inadequate information for unequivocal estimates of improvement in survival of the whole group of patients with hepatic metastases following chemotherapy. When
the high degree of patient selection necessary before administration of hepatic artery infusion is considered, it is clear
that the data on response to this procedure would not necessarily apply to patients with hepatic metastases as a whole.

New directions of improving treatment results
    Because of the limited improvement of therapeutic benefit
by hepatic arterial infusion, methods were developed to increase drug action or exposure time. The concept of *biochemical modulation* has been involved with sequential or concurrent
use of agents which modify the action of fluoropyrimidines.
Examples are the addition of allopurinol to modulate 5-FU
toxicity, permitting a doubling of the maximum tolerated
dose[28] or delayed uridine rescue[29]. Also attempts to improve

Table 1. Hepatic artery infusion chemotherapy with 5-FU or its analogues for liver metastases of colo-rectal origin.

Report	No. of evaluated patients	Response rate (%)	Median survival (months)
Sullivan et al 1965[12]	39	62	19
Brennan et al 1967[13]	13	70	=
Burrows et al 1967[14]	121	59	=
Watkins et al 1970[15]	82	73	15
Massey et al 1971[16]	10	42	11
Freckman 1971[17]	271	36	12
Tandon et al 1973[18]	67	64	8
Cady et al 1974[6]	51	71	16
Buroker et al[+] 1976[19]	21	35	8
Ansfield et al 1978[7]	521	> 60	8
Ariel et al 1978[20]	65	60	13
Petrek et al 1979[21]	24	=	9
Grage et al* 1979[10]	31	34	11
Reed et al 1981[22]	88	73	10
Smiley et al 1981[23]	110	26	8
Ensminger et al 1982[24]	60	83	21
Balch et al 1983[25]	81	88	26
total	1655	average 59	average 12

* randomized vs. i.v. 5-FU
+ after prior systemic 5-FU

the activity of 5-FU has been attempted by the addition of
PALA (by inhibiting of *de novo* pyrimidine synthesis[30,31]) or
sequential methotrexate by synergism[32,33]. These strategies
have not proved conspicuously successful to date.

Increasing drug exposure

As was shown in a pharmacokinetic model, concentration of
drug in the arterial watershed is inversely related to the
blood flow rate through the infused artery (assuming high total
body clearance). Decreasing the blood flow rate by 90% should
increase the arterial concentration of drug by about tenfold[34].
Many methods to decrease arterial blood flow have been described such as: hepatic artery ligation[35], infusion of vasocon-
stricting agents[36], and microspheres[37]. Results to date, however, are limited.
New impetus has been given to long-term drug exposure using a
totally implantable drug infusion pump as recently reported in
Phase II trials with promising results[24].

THE STEP TO ISOLATED LIVER PERFUSION

All described methods have one starting point. One attempts
to expose the tumor to more drug than otherwise possible. Efforts have been devoted to generate cytotoxic drug levels in
the target organ with lower, non toxic systemic drug levels;
i.e. dose limiting toxicity should be regional (liver), rather
than systemic (bone marrow and gut). This is the practical use
of the steep dose-response relationship of antitumor agents as
depicted in Fig. 3.
The creation of high local concentrations can be seen as high
dose chemotherapy with high local effects combined with relatively low systemic effects; the latter is also the effect
which can be observed after systemic administration of the
antitumor agent in low doses. To exploit this more readily
methods have been developed to isolate the hepatic circulation thus increasing drug dose without unacceptable toxicity.

298

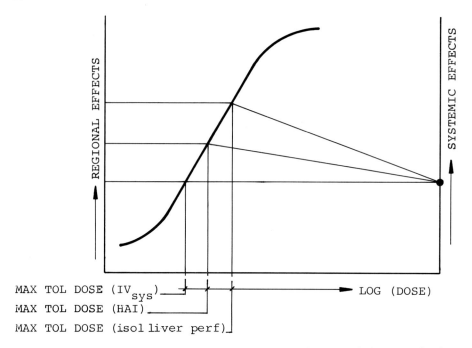

FIGURE 3. Regional cancerchemotherapy allows the use of the upper region of the steep dose-response relationship observed after systemic administration of a given antitumor agent.

In animals the techniques of hepatic vascular isolation have been shown to be technically difficult and numerous problems have been encountered[38].

We developed an easy applicable technique of isolated liver perfusion for one hour in pigs with the use of a specially developed intracaval shunt. Since the pig has a hepatic physiology and anatomy similar to the human these studies provide useful information as to the clinical applicability; supplementary information was obtained to evaluate the rational of maximizing dose by isolated liver perfusion.

The Leiden experience with isolated liver perfusion

Yorkshire pigs with an average weight of 24 ± 4 kg were used throughout the study. The operative technique which proved successful employed a double-lumen intracaval shunt made of flexible silastic with a length of 18 cm and a diameter of 1 cm. After introduction into the inferior vena cava this shunt allows complete collection of hepatic venous blood while permitting undisturbed flow from infra - to suprahepatic caval vein. Isolation was established after tighting a vascular tourniquet around the suprahepatic caval vein and clamping coeliac axis and gastric vessels. Perfusion was performed through the common hepatic artery (Figure 4). The portal flow was shunted, during perfusion, to the inner channel of the intracaval shunt. This technique of isolated liver perfusion proved to be safe and resulted in uniformous survival if applied without the use of chemotherapy (an extensive report on the technique is given by Van de Velde et al[39]).

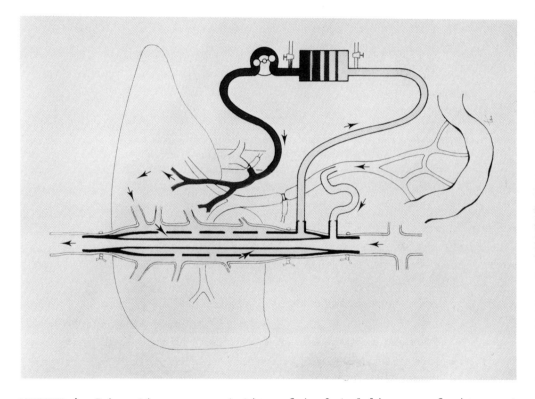

FIGURE 4. Schematic representation of isolated liver perfusion.

During one hour normothermic low flow perfusions, various dosages of 5-FU (20-40-80 mg/kg body weight) were administered to the isolated circuit. Samples were taken from blood (isolated and systemic circuit), bile and liver by wedge biopsy, at various intervals during and after perfusion for 5-FU analysis. Concentrations of 5-FU were determined by High Performance Liquid Chromatography (HPLC) according to a standardized method[40]. The measured concentrations were compared with those after hepatic artery infusion (without isolation of the liver) and with intravenous (jugular vein) administration.

Since the most extensive clinical experience with hepatic arterial infusion of 5-FU has been reported by Ansfield and associates[7] with a dose of 20 mg/kg, this dose was adopted for our first set of experiments. With this dose toxic reactions were observed in 30% of pigs without toxic deaths. In the initial series of Ansfield using an intravenous loading course, a 3% incidence of toxic death was observed[42].

The results of HPLC assays from blood samples from the general circulation are shown in Figure 5.

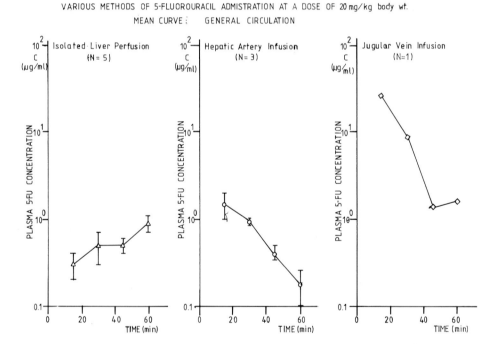

VARIOUS METHODS OF 5-FLUOROURACIL ADMISTRATION AT A DOSE OF 20 mg/kg body wt.
MEAN CURVE: GENERAL CIRCULATION

FIGURE 5.

An average plasma concentration of 0.5 µg/ml 5-FU was found during isolated liver perfusion. This represented 0.2% of the concentration measured in the isolated circuit. This extremely low leakage from the isolated liver circuit to the general circulation was confirmed by peripheral measurements of Tc^{99m} labeled erythrocytes given to the isolated circuit. This indicates that vascular isolation of the liver was indeed established. The slope in the two 5-FU curves for non-isolated administration indicates extensive total body clearance. The higher excretion of 5-FU in bile as represented in Figure 6 during isolated liver perfusion is in agreement with the larger supply of 5-FU to the liver. Despite the much higher concentration of the perfusate, the assays performed on liver tissue after wedge biopsies show no difference in favour of local-regional administration methods (Figure 7).

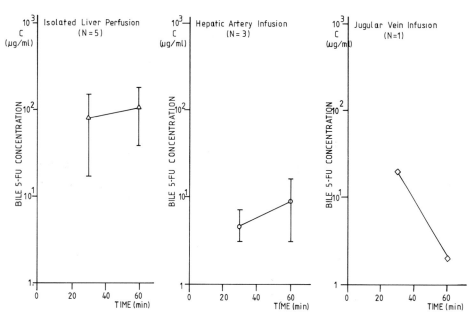

VARIOUS METHODS OF 5-FLUOROURACIL ADMINISTRATION AT A DOSE OF 20 mg/kg body wt.
MEAN CURVE: BILE

FIGURE 6.

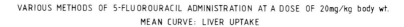

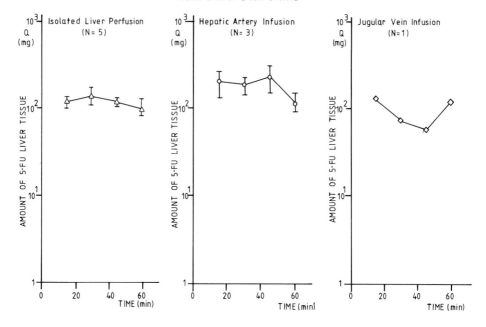

FIGURE 7.

Except for the much lower systemic concentration of 5-FU no
clear advantage of isolated liver perfusion as judged from
5-FU assays was observed in the 40 mg/kg body weight set of
experiments (Figures 8, 9 10).

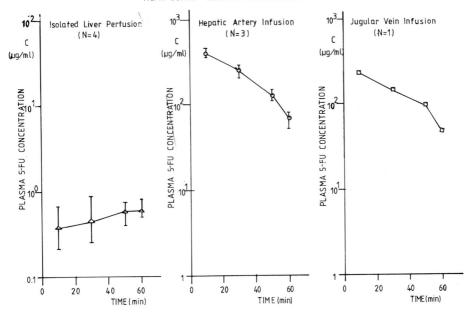

FIGURE 8.

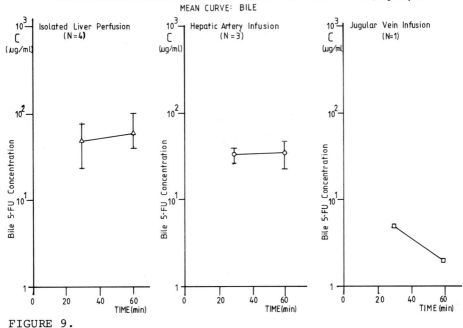

FIGURE 9.

304

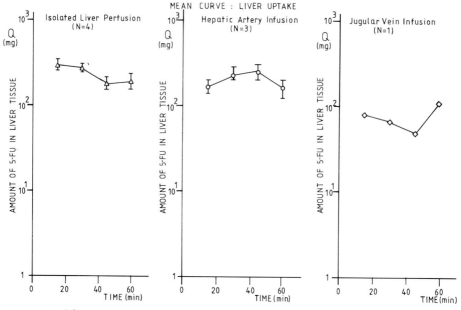

FIGURE 10.

At a dose of 80 mg/kg body weight, increases in concentration with isolated liver perfusion are clearly demonstrated (Figs. 11, 12, 13).

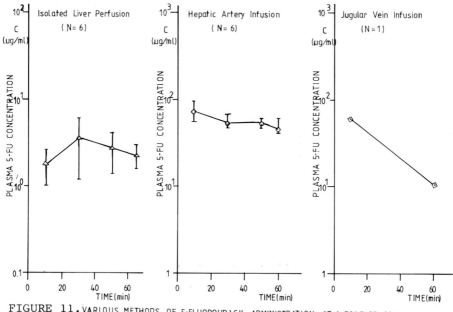

FIGURE 11. VARIOUS METHODS OF 5-FLUOROURACIL ADMINISTRATION AT A DOSE OF 80mg/kg body wt.
MEAN CURVE: GENERAL CIRCULATION

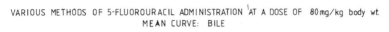

VARIOUS METHODS OF 5-FLUOROURACIL ADMINISTRATION AT A DOSE OF 80mg/kg body wt.
MEAN CURVE: BILE

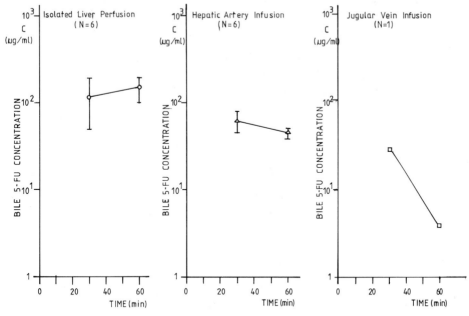

FIGURE 12.

VARIOUS METHODS OF 5-FLUOROURACIL ADMINISTRATION AT A DOSE OF 80mg/kg body wt.
MEAN CURVE: LIVER UPTAKE

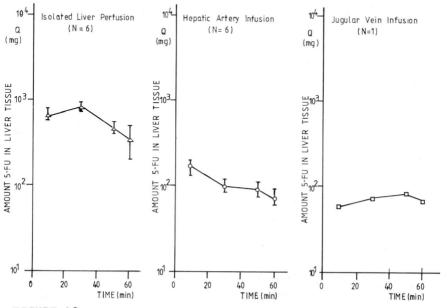

FIGURE 13.

The systemic concentration during isolated liver perfusion remains low. This dose is obviously too toxic after non-isolated administration. This large supply of 5-FU by isolated perfusion is translated to high 5-FU excretion by the liver and a significant higher uptake in liver tissue. It seems, therefore, that four times the conventional dose of 5-FU (4 x 20 mg/kg body weight) gives a measurable difference in amount of 5-FU in the target organ whereas systemic concentrations remain low.

How were these findings related to toxicity

Clinically 5-FU toxicity is for the major part confined to the gastrointestinal tract. The (infant) pig used in these studies has a gut length of approximately 15 meters. They were very susceptible to adhaesion formation, strangulation and invagination.

The three pigs which were treated by peripheral vein infusion died at day 21 (20 mg/kg: ileus without histological deviation of the gut), day 10 (40 mg/kg: ileus with gut infarction) and day 4 (80 mg/kg: no histological deviations but renal failure with urea 9.9 mmol/l, creatinine 769 μmol/l postoperatively. The animals treated by H.A.I. at a dose of 20 mg/kg and 40 mg/kg all survived without signs of gastrointestinal toxicity. A dose of 80 mg/kg body weight evidently was too toxic. Uniformly death at an average of 3.5 days postoperatively was observed. These data strongly suggest a clear dose-toxicity relation.

Isolated liver perfusion resulted in one postoperative death at day 58 as a result of pneumonia in the group treated with 20 mg/kg body weight. No deaths were seen in the 40 mg/kg dose group and 3/6 postoperative deaths occurred in the 80 mg/kg group (one gut malrotation day 2 postoperative, one gut invagination day 7 postoperative and one accidental loss due to an open connection of the carotid artery line). Also, within this group, toxicity may be responsible for some early deaths. The concentration of 5-FU in the isolated circuit averaged 1311 μg/ml in the 80 mg/kg dose group. After termina-

tion of the isolated liver perfusion no washout was performed
so that a minimal dose of 20 mg 5-FU/kg was released systemically. The drug released combined with the major operation is
likely responsible for the death rate. Presently, we always
perform a washout after perfusion so that only 6% of the perfusate volume enters the systemic circulation as is assessed
by Tc^{99m} assays. Hopefully this will result in better survival rates at high dose isolated liver perfusion.

These data indicate three major points:

1. Isolated liver perfusion with high dose 5-FU is feasible
   in an animal model which is anatomically and physiologically related to man.
2. Liver uptake in high dose isolated liver perfusion of 5-FU
   is significantly increased compared to other routes of administration.
3. Toxicity is related to the route of administration and so-
   far is confined to the gastrointestinal tract. After washout this toxicity seems to be diminished.

*How do these results relate to tumor control in the clinical
situation*

The initial clinical investigations of 5-FU demonstrated
frightening and frequently lethal toxicity establishing narrow therapeutic margin of this agent[43,44]. The main impact
after 20 years of intense investigation is that much has been
learned to reduce toxicity and optimize the limited therapeutic benefit. The aim of isolated perfusion is to create a
much higher dose than otherwise possible in liver metastases.
A major drawback of the experiments described above is that
metastases were not present and results cannot be translated
into improvement of survival. Our results indicate high concentrations of 5-FU within liver cells (about half of the
total amount administered) during liver perfusion. Thus far
no clear relationship has been established between tumor effect and intracellular concentration of 5-FU or its metabolites. Examination of the activities of several enzymes involved in 5-FU metabolism[45-50], of inhibition of DNA synthesis in the presence of 5-FU[51,52], of FdUMP and dUMP pools

following drug administration[53-55], and incorporation of 5-FU into RNA[56-58] revealed the numerous parameters involved in 5-FU cytotoxic action.

A unified mechanism for 5-FU action may not exist. It appears possible that the biochemical determinants of 5-FU vary in different cells as a result of differing susceptibilities to potential cytotoxic events and variation in 5-FU metabolism. Processes of activation (anabolic pool) and of degradation (catabolic pool) have been investigated, and several authors have pointed out the importance of the catabolic pathway to explain therapeutic failures with 5-FU[59-61]. Therefore observations of a fourfold higher uptake of ^{14}C-labeled 5-FU (15 mg/kg) as compared to other routes of administration[62] does not suggest automatically important clinical implications at these low doses, since no estimation of degradation of 5-FU can be made.

Our present efforts to test the efficacy of high dose isolated liver perfusion are devoted to (1) measurement of the metabolites of 5-FU and (2) testing isolated liver perfusion in a rat model with liver metastases of colonic origin.

ARE CLINICAL STUDIES WITH ISOLATED LIVER PERFUSION REALISTIC?

In terms of technical feasibility it seems reasonable to start Phase I studies with isolated liver perfusions in humans. We therefore developed a number of shunts suitable for clinical use. Aigner and coworkers from W. Germany demonstrated feasibility already with clinical isolated liver perfusion using a dose of 300 - 1000 mg 5-FU with promising results[63,64]. Case selection for this major operation is needed. A randomized Phase II study at a dose yet to be determined will be needed to determine if isolated liver perfusion is worth the efforts of the investigator and the patient with liver metastases.

Only by testing hypotheses will cancer research progress. In isolated liver perfusion dose-effect relation is the hypothesis to be tested. Especially if better drugs, even with high systemic toxicity, are developed, a clinical method of application has successfully been developed. These drugs may be used either alone or in combination with other treatments.

REFERENCES

1. Frei E III, Canellos GP. 1980. Dose: a critical factor in cancer chemotherapy. Am J Med 69: 585-594.
2. Southers Research Institute. Informal Reports to the Division of Cancer Treatment of the National Cancer Institute, Birmingham, Alabama, 1971-1982.
3. Ansfield F, Klotz J, Nealon T, et al. 1977. A Phase III study comparing the clinical utility of four regimens of 5-fluorouracil. A preliminary report. Cancer 39: 34-40.
4. Healy JE. 1965. Vascular patterns in human metastatic liver tumors. Surg Gynecol Obstet 12: 1187-1193.
5. Chen HSG and Gross JF. 1980. Intra-arterial infusion of anticancer drugs: theoretic aspects of drug delivery and review of responses. Cancer Treat Rep 64: 31-40.
6. Cady B, Oberfield RA. 1974. Regional infusion chemotherapy of hepatic metastases from carcinoma of the colon. Am J Surg 127: 220-227.
7. Ansfield IJ, Ramirez G. 1978. The clinical results of 5-fluorouracil intra hepatic arterial infusion in 528 patients with metastatic cancer. In: Ariel IM, ed., Progress in clinical cancer, vol. 7. New York, Grune & Stratton, pp. 201-206.
8. Huberman MS. 1983. Comparison of systemic chemotherapy with hepatic arterial infusion in metastatic colorectal carcinoma. Semin Oncol 10: 238-248.
9. Cotino H, Zwaveling A. 1976. Treatment of experimental liver tumors by continuous intra-arterial chemotherapy. Eur J Cancer 12: 177-180.
10. Grage TB, Vassipoulos PP, Shingleton WW, et al. 1979. Results of a prospective randomized study of hepatic artery infusion with 5-fluorouracil versus intravenous 5-fluorouracil in patients with hepatic metastases from colorectal cancer. A central Oncology Group study. Surgery 86: 550-555.
11. Davis HL. 1982. Chemotherapy of large bowel cancer. Cancer 50: 2638-2646.
12. Sullivan RD and Zurek WZ. 1965. Chemotherapy for liver cancer by protacted ambulatory infusion. JAMA 194: 481-486.
13. Brennan MJ, Talley RW, Drake EH et al. 1967. 5-Fluorouracil treatment of liver metastases by continuous hepatic artery infusion via Cournand Catheter. Ann Surg 158: 405-419.
14. Burrows JH, Talley RW, Drake et al. 1967. Infusion of fluorinated pyrimidines into hepatic artery for treatment of metastatic carcinoma of the liver. Cancer 20: 1886-1892.
15. Watkins E Jr, Khazei AM, Nahra KS. 1970. Surgical basis for arterial infusion chemotherapy and disseminated carcinoma of the liver. Surg Gynecol Obstet 130: 580-605.
16. Massey WH, Fletcher WS, Judkins MP, et al. 1971. Hepatic artery infusion for metastatic malignancy using percutaneously placed catheters. Am J Surg 121: 160-164.
17. Freckman HA. 1971. Chemotherapy for metastatic colorectal liver carcinoma by intra-aortic infusion. Cancer 28: 1152-1160.
18. Tandon RN, Bunnell IL, Copper RG. 1973. The treatment of

310

metastatic carcinoma of the liver by the percutaneous selective hepatic artery infusion of 5-fluorouracil. Surgery 73: 118-121.

19. Buroker T, Samson M, Correa J, et al. 1976. Hepatic artery infusion of 5-FUDR after prior systemic 5-fluorouracil. Cancer Treat Rep 60: 1277-1279.

20. Ariel IM, Padula G. 1978. Treatment of symptomatic metastatic cancer to the liver from primary colon and rectal cancer by intra-arterial administration of chemotherapy and radioactive isotopes. In: Ariel IM, ed., Progress in clinical cancer, vol. 7. New York, Grune & Stratton, pp. 247-254.

21. Petrek JA, Minton JP. 1979. Treatment of hepatic metastases by percutaneous hepatic arterial infusion. Cancer 43: 2182-2188.

22. Reed ML, Vaitkevicus VK, Al-Sarraf M, et al. 1981. The practicality of chronic hepatic artery infusion therapy of primary and metastatic hepatic malignancies: Ten year results of 124 patients in a prospective protocol. Cancer 47: 402-409.

23. Smiley S, Schouten J, Chang A, et al. 1981. Intra hepatic infusion with 5-FU for liver metastases of colorectal carcinoma. Proc Am Soc Clin Oncol 22: 391.

24. Ensminger W, Niederhuber J, Gyves J, et al. 1982. Effective control of liver metastases from colon cancer with an implanted system for hepatic arterial chemotherapy. Proc Am Soc Clin Oncol 1: 94.

25. Balch CM, Urist MM, Soong SJ, McGregor M. 1983. A prospective Phase II clinical trial of continuous FUDR regional chemotherapy for colorectal metastases to the liver using a totally implantable drug infusion pump. Ann Surg 198: 567-573.

26. Jaffe BM, Donegan WL, Watson F, et al. 1968. Factors influencing survival in patients with untreated hepatic metastases. Surg Gynecol Obstet 127: 1-11.

27. Bengmark S, Hafstrom L. 1969. The natural history of primary and secondary malignant tumors of the liver. 1. The prognosis for patients with hepatic metastases from colonic and rectal carcinoma by laparotomy. Cancer 23: 198-202.

28. Howell SB, Wung WE, Taetle R, et al. 1981. Modulation of 5-fluorouracil toxicity by allopurinol in man. Cancer 48: 1281-1289.

29. Martin DS, Stolfi RL, Swayer RC, et al. 1982. High-Dose 5-Fluorouracil with delayed Urine 'Rescue' in Mice. Cancer Res 42: 3964-3670.

30. Rubin J, Purvis J, Britell JC, et al. 1981. Phase II study of PALA in advanced large bowel carcinoma. Cancer Treat Rep 65: 335-336.

31. Ardalan B, Jamin D, Jayaram HN, Presant CA. 1984. Phase I study of continuous infusion PALA and 5-FU. Cancer Treat Rep 68: 531-534.

32. Cadman F, Davis L, Heimer R. 1979. Enhanced 5-fluorouracil nucleotide formation following methotrexate: Biochemical explanation for drug synergism. Science 205: 1135-1137.

33. Browman GP. 1984. Clinical application of the concept of Methotrexate Plus 5-FU Sequence Dependent. 'Synergy'. How

good is the Evidence? Cancer Treat Rep 68: 465-470.
34. Ensminger WD, Gyves JW. 1984. Regional cancer chemotherapy. Cancer Treat Rep 68: 101-115.
35. Ramming KP, Sparks FC, Eilbert FR, et al. 1976. Hepatic artery ligation and 5-fluorouracil infusion for metastatic colon carcinoma and primary hepatoma. Am J Surg 132: 236-242.
36. Iwaki A, Nagasue N, Kobayoshi M, et al. 1978. Intra-arterial chemotherapy with concomitant use of vasoconstrictors for liver cancer. Cancer Treat Rep 62: 145-146.
37. Dakhil S, Ensminger W, Cho K, et al. 1982. Improved regional selectivity of hepatic arterial BCNU with degradable microspheres. Cancer 50: 631-635.
38. Boddie AW Jr, Booker L, Mullins JD, et al. 1979. Hepatic hyperthermia by total isolation and regional perfusion in vivo. J Surg Res 26: 447-457.
39. Van de Velde CJH, Kothuis BJL, Barenbrug HWM, et al. 1984. A successful technique of in vivo isolated chemotherapeutic liver perfusion in the pig with survival. Submitted for publ. J Surg Res.
40. Tjaden UR, De Bruin EA, Van de Velde CJH, et al. 1984. Determinations of 5-Fluorouracil and related compounds by High Performance Liquid Chromotography. Submitted for publ. J Chromatogr Biomed Appl.
41. Ramirez G, Ansfield FJ. 1982. Chemotherapy of liver metastases. In: Weiss L, Gilbert HA, Hall GK, eds., Boston, Med Publ, pp. 348-359.
42. Ansfield FJ, Curreri AR. 1959. Further clinical studies with 5-fluorouracil. J Natl Cancer Inst 22: 497-507.
43. Curreri AR, Ansfield FJ, McIver FA, et al. 1958. Clinical studies with 5-fluorouracil. Cancer Res 18: 478-484.
44. Vaitkevicus VK, Brennan MJ, Bechet VL, et al. 1961. Clinical evaluation of cancer chemotherapy with 5-fluorouracil. Cancer 14: 131-152.
45. Danenberg PV, Langenbach RJ, Heidelberger C. 1974. Structures of reversible and irreversible complexes of thymidilate synthetase and fluorinated pyrimidine nucleotides. Biochemistry 13: 926-933.
46. Everson R, Kessel D, Hall T. 1970. Enzymatic determinants of responsiveness of the LPC-1 plasma cell neoplasm to fluorouracil and fluorodeoxyuridine. Biochem Pharmacol 19: 2932-2934.
47. Kessel D, Hall T, Reyes P. 1969. Metabolism of uracil and 5-fluorouracil in P-388 murine leukemia cells. Mol Pharmacol 5: 481-486.
48. Kessel D, Wodinsky I. 1969. Thymidine kinase as a determinant of the response to 5-fluoro-2-deoxyuridine in transplantable murine leukemias. Mol Pharmacol 6: 251-254.
49. Nahas A, Savlov ED, Hall TC. 1974. Phosphoribosyltransferase in colon tumor and normal mucosa as an aid in adjuvant chemotherapy with 5-FU. Cancer Chemother Rep 58: 909-912.
50. Reyes P, Hall TC. 1969. Synthesis of 5-fluorodeoxyuridine 5'-phosphate a pyrimidine phosphoribosyltransferase of mammelian origin. II. Correlation between tumor levels of the enzyme and the 5-fluorouracil-promoted increase in

survival of tumorbearing mice. Biochem Pharmacol 18: 2587-2590.

51. Klubes P, Connelly K, Cerna I, Mandel H. 1978. Effects of 5-fluorouracil on 5-fluorodeoxyuridine 5'-monophosphate and 2-deoxyuridine 5'-monophosphate pools, and DNA synthesis in solid mouse L1210 and rat Walker 256 tumors. Cancer Res 38: 2325-2331.

52. Myers CE, Young RC, Chabner BA. 1976. Kinetic alterations induced by 5-fluorouracil in bone marrow, intestinal mucosa and tumor. Cancer Res 36: 1653-1658.

53. Ardalan B, Buscaglia M, Schein PS. 1978. Tumor 5-fluorodeoxyridilate concentration as a determinant of 5-fluorouracil response. Biochem Pharmacol 27: 2009-2013.

54. Myers CE, Young RC, Chabner BA. 1975. Biochemical determinants of 5-fluorouracil in vivo: the role of deoxyuridilate pool expansion. J Clin Invest 56: 1231-1238.

55. Myers CE, Young RC, Johns DG, Chabner BA. 1974. Assay of 5-fluorodeoxyuridine 5'-monophosphate and deoxyuridine 5'-monophosphate pools following 5-fluorouracil. Cancer Res 34: 2683-2688.

56. Wilkinson DS, Pitot HC. 1973. Inhibition of ribisomal ribonucleic acid maturation in Novikoff hepatoma cells by 5-fluorouracil and 4-fluorouridine. J Biol Chem 248: 63-68.

57. Wilkinson DS, Tisty TD, Hanas RJ. 1975.The inhibition of ribosomal RNA synthesis and maturation in Novikoff hepatoma cells by 5-fluorouridine. Cancer Res 35: 3014-3020.

58. Mandel HG. 1981. The target cell determinants of the antitumor actions of 5-FU: DoesFU incorporation into RNA play a role? Cancer Treat Rep 65: 63-71.

59. Chaudhuri NK, Mukherjee KL, Heidelberger C. 1958. Studies of fluorinated pyrimidines (VII): the degradative pathway. Biochem Pharmacol 1: 328-341.

60. Mukherjee KL, Boohar J, Wentland D. 1963. Studies on fluorinated pyrimidines (XVI). Metabolism of 5-fluorouracil-2-C^{14} and 5-fluoro-2'-deoxyuridine-2-C^{14} in cancer patients. Cancer Res 23: 39-66.

61. Sadee W, Wong CG. 1977. Pharmacokinetics of 5-fluorouracil: inter-relationship with biochemical kinetics in monitoring therapy. Clin Pharmacokinet 2: 437-450.

62. Stone RT, Jabour A, Wilson SE, Rangel DM. 1980. Uptake of 5-fluorouracil during isolated perfusion of the canine liver. J Surg Oncol 13: 347-353.

63. Aigner K, Walther H, Tonn J, et al. 1983. First experimental and clinical results of isolated liver perfusion with cytotoxics in metastases from colorectal primary. In: Rentchnick P, Senn HJ, eds., Recent results in cancer research, vol. 86. Berlin, Springer Verlag, pp. 99-102.

64. Aigner KR, Tonn JC, Walther H, et al, 1984. The isolated liver perfusion technique for high-dose chemotherapy of metastases from colorectal cancer. Two years' clinical experience. In: Van de Velde CJH, Sugarbaker PH, eds., Liver metastasis. The Hague, Martinus Nijhoff, Chapter 29.

THE USE OF MICROSPHERES IN THE TREATMENT OF LIVER
METASTASES

J.G. McVie, J.M.V. Burgers, C. Hoefnagel and E. Tomlinson,

1. INTRODUCTION

It is a sad fact that the last ten years has seen no major
improvement in the medical treatment of liver metastasis. Hopes
for new superactive agents have been dashed in a wave of reality,
emphasized by the increased attention to the development of
safer analogues of existing drugs and better ways of targeting
the same. It has to be admitted that the use of either of those
aforementioned manipulations will at best only produce a small
increment in therapeutic ratio. Any such improvement however in
the field of cytostatic therapy is welcome as there is no other
comparable area where the margin between toxicity and effect is
so fine. Until a suitable tumor-specific target is identified,
unique and novel anti-tumor drugs will probably continue to be
stumbled on by chance. Until such time as an active new compound
is found, it seems appropriate to continue to improve the delivery
of the existing compounds to the required site, in the hope that
increased dose of the drug at the site of action will result in
an increased antitumor effect. The evidence for such dose-response
effect is in fact rather weak except perhaps for 5-fluorouracil
and coloncancer, and doxorubicin and softtissue sarcomas.

2. WHAT ARE MICROSPHERES?

At a recent international meeting, the first to address the
area of microspheres, it was commonly agreed that a microsphere
was a particle of between 0.02-300 /u, the core material of which
encompassed a range of biodegradable matrices such as lipoprotein,

gelatin, albumin, starch and ethylcellulose. Microspheres are
solid and monolithic and they can be used to carry a variety
of substances. They can for instance carry a cytostatic drug or
a radioisotope, or they can carry a combination of a magnetic
metal plus a cytostatic, or a cytostatic plus an immunoglobulin,
or a magnetic substance and a variety of immunoglobulins.
Microspheres can be used as carriers for a variety of drugs
delivered in a variety of different ways, e.g. intraperitoneally,
intravenously, intramuscularly, intra-arterially, into lymphatics
or directly into a joint or an eye or a tumor. In order to target
to liver metastases, two main routes of injection have been
suggested: intravenously for small particles up to 2/u - these
particles escape through lungs and they end up in the reticuloendothelial system or monocyte phagocytic system and then may
release their loaded drug; or else more commonly microspheres
of a larger size may be injected intra-arterially with the aim
of reaching a high dose directly at the target.

3. WHY MICROSPHERES?

Microspheres are probably the most stable delivery system yet
developed (1). Microspheres can be sterilized, can be freeze-
dried and stored, they have a shelf life which is of practical
value for the pharmacist and clinician (in contradistinction
to the majority of liposomes). Release from microspheres is
predictable and dependable; microspheres have a capacity for
high uptake of drug (payload), and they can be used for the
carriage of water-insoluble or water-soluble drugs. They are to
a large extent non-allergenic, in other words they do not provoke
allergic reactions in the host, and they have bio-compatible
surface properties and most indeed are bio-degradable within
a short space of time.

4. WHAT IS TARGETING?

Targeting implies a degree of concentration of the drug to be
applied at the organ or preferably at the tumor within an organ

at higher concentration than in the organs of most likely toxicity. The present generation of cytostatic drugs suffer from a variety of problems. Some have solubility problems, some have low absorption characteristics with high protein binding, many are short-lived in the plasma, and have large volumes of distribution. A good example is adriamycin which has a hypothetical volume distribution of over 500 litres and therefore is diluted very rapidly through body water. These molecules are often large and have difficulty in transversing all the anatomical or cellular barriers which protect the tumor. In the absence of unique targets, as mentioned above, targeting relies on mechanical tricks such as catheterisation of the arteries leading to organs, or else the localisation of drug-carrying spheres by the use of externally applied magnets which attract inbuilt ferrous particles for instance, or perhaps, for the future, the increased adhesion of microspheres to tumor cells may be arranged by mediation through a monoclonal antibody raised against tumor-associated antigens.

5. APPLICATIONS OF MICROSPHERES TO LIVER METASTASIS

The first and most widely used application of microspheres is in the detection of liver metastasis. Radioisotope-labelled microspheres have been used for many years now to detect space-occupying lesions in the liver. Lately quantitative hepatic artery perfusion scintigraphy has been refined so that by the means of arterial injection, elegant angiograms can be achieved (2), and with the use of quantitative gamma-camera equipment an assessment can be made of the relative uptake of microspheres within tumor capillary bed and normal liver. There is a general agreement that in around 80% of liver metastases the extra capillary network (perhaps provoked by release of angiogenesis factors by tumors) causes the holdup of 20 μ microspheres in a six- to tenfold concentration over the normal adjacent liver. This has been the basis of the work which my group has mainly addressed, i.e. the targeting of microspheres of 20 μ loaded

with cytostatic drugs, directly through the hepatic artery. It
is clear that the increased concentration of microspheres to
liver metastases is a) not universal, b) does not hold for lar
tumors (10 cm or greater), and c) is liable to variation and
subsequent shunting if more microspheres are injected sequentially too closely after each other. The present work which wi.
be further sketched later in this chapter, has mainly been
related to the drug-release characteristics of the microsphere:
in an attempt to perfect a drug-delivery system which gives a
constant release of intact drug for a particular length of tim

Larger microspheres (40 μ) are being used mixed with cytostatic drugs in a variety of trials in the hope that by blockiı
arterial capillary junctions a drug included in the mixture wi.
be rapidly taken up from capillaries due to the induced stasis
(3). Even larger microspheres (200 μ) have been used with
incorporated mitomycin to induce part infarction in tumor tissı
and part anti-tumor lysis (4). Microspheres have also been usec
to target a radioisotope like ^{32}P (5), and the potential exists
for the application of monoclonal antibodies against cellsurfac
components of tumor cells in liver (6) - examples might be
alpha-foetoprotein, carcinoembryonic antigen and tumor-related
glycoproteins.

6. MANUFACTURE OF MICROSPHERES

Microspheres can be made simply by producing water in oil
emulsions followed by stabilisation with the use of heat, or
of one of a variety of crosslinking agents. The choice of
stabilisation is important because anthracyclines are destroyed
by heat, and therefore require to be built in to albumin microspheres, using a chemical crosslinker. We have used 2,3-butadio
or glutaraldehyde. Methotrexate on the other hand is inactivate
by the use of the latter technique and therefore should be
built in to microspheres by the use of heat. Microspheres can
also be manufactured by polymerisation and coacervation. This
can lead to microspheres of similar size but of dissimilar

molecular weight. This must be carefully controlled as molecular weight is as important as microsphere diameter in determining the clearance of microspheres. Up until now methotrexate, doxorubicin, actinomycin, L-asparaginase, mitomycin, 5-fluorouracil, bleomycin, BCNU, have all been successfully incorporated into a microsphere delivery system. Albumin has been favoured by most investigators as the carrier material of choice, probably due to the high payload possible (up to 35% of the weight of the carrier can be drug), and because the release characteristics of intact drugs from albumin microspheres have been more extensively studied than for other materials. We have succeeded in producing microspheres of uniform size and then confirmed the importance of size in determining not only distribution in the body, as mentioned previously, but the rate of release of drugs under steady-state conditions. Important factors which influence size include the design of the manufacturing vessel, the nature of the oilbase used, the stirring speed of the water in oil emulsion, the amounts of oil, albumin and aqueous phase volume, the use of surfactants, and the presence or absence of chemical crosslinkers (7).

Microspheres can be lyophilised and stored for many months without deterioration in their properties. On reconstitution they will swell due to the uptake of water, and this will result in an increase in diameter of 40% if the microsphere is pure albumin. Drug-containing microspheres however swell in a linear fashion dependent on the size of the freeze-dried microspheres. 5 micron bearing microspheres will increase in size by 25%, whereas 35-40/u microspheres will increase by 80% of their diameter. As it is the reconstituted microsphere diameter that determines the fate of the spheres, this factor has to be borne carefully in mind.

7. DRUG RELEASE

As the advantage of drug-containing microspheres over a mixture of empty microspheres and drugs is the control of release of the drug and therefore the control of exposure of target tissue to the drug, we have carefully considered the factors which affect these parameters by using a simple equation:

$$Q_t = Ae^{-\alpha t} + Be^{-\beta t} + C$$

where Q_t = amount of drug in the microspheres at time t
  A,B = constants of the fast and slow release of drug from the microspheres, respectively
  α,β = rate constants of the fast and slow release, respectively
  C = amount of drug remaining in the microspheres after reaching the detection limit of the drug in the eluent

The mutually dependent constants A, B, C, α and β can be calculated using a computerized least squares procedure with 95% confidence limit and by the "best fit" straight lines through all data points of the plot of the amount of drug in the spheres against time. The mentioned constants characterize completely the fast and slow processes of release of built-in drug from the microspheres.

Analyzing release data of various drug-containing microspheres reveals that:

1. If identically sized microspheres are more stabilised (by raising the concentration of crosslinker (glutaraldehyde) and/or by raising the time of stabilisation), then (i) the amount of drug released in the fast process (determined by A and α) lowers, (ii) the amount of drug released in the slow process is raised (B is raised), while the release in this process becomes slower, and (iii) the amount of drug remaining in the spheres increases.
2. If the amount of drug in the microspheres is raised, then (i) the amount released in the first process increases,

although the release becomes slower, (ii) the amount in the second, slow process is raised while release is getting more sustained and (iii) C, the amount remaining, increases.

3. If the diameter of the microspheres is raised (from 7.5 up to 36/u), then (i) the amount of drug released in the fast process is uninfluenced, (ii) the amount released in the slow process increases and becomes slower with decreasing diameter of the spheres, and (iii) the amount of drug remaining in the microspheres drops to zero with smaller sized microspheres. This indicates that release of drug from the microspheres is diffusion-controlled.

4. Using 2,3-butadione as crosslinking agent, comparable results were obtained for the release from the microspheres.

In general it has been found that for highly water-soluble organic polar drugs their release from chemically stabilised albumin microspheres is biphasic, with a large burst effect taking place. This effect can constitute between 40 and 93% of the initially incorporated drug. The burst effect is extremely reproducible for any given set of manufacturing conditions and is found to be dependent upon the extent of denaturation.

Although the release of less polar drugs from albumin microspheres showed a biphasic release profile, it has been found that the burst effect of these compounds is much lower.

The burst can be avoided by pretreatment of the microspheres (ultrasonication in aqueous media followed by removal of the supernatant). This leads to a release profile similar to normal microspheres (i.e. microspheres without presonication) but without the burst phenomenon.

One of the most important features of the drug release study is that glutaraldehyde, because of the more favourable experimental conditions (particularly the shorter crosslinking times needed and the lower amount of crosslinking agent), is the crosslinker of choice.

The findings obtained from studies of the release of model compounds can be used to predict the release of cytostatics

incorporated in albumin microspheres with respect to extent of
stabilisation, microsphere size and amount of cytostatic
present in the microspheres. Further release studies with a
variety of cytostatic compounds are currently in progress.

8. CLINICAL POTENTIAL

There are no clinical results on the application of intra-
arterial drug-loaded albumin microspheres, at least in the
20μ range. As such spheres however can be easily labelled
with radioisotopes, a variety of gamma-camera studies have been
done to study dose distribution not only after intra-arterial
but also after intravenous injection. These studies confirm the
in vitro characteristics of microspheres, but the finding of
20% of patients who have either no increased uptake of microspheres in their liver metastases, or else a high degree of
arterio-venous shunting, underlines the need for screening of
patients prior to application of this therapy. This caveat
applies equally for the administration of cytostatic drugs
mixed with starch microspheres and this is backed up by actual
clinical results. These starch microspheres are 40μ in
diameter and have a much shorter halflife than those made of
albumin, being broken down by plasma enzymes within 10 minutes
of administration. A variety of drugs have been administered
with starch microspheres (not within the spheres), and the
pharmacokinetic advantage for the technique has been proved
conclusively, e.g. for bischloroethylnitrosourea (BCNU) and
mitomycin by the Ann Arbor group. This group showed that 9×10^6
microspheres/ml injected into the hepatic artery reduced hepatic
flow by 80 to 100% over a period of 15 minutes. Giving 50 mg/m^2
of BCNU mixed with microspheres produced a reduction in leakage
of BCNU through the liver into the systemic circulation of
between 30 to 90% in 5 patients (7). In a further 10 patients
this group studied mitomycin in the same model and this showed
the same degree of protection of the systemic compartment when
10 mg/m^2 mitomycin was given together with 90×10^6 microspheres

(8). Reducing the number of microspheres to 36 x 10^6 did not significantly alter the degree of retention of mitomycin in the liver (the mean reduction in systemic exposure was around 35%), although in all patients studied there was a wide individual difference. Although these pilot studies were carried out to test the feasibility of the technique and the pharmacological hypothesis, clinical observations were made concurrently and although no major clinical responses were noted, toxicity was minor, consisting of a minimal myelosuppression, transient liver pain and reversible elevation of liver transaminases. A randomised trial is now under way in several centres in America and in Scandinavia to test mitomycin plus starch microspheres as a device delivered through the hepatic artery for the treatment of liver metastases.

The major experience in the use of chemo-embolisation, that is large 200/u ethylcellulose microspheres containing mitomycin, comes from Japan (9). Although no pharmacological data has been published to support the use of these spheres in the treatment of liver metastases, this group has done studies on the release of mitomycin after injection of the drug, alone or encapsulated, into the renal artery for the treatment of primary renal cancers. The advantage in the experimental system amounts to around 40% sparing of potential toxicity. Although there is a wide experience in the treatment of metastatic hepatic lesions and indeed primary hepatoma, these results are included in a large study of 285 patients who are suffering from a mixed bag of tumors. Therapeutic results are not given by tumor type; what is clear however is that toxicity is minor and mostly results from infarction of the target organ. Overall tumor response rates were 3% complete response and 33% partial response in a total of 211 evaluable patients. There was a higher scoring of response for the palliation of symptoms such as pain and bleeding.

At the other end of the range, a Japanese group has studied small albumin microspheres (1.44/u) containing 0.15 mg

adriamycin per mg of microspheres   after intravenous injection
into rats bearing liver metastases of AH7974 tumor (9).
The vein used was the portal vein or the tail vein, the former
producing consistently higher levels of the drug in liver and
lower levels in heart, lung, spleen and kidney. Release of
adriamycin from the albumin microspheres was unaffected by the
route of administration and the best antitumor results were
achieved by the intraportal route. Neat adriamycin in the same
dose administered intraportally produced no prolongation of survival nor did empty microspheres. In fact the microspheres
containing adriamycin produced 150% tumor-over-control values
with 2 longterm survivors out of 10 rats. This study confirms
the possible selective nature achievable by this technique and
encourages further clinical applications.

That therapeutic advantage can also be exploited by the
radiation therapist and indeed pilot studies of yttrium delivered
into the hepatic artery of tumor-bearing animals showed improved
results when injected within microspheres (17.5/u, styrene-
divinyl benzene copolymeric ion-exchange resin microspheres) (10)
The calculated mean increase in therapeutic ratio achieved by
this technique was 2.9. Preparations of ion-exchange microspheres
containing ^{32}P have also been tested for pharmaceutical propertie
but therapeutic tests remain to be carried out (5).

10. CONCLUSION

The use of microspheres to target cytostatic drugs or radiatio
therapy is a practical and proven device which, if applied on a
pharmacological basis, should result in a modest increment of
therapeutic ratio. Second order targeting has been achieved by
the injection of these particles into the hepatic artery or the
portal vein in appropriate model systems and, depending on the
microvasculature of the target tumor, an increased dose of the
drug or radioisotope can be safely delivered. Further improvement
of the specificity of the device by incorporation of metals will
probably be of little relevance to the treatment of liver

metastases, as the direction of magnetic fields over this organ will be too complex. It may be possible however to produce a "smart" microsphere in the future which will interact with a surface component of tumor cells via monoclonal antibody and thus produce real selectivity, perhaps also a trigger for intracellular uptake of appropriately sized particles which will then discharge their toxic load within the cells. Further improvement of microsphere therapy for liver tumors must await the evolution of better cytostatic agents.

REFERENCES

1. Tomlinson E, McVie JG. 1983. New directions in cancer chemotherapy 2. Targeting with microspheres. Pharmacy International 4, 11:281-4.
2. Ziessman HA, Thrall JH, Gyves JW, Ensminger WD, Niederhuber JE, Tuscan M, Walker S. 1983. Quantitative hepatic arterial perfusion scintigraphy and starch microspheres in cancer therapy. J Nucl Med 24:871-875.
3. Dakhil S, Ensminger W, Cho K, Niederhuber J, Doan K, Wheeler R. 1982. Improved regional selectivity of hepatic arterial BCNU with degradable microspheres. Cancer 50:631-635.
4. Nemoto R, Kato T. 1984. Microencapsulation of anticancer drug for intra-arterial infusion and its clinical application. In Microspheres and drug therapy; eds. E Tomlinson, JG McVie, L Illum, SS Davis, Elsevier, Amsterdam.
5. Zielinski FW, Kasprzyk M. Synthesis and quality control testing of ^{32}P labeled ion exchange resin microspheres for radiation therapy of hepatic neoplasms. Int J Appl Radiat Isot 34, 9:1343-1350, 1983.
6. Kemshead JT, Gibson FJ, Ugelstad J, Rembaum A. A flow system for the in vitro separation of tumour cells from bone marrow using monoclonal antibodies and magnetic microspheres. 1983. Proc of AACR 24 : 217.
7. Tomlinson E. 1983. Microsphere delivery systems for drug targeting and controlled release. Int J Pharm Tech and Prod Mfr 4, 3:49-57.
8. Gyves JW, Ensminger WD, Van Harken D, Niederhuber J, Stetson P, Walker S. 1983. Improved regional selectivity of hepatic arterial mitomycin by starch microspheres. Clinical Pharmacology and Therapeutics 34, 2:259-265.
9. Morimoto Y, Sugibayashi K, Kato Y. 1981. Drug-carrier property of albumin microspheres in chemotherapy V. Antitumor effect of microsphere-entrapped adriamycin on liver metastasis of AH 7974 cells in rats. Chem Pharm Bull 29, 5:1433-1438.
10. Chamberlain MN, Gray BN, Heggie JCP, Chmiel RL, Bennet C. 1983. Hepatic metastases - a physiological approach to treatment. Br J Surg 70:596-598.

SURGICAL TECHNIQUES IN THE MANAGEMENT OF HEPATIC METASTASES

TECHNIQUES OF HEPATIC SURGERY FOR METASTATIC CANCER

P.H. SUGARBAKER, R.T. OTTOW

In previous chapters the indications and results of surgery for metastatic cancer have been presented. Authors have discussed at length
the clinical and research problems associated with treating metastatic
disease to the liver. From this discussion the following four concepts
should be considered when one reviews a patient with hepatic metastases.
1) Surgical resection of metastatic cancer must be considered as a
treatment option in selected patients. 2) Hepatic resection, be it
lobectomy or wedge resection, is as safe as many other surgical
procedures routinely performed. 3) The indications for hepatic
surgery for metastatic cancer are being expanded; if effective local-
regional adjuvants are found these indications may markedly increase.
4) Patients who are made clinically disease free as a result of
surgery live longer than untreated or chemotherapy treated patients.
It is possible that many patients, even though not cured by hepatic
resection, are helped by preventing the cascade phenomenon. That
is, systemic metastases from the hepatic metastases would be prevented.

Preoperative work-up prior to contemplating surgery for hepatic
metastatic disease includes laboratory and radiologic tests undertaken
to prove that metastatic disease is confined to the liver. Full lung
tomography, Barium enema, intravenous pyelogram, bone scan and CT
scan must show no extra hepatic malignancy.

Selective hepatic angiography is performed prior to surgery to define the hepatic arterial anatomy. Obtaining a late film sequence
following celiac injection allows one to delineate the portal venous
anatomy. Occasionally, large hepato-duodenal nodes from metastatic
tumor that encroach on the portal vein are suspected from this study.

CT scan with EOE-13 liver contrast is of great help in planning
the resection (see chapter on Liver Contrast Agents). Because the

EOE enhanced CT scan clearly shows the hepatic and portal veins and
their relationship to tumor nodules, it can be of great help in
determining resectability and in defining the proper operation.
If EOE CT shows involvement of a major branch of the hepatic veins
hepatic lobectomy rather than metastatectomy is the safest way of
removing the tumor nodule.

Occasionally hepatic venography may be indicated to show the
relationship of a tumor nodule to the hepatic veins. However,
such studies generally show narrowing of veins from external compression rather than tumor invasion into the veins. It is usually
impossible to determine whether or not hepatic venous invasion is
present prior to surgical exploration and direct visualization.
Likewise, contrast radiography of the inferior vena cava is seldom
helpful in determining invasion of this structure by hepatic metastases. Frequently a large tumor mass in the right lobe of the liver
will cause compression of the inferior vena cava. It is unusual to
see direct invasion of the vena cava by cancer; even if the vena
cava is markedly narrowed, exploraton is indicated to determine
whether or not frank invasion is present. Likewise, evidence of
compression of the right kidney by tumor arising in the right lobe
of the liver should not be interpreted as indicating an inoperable
situation. We have not seen invasion of the kidney itself although
we have observed tumor extension into Gerota's fascia. In any
event, the right kidney can be sacrificed along with the right
adrenal gland if necessary to achieve a negative margin of resection.
Invasion of the right or left hemidiaphragm is not unusual. Resection
of a portion of the diaphragm along with the tumor deposit should be
undertaken.

Operative Approach to Right or Left Hepatic Lobectomy: The incisions described for performing a hepatic lobectomy are shown in
Figure 1. For both right and left hepatic lobectomy we prefer an
oblique incision through the seventh or eight intercostal space.
The incision starts in the midline abdomen and allows a thorough
exploration prior to an incision into the thoracic cavity. The
operative site of a previous primary large bowel tumor should be
explored. A careful examination of the pelvis should be performed
in order to rule out pelvic implants from peritoneal carcinomatosis.

326

FIGURE 1. Incisions used for hepatic surgery. The preferred incision for a right hepatic lobectomy is a right thoracoabdominal incision. This incision plus a radial division of the diaphragm down to the hepatic veins provides excellent visualization of the anterior and especially posterior portion of the right liver. It also allows the operating surgeon to place his nondominant hand beneath the liver so that as the parenchyma is transected the structures to be divided are placed on stretch. Also, this means that the field of dissection is pulled up out of the abdomen for optimal visualization. Alternatively, a right subcostal incision may be utilized. This should only be used for wedge excisions. If more generous exposure must be obtained a T extension into the right chest can be performed. An alternative incision that gives wide exposure is the partial median sternotomy. This is especially good for a left hepatic lobectomy. From Ottow RT, August DA, Sugarbaker PH: Surgical therapy of hepatobiliary tumors. In: Bottino JC, Opfell R, Muggia F (eds), Therapy of Neoplasms Confined to the Liver and Biliary Tracts. Boston:Martinus Nyhoff, 1984.

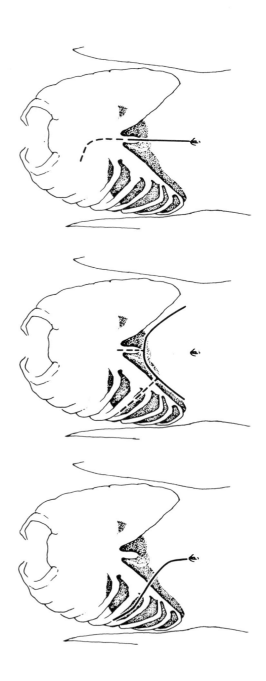

The retroperitoneum should be assessed as thoroughly as is possible from the anterior portion of the abdomen. Finally, when the surgeon is convinced that the viscera and retroperitoneum are free of tumor, the liver itself should be carefully examined by bimanual palpation. The relation of the tumor to the portal vein and the confluence of vena cava and hepatic veins is of critical importance. Small tumor nodules at the periphery of the liver can be removed by a wedge resection. Large or centrally located metastases are treated by a lobectomy.

Prior to opening the chest cavity one must carefully check the hepatic and celiac lymph nodes. If any are enlarged and firm a cryostat section must be obtained. In our experience, a frequent cause for cancelling intraoperatively a hepatic resection is involvement of these node groups. Intraoperative sampling of normal appearing hepatic and celiac (and if the chest is opened mediastinal) lymph nodes utilizing frozen section diagnosis in search of microscopic secondary nodal metastases prior to undertaking a hepatic resection may also be indicated. This may permit exclusion of patients who will develop subsequent nodal disease despite seemingly curative hepatic resection.

If no disease is found outside of the liver, the right chest is opened and the costal cartilage divided. A radial incision in the diaphragm in the direction of the hepatic veins is made. The entire hemidiaphragm down to the level of the hepatic veins does not need to be divided. Usually, a 3-4 cm incision into the diaphragm exposes the hepatic veins quite clearly.

In order to transect the liver in a relatively bloodless fashion, several preliminary steps need be taken. A self retaining retractor should be positioned within the abdomen and chest so that the operative field is widely exposed and completely stabilized. The dissection is begun by dividing the attachments between liver and diaphragm. For a right hepatic lobectomy it is easiest to start in the area of the hepatic veins and work towards the right. In this procedure the attachments to tne left lobe of the liver should be left completely intact. The converse is true for a left hepatic lobectomy.

The liver is next reflected off of the vena cava to either the right or left. In a right hepatic lobectomy, one to eight branches of the

veins that go directly from caudate lobe to vena cava must be isolated and divided. Similarly, on the left side, one or two branches
going directly from the liver to the vena cava should be secured.
After the attachments are divided and the vessels from caudate and
quadrate lobes directly into vena cava are secured, the liver has
markedly increased mobility (Figure 2).

At this point the liver may be reflected superiorly and the portal
dissection commenced. In a right hepatic lobectomy the right duct
and right hepatic artery are isolated, ligated and divided. A convenient way to locate these structures is to remove the gallbladder
and trace cystic duct back to common duct and cystic artery to right
hepatic artery. In a right hepatic lobectomy the gallbladder should
always be removed. Division of the right duct and right hepatic
artery permits visualization of the right portal vein which lies
directly beneath the artery and duct. Alternatively a tourniquet
may be placed around the hepatic artery and portal vein to inter-
rupt flow. This is preferred if a large tumor causes poor exposure
of the porta-hepatis.

After gaining control of the right or left portal vein, a line of
demarcation through the liver becomes evident. Using electrocautery,
a line approximately 1 cm into darkened parenchyma is marked out
(Figure 3). This marks for the surgeon the proposed line of liver
transection and avoids disorientation during the later parenchymal
dissection. To divide the liver parenchyma we use the ultrasonic
dissector (Figure 4-6). Lacking this instrument the liver parenchyma
can be divided with a blunt instrument (cannula of a sucker, knife
handle) or the finger fracture method. Small biliary radicals and
vessels and ducts are secured with tantalum clips (these do not
produce artifacts on follow-up NMR or CT scan) or ligated with sutures.
The larger branches of the portal vein and the major hepatic veins
are secured by ligation in continuity prior to their division.
Large ducts should also be suture ligated. On the posterior aspect
of the liver Glisson's capsule is divided with electrocautery to
deliver the specimen. Figure 7 shows the procedure completed. We
do not cover the cut liver surface or attempt to approximate the cut
edges of the liver.

The area is copiously irrigated. A Tenckhoff catheter is placed

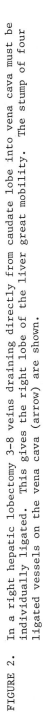

FIGURE 2. In a right hepatic lobectomy 3-8 veins draining directly from caudate lobe into vena cava must be individually ligated. This gives the right lobe of the liver great mobility. The stump of four ligated vessels on the vena cava (arrow) are shown.

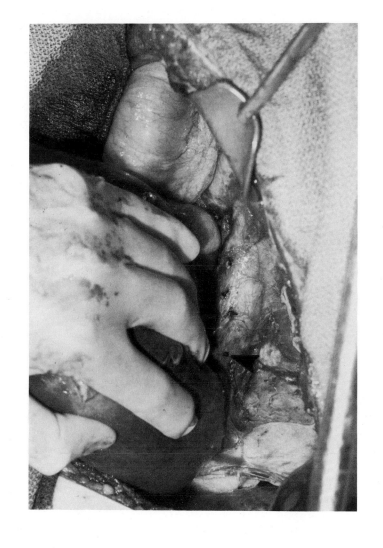

330

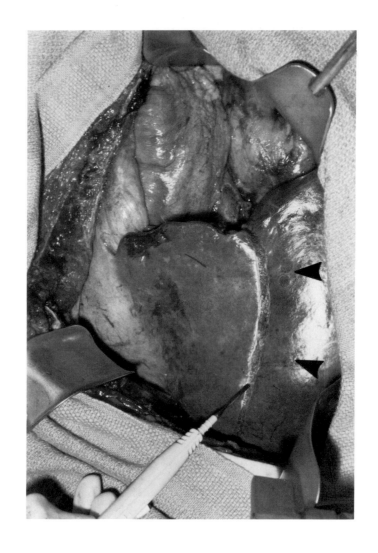

FIGURE 3. A line of demarcation (arrows) of the liver is seen following ligation of right hepatic artery and right portal vein. The parenchyma is transected just 1 cm into the devascularized tissue. Electro-cautery is used to mark the line of transection.

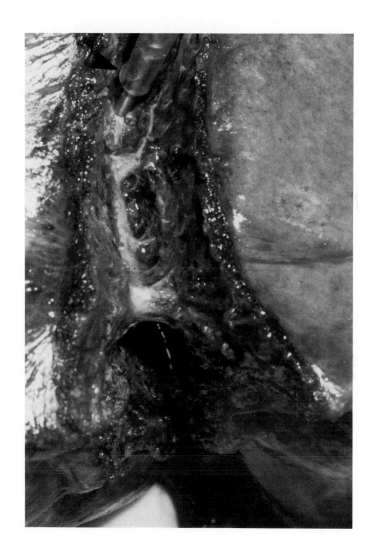

FIGURE 4. Transection of liver parenchyma with the ultrasonic dissector (arrow). This instrument fragments liver tissue from around vessels and ducts so they can be clearly visualized.

332

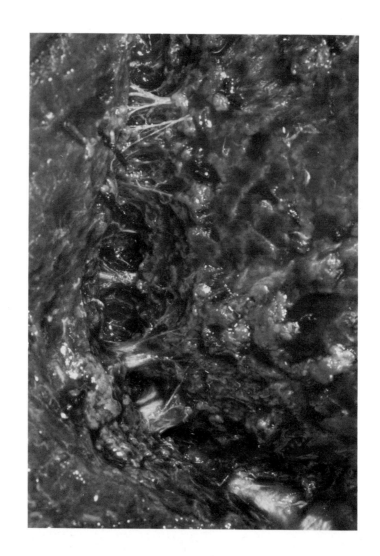

FIGURE 5. In dissecting through the hepatic parenchyma large, medium and minute vessels and ducts are encountered. The small structures are divided with electrocautery. Five to eight individual structures are dissected free of parenchyma and then secured.

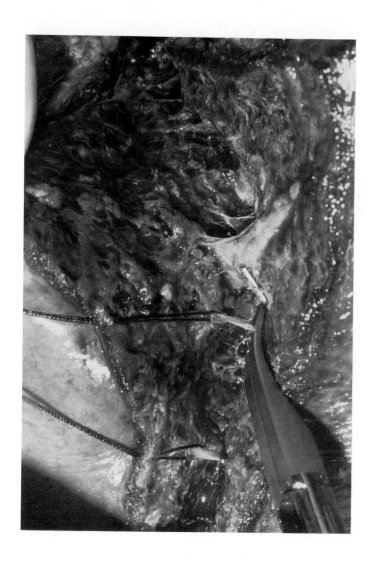

FIGURE 6. On the patient side of the parenchymal dissection vascular and ductal structures are ligated with sutures. On the specimen side metal clips are used to conserve time.

334

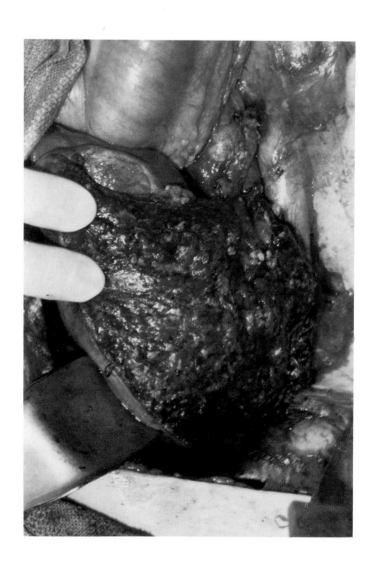

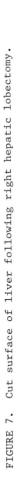

FIGURE 7. Cut surface of liver following right hepatic lobectomy.

into the abdominal cavity and a closed system suction drain beneath
the hemidiaphragm. A tube thoracostomy is placed in the chest. The
diaphragm is closed, the costal margin is secured with wire, and the
chest and abdominal closures proceed in a routine fashion.

In the immediate postoperative period we lavage the peritoneal cavity
with a peritoneal dialysate solution until drainage is clear. Intra-
abdominal infusions of fluid are continued on a two hour, six hour,
and 24 hour basis until the seventh postoperative day. These intra-
abdominal irrigations are used to prevent blood accumulation within
the abdomen. The chest tube is generally removed on the seventh
postoperative day when peritoneal lavage ceases. We do not use
intra-abdominal drains other than the Tenckhoff catheter and closed
suction drain thinking that they are more likely to introduce infection
into the abdominal cavity than to facilate drainage of bile and
blood. Technical requirements of hepatic lobectomy are listed in
Table 1. The resections most commonly performed are shown in Figure 8.

Technique of Metastasectomy: Prior to beginning the parenchymal
dissection the foramen of Winslow must be clearly identified. A non-
crushing vascular clamp may be used to intermittently occlude the
portal structures while dissecting through liver. Attempting to stay
approximately 1 cm from each metastasis, they are removed with a clear
margin. Inflow occlusion of the liver is limited to 30 minutes. This
period can safely be extended, possibly up to 60 minutes. Vessels are
tied or electrocauterized in the surrounding liver; a gelfoam plug is
placed within the defect to encourage blood clotting. It is especially
important to check for bile leaks upon removal of the gelfoam; if noted
they should be suture ligated. Bile leaks following metastatectomy of
large tumor deposits have occurred in several patients. They may require postoperatively percutaneous external drainage for a prolonged
period of time.

The Ultrasonic Dissector: The Cavitron Ultrasonic Aspiration Device
(CUSA) consists of a hollow Titanium probe, oscillating longitudinally
at a frequency of about 23 kilo hertz over a range of about 100 microns.
The tip is shown in Figure 4. The oscillating movement selectively
fragments liver parenchyma, leaving the vessels and ducts intact so
that they can easily be clipped, tied or cauterized. Parenchyma and
blood are aspirated through the probe, and additional suction apparatus

336

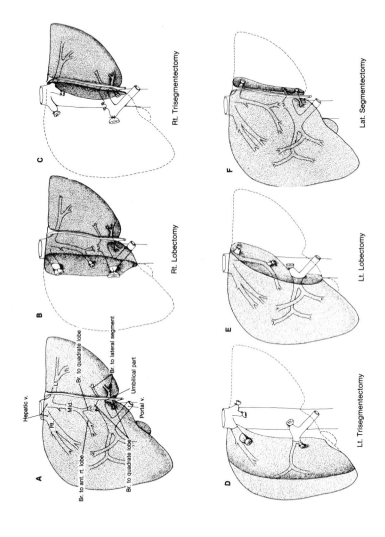

FIGURE 8. The hepatic resections most commonly performed include the right lobectomy, right trisegmentectomy, left trisegmentectomy, left lobectomy and left lateral segmentectomy. From Ottow RT, August DA, Sugarbaker PH: Surgical therapy of hepatobiliary tumors. In: Bottino JC, Opfell R, Muggia F (eds) Therapy of Neoplasms Confined to the Liver and Biliary Tracts. Boston:Martinus Nyhoff, 1984.

keeping the field clear at all times. Bleeding from small vessels in a normal liver is prevented by CUSA dissection facilitating a dry operating field. Continuous irrigation with saline provides cooling of the tip and helps in aspiration. Technical requirements for optimal CUSA dissection are noted in Table 2.

TABLE 1. Technical Requirements of Hepatic Lobectomy

1. Wide exposure through a thoraco-abdominal incision utilizing a self retaining retractor.

2. Complete mobilization of the liver lobe to be removed.

3. Preliminary ligation of the right (left) hepatic artery and right (left) protal vein.

4. Systemic hypotension during hepatic transection.

5. Elevation of the liver to place traction on intraparenchymal structures during hepatic transection.

6. Hepatic dissection which allows ligation of vessels within the parenchyma prior to their division.

7. Closed system drainage.

TABLE 2. Technical Requirements of CUSA Dissection - Cavitron Ultrasonic Surgical Aspirator

1. Field in which CUSA dissection is used must be dry - extravasated blood interferes with function.

2. The instrument must be moved slowly over the surface of the tissue.

3. Once medium and large vessels are visualized, one must take care to avoid direct contact with the CUSA tip.

4. Hemostasis is achieved on the smaller vessels.

5. One must maintain traction on the parenchyma being divided.

Postoperative Care: Liver resection is usually well tolerated, but complications do occur. Subphrenic abcess can often be managed in consultation with the interventional radiologist by percutaneous CT or ultrasound guided drainage. Some small amount of biliary fluid leaking postoperatively occasionally occurs; it usually stops spontaneously because the biliary network is a low pressure system. Postoperatively many patients show transient jaundice. The SGOT often shows a sharp peak just after resection; the alkaline phosphatase is often elevated for months, even years after resection. In the first postoperative week serum albumin levels may be depressed and prothrombin times often elevated. Albumin should be given along with fresh frozen plasma when indicated. Parenteral Vitamin K given preoperatively may be helpful. In noncirrhotic patients regeneration starts in a matter of days and is complete in two to four months. Cirrhotic livers do not show regeneration.

TECHNIQUE OF HEPATIC INFUSION CHEMOTHERAPY

P.H. SUGARBAKER, P.D. SCHNEIDER

The arterial blood supply to the liver is reported to be
"normal" in only about half of the general population. Placement
of hepatic artery catheters is dependent on an accurate knowledge
of this anatomy. Arteriography through the celiac and superior
mesenteric artery must be performed to plan the surgical approach.
In a review of hepatic arterial anatomy by Edwards, MacArthur and
Malone they found the entire hepatic artery coming from the celiac
axis in 55% of patients (Table 1). There was a replaced left hepatic
artery from the left gastric in 10% of patients. "Replaced" indicates
that the major arterial blood supply to the left lobe of the liver
was through the left gastric artery, while "accessory" left hepatic
artery identifies a small vessel present in addition to the major
arterial blood supply to the left lobe of the liver. A replaced
right hepatic artery from the superior mesenteric occurred in approximately 11% of patients. An accessory left hepatic artery is
seen from the left gastric in 8% of patients and an accessory right
hepatic from the superior mesenteric in 7% of patients. The entire
hepatic was reported to come from the superior mesenteric in 4.5% of
patients. Another problem to catheter insertion is the early branching of the left hepatic artery from the common hepatic. These variations in the vascular anatomy of the liver will be presented and
the surgical approach to catheter insertion will be presented.
Entire Hepatic From Celiac Axis – Normal Anatomy.

When the hepatic artery with right, middle and left branches
comes off the celiac axis, the infusion catheter is inserted throught
the gastroduodenal artery (Figure 1). The beaded tip of the catheter should sit just inside the gastroduodenal artery as it enters

340

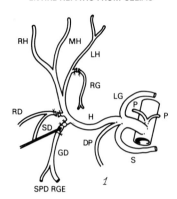

ENTIRE HEPATIC FROM CELIAC

1

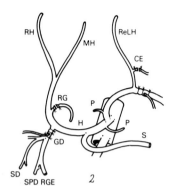

**REPLACED LEFT HEPATIC
FROM LEFT GASTRIC**

2

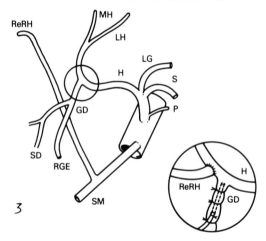

**REPLACED RIGHT HEPATIC
FROM SUPERIOR MESENTERIC**

3

FIGURE 1.   "Normal" hepatic arterial anatomy. The hepatic artery and
all its branches are off the celiac artery.

FIGURE 2.   Replaced left hepatic artery from the left gastric artery.
This anatomic situation requires dual catheter insertion.

FIGURE 3.   Replaced right hepatic artery from the superior mesenteric
artery.

TABLE 1. Sources of the Hepatic Arteries and Percent of Patients
Showing the Anatomy.

1. Entire hepatic artery from the celiac (55%).

2. Replaced left hepatic from left gastric (10%).

3. Replaced right hepatic from superior messenteric (11%).

4. Accessory left hepatic from left gastric (8%).

5. Accessory right hepatic from superior mesenteric (7%).

6. Entire hepatic from superior mesenteric (4.5%).

From Edwards, MacArthur and Malone: Operative anatomy of abdomen
and pelvis. Lea & Feliger, 1975, p 166.

the common hepatic. It is extremely important that the hepatic
artery be dissected along its course up into the liver so that
small branches off this vessel to the stomach, pancreas and duodenum
that are distal to the gastroduodenal artery are ligated and divided.
A superior duodenal, a right duodenal and a right gastric artery are
commonly seen. Failure to ligate visceral branches of the hepatic
artery distal to the point of catheter insertion may result in
severe duodenitis and gastritis and prevent adequate, safe drug
delivery.

Replaced Left Hepatic Artery From the Left Gastric Artery.

In this anatomic situation there are two distinct vessels supplying the liver with arterial blood. This requires the use of a two
catheter system. Two infusion pumps may be used or the dual infusion
pump from Infusaid Corporation may be utilized. To perfuse the
right lobe of the liver the gastroduodenal artery is again cannulated.
To infuse the left lobe of the liver the left gastric artery is
canulated just distal to the take-off of the replaced left hepatic
artery. Small branches from this vessel to the stomach and esophagus
distal to the site of catheter insertion must be ligated and divided
(Figure 2). The surgical approach to the replaced left hepatic
artery is generally through the lesser omentum. Problems with ischemia in the gastric wall following ligation of the left gastric
artery have not been seen.

Replaced Right Hepatic Artery From the Superior Mesenteric Artery.

When the right hepatic artery comes off the superior mesenteric there are usually no branch vessels suitable for catheter insertion along its course. Also the vessel runs just posterior to the pancreas and access to the replaced right hepatic artery where branches may occur is difficult or impossible. If the replaced right hepatic artery can be dissected out over several inches it should be ligated proximally and the distal portion anastomosed end to side to the left hepatic artery. Catheter insertion can be performed through the gastroduodenal artery (Figure 3). Alternatively, a Holter tip catheter can be placed directly into the replaced right hepatic artery for infusion of this vessel. In our experience this has resulted in a high incidence of arterial thrombosis weeks to months following the insertion of the catheter. We do not recommend this technique presently. Alternatively, prosthetic material can be sewn onto the replaced right hepatic artery and infusion is then performed through the prosthetic graft.

Accessory Left Hepatic Artery From the Left Gastric Artery.

If there is an accessory blood supply to a lobe of the liver we recommend ligation of the accessory vessel. If an accessory left hepatic artery comes off the left gastric it should be ligated. The infusion catheter would then be inserted into the gastroduodenal artery as described above (Figure 4).

Accessory Right Hepatic Artery From the Superior Mesenteric Artery.

The accessory vessel is ligated as it enters the liver and the pump is placed into the gastroduodenal artery (Figure 5).

Entire Hepatic Artery From the Superior Mesenteric Artery.

In this anatomic situation one carefully searches in an around the head of pancreas and second portion of the duodenum for a vessel of sufficient size to allow catheter insertion (Figure 6). If a vessel of sufficient size cannot be found then the Holter tip catheter must be inserted directly into the vessel. Alternatively a small caliber vascular prosthesis can be sutured end to side of the replaced hepatic artery and infusion be performed through the vascular prosthesis.

Early Branching of the Hepatic Artery.

This is not an uncommon finding. It is seen in approximately 20% of patients and presents a special problem in that drug infused through the gastroduodenal artery will only treat the right side of the liver. In this situation we recommend ligation of the gastroduo-

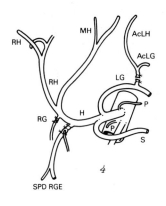

ACCESSORY LEFT HEPATIC FROM LEFT GASTRIC

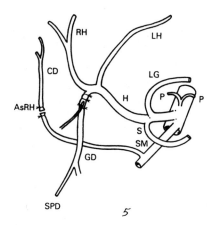

ACCESSORY RIGHT HEPATIC FROM SUPERIOR MESENTERIC

ENTIRE HEPATIC
FROM SUPERIOR MESENTERIC

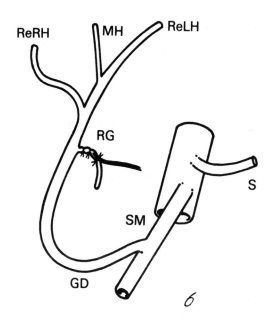

FIGURE 4. Accessory left hepatic artery from the left gastric artery. The accessory vessel is simply ligated.

FIGURE 5. Accessory right hepatic artery from the superior mesenteric artery. The accessory vessel is simply ligated.

FIGURE 6. Entire hepatic artery from the superior mesenteric artery. A side branch of the artery beneath the second portion of the duodenum is sought for catheter insertion.

denal artery and pump infusion through the splenic artery (Figure 7).
The common hepatic artery is traced back along the border of the pancreas until the celiac axis is found. The splenic artery is isolated
and the catheter inserted into the splenic artery. One must be
careful to dissect along the common hepatic artery up and to the
liver to make sure there are no side branches of this vessel that
have not been ligated and divided.

Portal Venous Catheterization Through the Inferior Mesenteric Vein.

In some protocols, after surgical removal of tumor from the
liver, portal venous catheterization has been used in an attempt to
prevent tumor proliferation from portal venous blood supply. The
initial efforts with portal venous catheterization were through
recanalization of the obliterated umbilical vein. However, this
maneuver is technically difficult. Sometimes it causes spliting of
the umbilical vein as it enters the portal venous system and hemorrhage. It cannot be performed 100% of the time. If a patient is
having a left colectomy the inferior mesenteric vein is usually
dissected free and we have found it easy to catheterize (Figure 8).
If a patient is having a right colectomy then catheterization of the
mid colic vein is to be recommended. If either of these vessels has
been destroyed with the previous surgery the venous blood supply is
sufficiently extensive that sacrifice of the other vessel and placement of a catheter can safely be performed. Also, the gastroduodenal
vein can be cannulated.

In general, catheterization of the hepatic veins has been well
tolerated; no portal venous thrombosis have to our knowledge been
reported. Further clinical trials to evaluate portal venous infusion
with or without hepatic artery ligation are necessary.

**EARLY BRANCHING
OF LEFT HEPATIC**

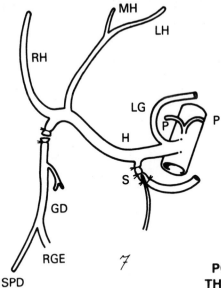

**PORTAL VENOUS CATHETERIZATION
THROUGH INFERIOR MESENTERIC VEIN**

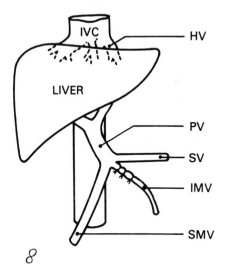

FIGURE 7.   Early branching of the left hepatic artery. The splenic
artery is used for catheter insertion.

FIGURE 8.   Portal venous catheterization through the inferior mesenteric
vein. Alternatively the obliterated umbilical vein, right
colic vein or gastroduodenal vein may be cannulated.

THE ISOLATED LIVER PERFUSION TECHNIQUE FOR HIGH-DOSE CHEMOTHERAPY OF METASTASES FROM COLORECTAL CANCER - TWO YEARS' CLINICAL EXPERIENCE

K.R. Aigner, J.C. Tonn, H. Walther, K.H. Link, K. Schwemmle

SUMMARY

In 33 patients with liver metastases (30 colorectal, 2 carcinoid, 1 hepatoma) the liver was completely isolated with a special cannulation system and perfused with 5-Fluorouracil at 40°C in an extracorporal circuit with a heart-lung-machine. The treatment was primarily performed in patients with extensive liver enlargement. Generally a 20% reduction of total liver volume as measured on CT-scan was noted. Median survival after isolated liver perfusion was 8 months. When isolated liver perfusion is followed by hepatic artery short-time infusion as a maintainance therapy, the actual median follow-up period in a group of 12 patients is 16,5 months.
Currently the most effective treatment of disseminated liver metastases of colorectal primary is supposed to be the intra-arterial infusion chemotherapy. As liver metastases are mainly vascularized by the hepatic artery (9), the intra-arterial infusion of cytotoxics provides a much higher concentration of the drug in tumors than can be achieved by systemic chemotherapy. In an attempt to avoid systemic cytotoxic side-effects and with regard to the close dose-response relationship (11) in cancer chemotherapy we developed a standardized technique for isolated perfusion of the liver.

Operative technique of isolated liver perfusion

Through an abdominal midline incision the liver, the hepato-duodenal ligament and vena cava are exposed. The hepatic artery and portal vein are both cannulated and perfused separately with arterialized blood. The venous hepatic outflow through a special catheter which is inserted from below the renal veins is collected by gravity in the oxygenator of the heart-lung-machine (Fig. 1). Two lateral openings in the double

channel perfusion catheter (Fig 2) collect the venous return from the
kidneys. The portal blood from the G.I. tract passes a hemofilter.which
only recently has been omitted without noticeable changes and enters
the porto-caval shunt tube which inserts in the perfusion catheter.
 The hepatic artery is perfused at a maximum flow rate of 300 ml/min,
the portal vein with 150-250 ml/min for 1 hour at a tissue temperature
of 40°C. Dosages of 5-Fluorouracil which is injected into the arterial
line of the extra-corporeal circuit, range between 750 and 1250 mg.
At the end of a one hour perfusion the liver is rinsed and thus remaining
drugs washed out of the vascular system. The catheters are withdrawn
stepwise and the vessels repaired with running sutures (1,3).
Postoperatively the patients were under intensive care for one night.
Two weeks later first results were controlled on CT-scan. Three months
after the perfusion CT-scan was repeated and in a small group of patients a tumor biopsy for histological examination was taken at a second-
look-operation. Serological liver enzymes and CEA were determined preoperatively, followed up postoperatively and controlled on hospitalization for second-look-operation.

Patients:

38 patients were submitted to isolated liver perfusion. 35 patients
had liver metastases of previously resected colo-rectal cancers, one
had extensive hepatoma, and two had carcinoid. For classification of
clinical stage in all patients total liver volumes and tumor volumes
were measured by CT-scan and not estimated by the surgeon during operation. At the time of operation there was no evidence of extrahepatic
metastases or local recurrence. 24 patients were divided into two
groups in order to find out whether isolated liver perfusion combined
with subsequent hepatic artery infusion was superior to isolated liver
perfusion alone. The treatment groups were compared with untreated
historical controls (7,14,16). Three patients had died within two weeks
after perfusion. The remaining, recently operated six patients, received combination treatment (perfusion and i.a. infusion) as well.
Their follow-up period does not exeed ten months yet (Fig. 6).

FIGURE 1

The isolated liver perfusion circuit and portocaval hemofiltration.

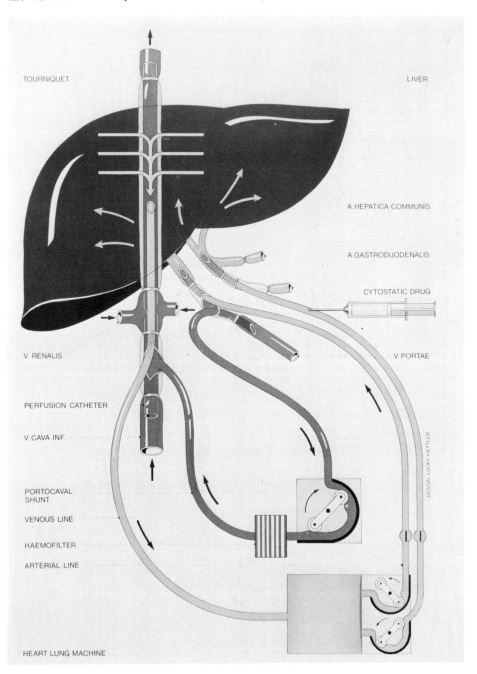

FIGURE 2

Double channel vena cava catheter for isolated liver perfusion.
The cannulation is performed below the renal veins.

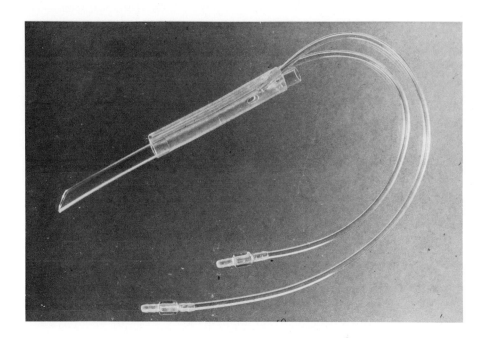

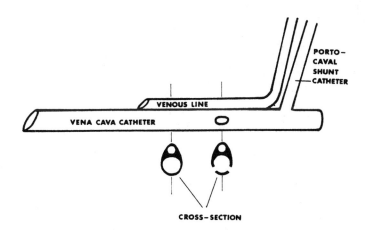

DOUBLE-CHANNELLED CATHETER FOR ISOLATED LIVER PERFUSION

Group 1:

Out of 12 patients treated exclusively with isolated liver perfusion, one patient was already under parenteral nutrition and three further patients had dysphagia due to extensive liver enlargement.As measured on CT-scan, in 5 patients the volume relationship between tumor tissue and liverparenchyma was below 50%, in 7 patients it amounted to 50% and more. Median liver volume as measured in CT-scan was 4 liters, median tumor volume 1,8 liters (1).

Group 2:

In these 12 patients the clinical staging concerning percentage of tumor involvement in the liver was comparable to that in group 1 (< 50% tumor involvement in 5 patients, ≥ 50% tumor involvement in 7 patients). After the isolated liver perfusion an 'Implantofix'[R]-catheter was inserted into the gastroduodenal artery (Fig. 3). Via the

subcutaneously placed reservoir of this catheter intra-arterial short-time infusions over a one-hour period on six consecutive days were repeated every four weeks (Table 1).

FIGURE 3
Implantofix[R] arterial catheter. A valve in the tip avoids occluding. The reservoir is implanted subcutaneously.

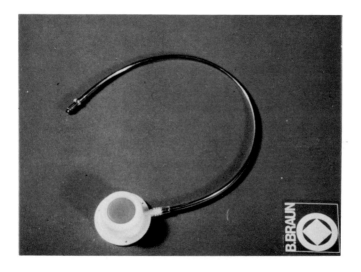

Table 1   Dose schedule for cytotoxic hepatic artery infusion
           in liver metastases of colorectal primary

Day	Drug	Dosage	Infusiontime
1	Mitomycin C	8 mg/m²	60 min
2	5-Fluorouracil (5-FU)	550 mg/m²	60 min
3	5-FU	550 mg/m²	60 min
4	5-FU	550 mg/m²	60 min
5	5-FU	550 mg/m²	60 min
6	5-FU	550 mg/m²	60 min

RESULTS

There was no clinical evidence of drug induced hepatitis. Generally
the serological liver enzymes SGOT and SGPT were elevated to about
80-100 U/l for at least one week. The most apparent finding is a decrease of the cholinesterase to low levels between 600 and 1200 U/l
for two or three weeks. After a short term postoperative elevation,
AP and LDH declined to values below the preoperative levels. There
is only a slight increase of serum bilirubin postoperatively - only
one patient had jaundice during five days. CEA, after an initial peak
in all patients showed a tendency to decline. In four patients CEA
levels changed to normal within 3 months after the perfusion.

Complications:

One patient died due to intractable bleeding two hours after
isolated liver perfusion combined with a hemihepatectomy. The tumor
had already encapsulated the vena cava. Antoher patient died from sep-
ticemia and respiratory disturbances six days after perfusion. The
third patient had renal failure two weeks postoperatively. His autopsy
showed a 90% tumor regression, 70% of the liver tissue had been involved
by metastases. In one patient a subdiaphragmatic abscess had to be
drained. In the last 25 patients treated there were no complications
due to the operative technique. Actually isolated liver perfusion is
a safe procedure and patients can be discharged within 10 days postoperatively.

<u>Drug levels</u>:

5-FU levels in the perfusion circuit as measured by HPLC ranged between
250 µg/ml at the beginning and about 50 µg/ml at the end of perfusion
time, which corresponds to peak levels in systemic treatment immediately after an intravenous bolus injection of the same amount of drug.

<u>Computed tomography</u>:

In the patient demonstrated in Figs. 4, 5, perfusion resulted in
extensive colliquation areas and volume reduction of a bulky tumor
in the left and of disseminated lesions in the right liver lobe.

FIGURE 4

Computed tomography before isolated liver perfusion. Metastases had
mainly involved the left liver lobe.

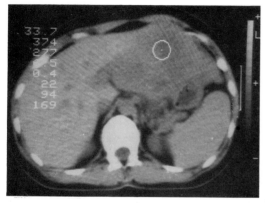

FIGURE 5

Three months after isolated liver perfusion in CT-scan the tumor is
replaced by necrotic tissue.

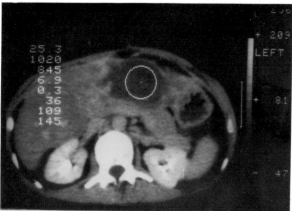

Most commonly immediately after isolated liver perfusion on CT-scan
there seems to be no alteration in tumor diameters, but only in tumor
density. Generally total liver volume decreased by 20% after one perfusion. Maximum liver volume reduction after combination treatment
(group 2) was 1.6 liters (30%).

Actual survival:

In group 1, treated by isolated liver perfusion alone median survival
was 8 months (Fig. 6) and no patient survived more than twelve months.
In the perfused livers tumor recurrence was observed 5 to 10 months
postoperatively.

Finally all patients had extrahepatic tumor growth in the peritoneum,
lungs or large bowel anastomosis. In group 2, treated by isolation
perfusion and subsequent hepatic artery short-time infusion, the median
follow-up is 16.5 months and only one patient died 12 months postoperatively. One patients is living 2.5 years without complaints.
His liver scan is unchanged. However, meanwhile one lung metastasis
and local tumor recurrence in the perineal scar   and pelvis occured.
Extrahepatic metastases were diagnosed in all patients that survived
more than twelve months.

DISCUSSION

Isolated cytostatic perfusion of the liver has been emphasized as an
alternative method for treatment of inoperable primary or metastatic
neoplastic disease. There have been a few attempts to isolate and perfuse the liver in the animal experiment (6,8,13,17,18). The basic
principles of cannulation have been similar in each working group. Our
innovations of previously described surgical technique have been cannulation of the vena cava from below the renal veins and hemofiltration of the portal blood (1,3). Using this technique with our catheter
(Fig. 2) cannulation of the superior vena cava system could be avoided,
in a manner similar to that describe in Chapter 25 by van de Velde et al.
and thus total operation time reduced.

The isolation perfusion model is supposed to be as efficient as the drug
that is used. It promises to be a most potent technique to administer
newly developed drugs or drug combinations at ultimate high doses while
systemic side effects such as bone marrow depression or renal toxicity
may be avoided. In case of 5-FU two mechanisms, inhibition of thymidi-

late synthetase and incorporation into RNA (10) appear capable of causing cell injury. Tumor toxicity in isolation perfusion is most probably caused by the effect on RNA function.

Although the predominant mode of action finally has not been clarified, the activity of 5-FU in isolated liver perfusion was demonstrated clinically. FUDR which has been widely used in continuous longterm infusions is converted to the active product 5-FdUMP by only a single enzyme, but lacks effects on RNA. For this reason and the high toxicity to normal tissues we have not used it in isolated liver perfusion. A high 'first pass extraction' in the liver parenchyma is not mandatory in the perfusion situation.

However, there might be an advantage using alcylating agents in high concentration. Therefore the efficacy of isolated liver perfusion cannot be estimated according to results in the 5-FU study alone. Mitomycin C for example which turned out to be highly effective in hepatic artery infusions (2, 15) for colorectal metastases warrants further investigation in isolated perfusion. The application of cis-platinum in perfusion of primary hepatomas might be of interest too since that drug was well tolerated in the animal model (to be published) and caused only moderate side-effects in isolated extremity perfusion for melanoma (4). Unfortunately at the time of diagnosis most hepatomas are already palpable far below the costal margin and thus make cannulation technique difficult.

In our hepatoma patient preoperatively the liver edge was palpable at the umbilicus. Four months after isolated 5-FU-perfusion tumor progression was noted and the patient died five months postoperatively. Most probably a single high dose perfusion treatment will not eradicate all cells of a solid tumor. For this reason local tumor recurrence was observed in the group of patients who had perfusion only and median survival would not exceed 8 months. On the other hand the extent of tumor cell kill, as mentioned above, strongly depends on the drug used, and in sensitive tumors there is a steep dose response relationship (11). As compared with untreated historical controls with extensive hepatic involvement in which median survival was 2.2 to 2.5 months (7,14) or 1.4 months (16), isolated liver perfusion prolongs life expectancy at a good quality of life without chemotherapeutic side-effects.

355

Fig. 6 Actual survival after isolated liver perfusion alone (——) and in combination with repeated hepatic artery infusion (——). Arrows indicate median survival and -follow-up.

●——— untreated controls,
▲——— alive, ——— dead

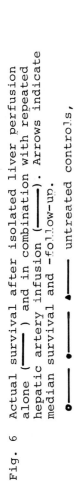

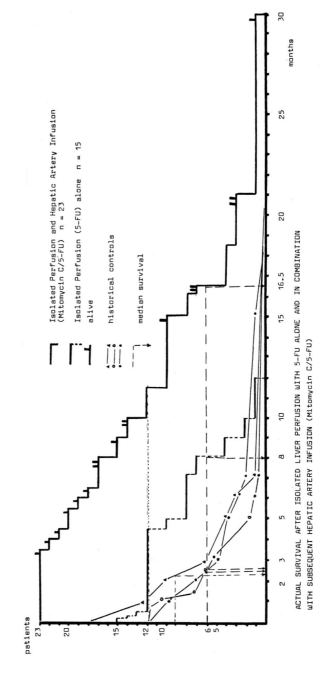

Isolated Perfusion and Hepatic Artery Infusion (Mitomycin C/5-FU) n = 23

Isolated Perfusion (5-FU) alone n = 15 alive

historical controls

median survival

ACTUAL SURVIVAL AFTER ISOLATED LIVER PERFUSION WITH 5-FU ALONE AND IN COMBINATION WITH SUBSEQUENT HEPATIC ARTERY INFUSION (Mitomycin C/5-FU)

In spite of the low response rate in systemic treatment of colorectal liver metastases (5,12) hepatic artery infusion as a maintainance therapy after isolated liver perfusion does prolong remission induction. We feel that short-time hepatic artery infusions over 60 minutes provide locally higher drug levels and thus higher response rates are noted (1,2). Although about 12 months after 'isolated perfusion - intra-arterial infusion' combination treatment (group 2), extrahepatic metastases have been documented as well, survival is prolonged as compared with group 1, treated with perfusion alone. Six patients out of group 2 died 11.5, 11.5, 15,16,16.5,19.5 months after the initial perfusion.

Since only in three of the surviving patients (6/12) tumor progression was diagnosed 13, 16 and 18 months after start of treatment it is obvious that remission intervals are longer when i.a. maintainance therapy is performed. Although the groups compared are rather small, survival rates seem to be significantly longer in the combined treated group.

Since in most of our perfused patients, extensive disease was documented on CT-scan, micrometastases to other organ sites such as lungs and bones have to be assumed. It has been pointed out (16) that the presence of concomitant metastases in other organs would not influence the lenght of survival of a patient already harbouring hepatic metastases.

Our patients, however, seem to be surpassed by their local recurrences or lung metastases several months after isolated perfusion, the growth of their hepatic metastases remaining stationary or suppressed. For this reason the most beneficial effect might be attained in patients suffering from only few metastases in one or both liver lobes where local resection in a second-look-operation may free the patient from visible tumors whereas micrometastases are supposed to be killed by regional chemotherapy.

REFERENCES

1. Aigner K.R., Walther H., Tonn J.C., Link K.H., Schoch P., Schwemmle K., : Die isolierte Lerberperfusion bei fortgeschrittenen Metastasen kolorektaler Karzinome. Onkologie 7, 13-21, 1984.

2. Aigner K.R., Walther H., Link K.H., Muhrer K.H., Filler R.D., Schwemmle K., Seuffer R., Schoch P., Petreje C., Tonn J.C., Müller H.: Die intraarterielle Zytostatikainfusion bei Lebertumoren. Med.Klinik 78, 774-778, No. 24, 1983.

3. Aigner K., Walther H., Tonn J.C., Krahl M., Wenzl A., Merker G., Schwemmle K.; Die isolierte Leberperfusion mit 5-Fluorouracil (5-FU) beim Menschen. Chirurg 53: 571-573, 1982.

4. Aigner K., Walther H., Tonn J.C., Wenzl A., Hechtel R., Merker G., Schwemmle K.: Regional perfusion with Cis-platinum and DTIC. In: Schwemmle K., Aigner K.: Recent Results in Cancer Therapy, Springer Verlag, Berlin, Heidelberg, New York 1983.

5. Ansfield F., Klotz J., Nealon T., Ramirez G., Minton J., Hill G., Wilson W., Davis H., Cornell G.: A phase III study comparing the clinical utility of four regimes of 5-fluorouracil. Cancer 39:4,1977.

6. Ausmann R.K.: Development of a technic for isolated perfusion of the liver. N.Y. STate J. Med. 61: 3993, 1961.

7. Bengmark S., Hafström L.: The natural history of primary and secondary malignant tumors of the liver. Cancer 23: 198-202, 1969.

8. Boddie A.W., Booker L., Mullins J.D., McBride C.J.: Hepatic hyperthermia by total isolation and regional perfusion in vivo. J. Surg. Res. 26: 447, 1979.

9. Breedis C., Young G.: The blood supply of neoplasmas in the liver. Am. J. Pathol. 30: 969, 1953.

10. Chabner B.: Pyrimidine Antagonistis in: B. Chabner: Pharmacologic Principles of Cancer Treatment. W.B. Saunders Company, Philadelphia. 183-212, 1982.

11. Frei E., Canellos G.P.: Dose: A critical factor in cancer chemotherapy. Am. J. Med. 69: 585-592, 1980.

12. Grage T.B., Vassilopoulos P.P., Shingleton W.W., Juber A.V., Elias E.G., Aust J.B. Moss S.E.: Results of a prospective randomized study of hepatic artery infusion with 5-fluorouracil versus intravenous 5-fluourouracil in patients with hepatic metastases from colorectal cancer: A Central Oncology Group Study. Surgery 86: 550, 1979.

13. Kestens P.J., Farrely J.A. Mc.Dermott W.V.: A technique of isolation and perfusion of the canine liver. J. Surg. REs. 2: 58, 1962.

14. Kinami Y., Miyazaki J.: The superselective and selective one shot methods for treating inoperable cancer of the liver. Cancer 41: 1720-1727, 1978.

15. Van Oosterom A.T., De Bruijn E.A. Langenber, J.P.: Intraarterial hepatic infusion of mitomycin C: clinical data and pharmacokinetic profiles. In: Mitomycin C, Ed.: M. Ogawa, M. Rozencweig M.J. Stacquet, Excerpta Medica 1982.

16. Pettavel J.: Arterial infusion chemotherapy for hepatic metastases. In: Schwemmle K., Aigner K.: Recent Results in Cancer Research. Vol. 86, Vascular, Perfusion in Cancer Therapy. Springer Verlag, Berlin, Heidelberg, New York 1983.

17. Skibba J.L., Condon R.E.: Hyperthermic isolation perfusion in vivo of the canine liver. Cancer 51: 1303-1309, 1983.

18. Van de Velde C.J.H., Tjaden U.R., Kothuis B.J.L.: Isolated Regional Liver Perfusion in the treatment of hepatic metastases. In: 'Liver Metastasis', van de Velde C.J.H., Sugarbaker P.H. (Eds), chapter 25, 1984.

METHODOLOGY IN THE CLINICAL STUDY OF HEPATIC METASTASES

C.J.H. van de Velde, C.H.N. Veenhof, P.H. Sugarbaker

Following the two day Symposium on Liver Metastasis held in Leiden, summarized in the preceeding chapters, a workshop was held in which most of the speakers of the Symposium were participants. The thoughts and conclusions of this workshop are presented in this chapter. The goals of the workshop were to reach a consensus on issues of importance to future collaborative research of hepatic metastases:

1. A staging system for patients with hepatic metastases
2. The criteria for response on treatment for hepatic metastases
3. The eligibility requirements for surgical resection of hepatic metastases
4. A "matrix" for future hepatic metastases treatment protocols

It was considered of great importance to clarify these aspects and to propose general rules to arrive at a common language in order to be able to compare various diagnostic and treatment protocols. These kind of protocols for randomized clinical studies are still considered as the only acceptable approach to patients with hepatic metastases as long as no effective standard treatment exists. Treatment off-protocol might often do more harm than be of profit to the patients.

STAGING OF HEPATIC METASTASES

All participants at the Workshop contributed in an attempt to find a mutually agreeable staging system. There was a special interest in the staging systems already in use designed by Dr. Pettavel, Dr. Gennari and others. The objective was to construct a *working system* by which to stage hepatic metastases, so that a common system could be used by all. There were two requirements for such a staging system:

1. It should be mutually agreeable to the group as a whole;
2. It should be simple enough for every day use.

The staging system should be considered a *proposed system*, that is, work in progress. If better prognostic information from analysis of large numbers of patients with hepatic metastases is made available, certainly this system should be revised. The system proposed at the Workshop should be called the

INTERNATIONAL STAGING SYSTEM FOR HEPATIC METASTASES

In Pettavel's staging system the major criterium by which patients are placed into three groups is the percent of liver replaced by cancer. Patient with stage I have less than 25 percent of the liver involved by tumor (P1). Stage II involves 26 to 75 percent of the liver (P2) and stage III more than 75 percent of the liver (P3) (Chapter 15)(Table 1).

Table 1
Staging According to Percent Hepatic Replacement by Tumor (PHR)

Stage   I : PHR less than 25%
Stage   II : PHR between 25% and 75%
Stage III : PHR more than 75%

The basic feature of Pettavel's staging system is the proportion of tumor contained within the liver. Participants in the Workshop adopted the PHR criterium. Descriptions of the effect of tumor on liver function tests were thought to be of indirect value. In the new International Staging System patients will be categorized by two additional clinical features. Those patients who have extra-hepatic disease will be designated by E. Patients who have symptoms will be designated by S. Therefore, a patient in the best treatment category will be designated as P1. This will include patients with less than 25 percent of the liver involved by tumor, no extra-hepatic disease and no symptoms of the hepatic metastases. A patient in the worst category would be P3 E S. P3 designating more than 75 percent of the liver involved by tumor, E the presence of extra-hepatic disease and S symptoms present. The stages of hepatic metastic disease defined by these clinical feature are shown in Table 2.

Table 2

Proposed International Staging System for Hepatic Metastases

Stage   0 : Curatively resected metastases
Stage   I : P1 (no E, no S)
Stage   II : P2 (no E, no S)
Stage III : P3 (no E, no S or Any P with E and/or S)

E : Concurrent extrahepatic disease
S : Symptomatic

Not included are other possibly important variables (Table 3). They include laboratory tests such as CEA, and alkaline phosphatase; the metastases being synchronous or metachronous; the size and number of nodules; nodules present in one or both lobes of the liver; grade of differentation; tumor vascularity; performance status of the patient. Rather than performance status patients would be categorized merely as symptomatic (S) or asymptomatic.
This staging system is to be used for patients only with colorectal malignancy.

Table 3

Variables not included in the Proposed Staging System

1. laboratory tests
2. metastases being synchronous or metachronous
3. size and number of metastatic nodules
4. unilobar or bilobar metastatic nodules
5. grade of differentation
6. degree of vascularity
7. performance status

It should be noted that this staging system is not a dynamic one. It makes an assessment at a single point in time. Although the workshop participants recognised the advantages of a system that would attempt to compute a doubling time of the tumor so that the rate of progression

of the disease could be established, this was thought to be too complicated for the every day use of the staging system.

It was also decided to add a stage 0 **to** indicate patients whose hepatic metastases had been potentially curatively resected (Table 2 and 4).
It was noted that in the future patients with resectable hepatic metastases may be further categorized according to: 1) margins positive or
negative; 2) the number of nodules that are resected; 3) the location
of nodules, unilobar or bilobar (Table 4).

Table 4
Prognostic Features in Stage 0 Patients (Resection with curative intent)

I   Prognostic Features of Value
     - margins of resection positive or negative
     - number of nodules resected
     - location of nodules, uni-versus bilobar
II   Prognostic Features of Undefined Value
     - Dukes' stage of primary tumor
     - metachronous or synchronous metastases
     - type of resection of the metastases (lobectomy vs. wedge resection)
     - grade of differentation of the metastases
     - size of the metastases
     - vascularity of the metastases
     - intraoperative bloodloss
     - method of detection of metastases

Variables not likely to have a prognostic implication were considered
the Dukes' stage of the primary tumor, whether the metastases were
synchronous or metachronous, the intraoperative bloodloss, the type of
resection performed (wedge resection or lobectomy), the grade of the
metastases, size of the metastases and method of detection of metastases (Table 4).

A problem with the staging of hepatic metastases concerns the liver
imaging techniques used to assess the percentage of hepatic parenchymal
replacement by tumor. At the workshop the group decided that selection

of a liver imaging technique was to be made by each institution depending upon their expertise and available equipment. Close cooperation of
oncologist and radiologist in this approximation of the percent of liver
involved by tumor is required. Either CT-scan of the liver, a liver
ultrasound or a radionuclide scan could be used.

The liver imaging technique used should be designated in the reporting.
It should be noted that if an ultrasound examination is used, there is
no permanent record of the size of the tumor metastases available for
review at a later date. Liver scintiscan and CT-scan would provide this.
Also serial angiography was thought to provide accurate information
under special circumstances in following the size of hepatic metastases.
An ideal way by which to serially assess changes of tumor volume would
be serial EOE-13 liver CT-scan with computerized reconstruction showing
the percentage of tumor in the liver.

RESPONSE CRITERIA

The workshop group accepted serial liver imaging studies to measure
response or progression of tumor. Tumors should be measured as the
largest of two dimensions on CT-scan, ultrasound or radionuclide scan.
CEA assays should be serially obtained but are not used as objective
criteria for evaluation of response. It was noted that if the CEA is
positive and the titer moves up or down, this is a signal of progression or regression of tumor. If the CEA is not elevated this laboratory test is unlikely to be of benefit. Some thought that serial biopsies of the liver might be an excellent way of monitoring response.
However, there is a marked sampling error which may result in inaccurate
assessments if this is used as a sole criterium. A second look surgery
procedure with biopsy of hepatic tumor nodules would give valuable information but was impractical to recommend.

Although the two most important endpoints are quality of life and survival, at this early stage in our studies it is essential that changes
in tumor size be reliably and regularly assessed. Serial assessment
would lead the clinician to establish progression, regression or stabilization of disease. At this workshop the definitions of progression

and regression from EORTC* protocols were reviewed and accepted:

1. Objective regression

   1.1 Complete response: disappearance of all symptoms and signs of clinically detectable tumor.

   1.2 Partial response: reduction of at least 50% of the sum of the products of the longest perpendicular diameters of the clearly measurable mass lesions.

   If hepatomegaly is the primary indicator, there must be at least a 30% reduction in the sum of the liver measurements below the costal marging at the midclavicular lines and at the xyphoid process.

   Measurements below the costal margin must always be made at the same distance from the median line of the abdomen.

   This distance must be indicated on the schema of the flow sheet. The reduction in the volume of the liver must also be accompanied by a trend to normalization of all pretreatment abnormalities in liver function.

   There may be no increase in any other indicator lesion and no new areas of malignant disease may appear.

2. Objectively stable: all of the following

   2.1 Insufficient regression of the primary lesion to meet the above criteria.

   2.2 < 25% increase in any measurable lesions

   2.3 no new areas of malignant disease

3. Objective progression: any of the following

   3.1 Increase in a measurable lesion by > 25%

   3.2 Appearance of new areas of malignant disease

It should be noted that these judgements only apply to disease contained within the liver. The frequency at which liver imaging studies, liver function tests and CEA assays should be performed was not determined at this time.

* European Organization For Research on Treatment of Cancer

ELIGIBILITY CRITERIA FOR RESECTION OF HEPATIC METASTASES FROM
COLORECTAL CANCER

The eligibility criteria for potentially curative surgical removal of
hepatic metastases stimulated a discussion in which many divergent
opinions were expressed. Dr. Cady (Boston, U.S.A.) thought patients who
have less than ten percent operative mortality and fewer than five nodules candidates for operative resection. He considered histologies
other than colorectal also candidates for resection. Mr. Taylor
(Southampton, UK) commented that the indications for liver resection in
England were limited to solitary metastases from colorectal malignancy.
Dr. Kemeny (California, U.S.A.) said that the resection criteria are
bound to change with the institution. Dr. Schiessel (Vienna, Austria)
mentioned that in a young or good risk patient he might advocate resection of up to a dozen nodules. He suggested that, if there was minimal
risk to the patient in terms of operative mortality because of the skill
of the operating team and the patients' young age and good health, resection of many metastases might be indicated. He even saw the resection of metastases as a reasonable palliative venture in selected
patients. Dr. Zwaveling (Leiden, The Netherlands) stated that in his judge-
ment three or less metastases confined to a single lob fit the resectability criteria. From the surgeons at Montpellier (France), a report
of resection of the right lobe of the liver in ten patients with diffused
liver metastases was conveyed. Following a delay, in which liver hypertrophy is allowed to occur, metastases on the left side were then removed.

In conclusion, the group was in agreement on some eligibility criteria
for surgical treatment. Solitary metastases should be removed and two
to three metastases in a single lobe. One metastasis in each lobe of
the liver was thought by approximately half the group to be an indication for resection, but considered a better candidate for medical treatment by the others.

ELIGIBILITY CRITERIA FOR NON-SURGICAL TREATMENT OF HEPATIC METASTASES

Also eligibility criteria for non-surgical treatment were discussed.
The Workshop consensus led to the three following criteria:
1. unresectable hepatic metastases
2. disease confined to the liver with a resected primary tumor
3. no chemotherapy or radiotherapy directed at the hepatic metastases
   unless more than one year ago.

MATRIX OF A HEPATIC METASTASIS PROTOCOL

In this session again the importance of delineating the objectives,
staging procedures, criteria for response, follow-up procedures and
statistical analysis of the data was stressed. These aspects were
considered to be essential in future protocols designed to compare
various treatment strategies or to test a hypothesis. A more general
discussion took place concerning some of these aspects.

PORTAL VENOUS INFUSION PROTOCOL

As an example of a hepatic metastasis protocol based on a well defined
objective and testing a hypothesis derived from histologic studies,
Dr. Gerard (Brussels,Belgium) presented the EORTC protocol 40794 (Clinical
trial on the treatment of liver metastases of colorectal origin by
hepatic artery ligation and portal infusion). He showed that after
hepatic artery ligation the major portion of a metastasis underwent
necrosis but that a rim of viable tumor remained, supplied (probably)
by portal venous blood. This hypothesis and the encouraging preliminary
results of Taylor (Southampton, UK) indicating a statistically significant improvement in survival by hepatic artery ligation and portal
venous infusion (5-FU), led to the ongoing EORTC protocol.

INTRA-ARTERIAL INFUSION PROTOCOL

As an introduction to the discussion concerning intra-arterial infusions
with or without implantable pump systems, Dr. Levin (Chicago) outlined
the three arm study in which a totally implantable pump system is used.

All patients have to undergo a laparotomy for staging and implantation
of the pump. Comparison is made between 1) systemic 5-FU (implanted pump
not in use), 2) intra-arterial FUDR, and 3) intra-arterial FUDR +
Mitomycin C plus systemic 5-FU. At progression of disease (intra- or
extrahepatic) all patients are treated intra-arterially with dichloro-
methotrexate. Mr. Taylor commented on the design of this trial. He pointed
out that it is absolutely essential to have patients included in a
no treatment control arm, so that the morbidity, toxicity and the treatment results can be established. Dr. Levin replied that in the United
States patients with hepatic metastases cannot be left untreated nowadays on ethical grounds. One of the reasons why every patient has a
pump implanted was to have the possibility to evaluate the complications
associated with this procedure, and to settle once and for all the
utility of implantable pumps. The general consensus of the group was
that implantable pump systems still have to prove their value even
though many reports already suggest a good palliative effect by locoregional chemotherapy and/or embolisation. The Workshop group also
agreed that this can only be reached by means of prospective randomized
trials. It questioned the design of this three arm study because of
the expenses involved, the complication rate and toxicity to be expected from intra-arterial FUDR and the failure to include a no treatment
control group.

NEED FOR DETERMINING SITES OF TREATMENT FAILURE

A further item of discussion was the site of treatment failure in
patients given loco-regional treatments. It is not clear which sites
are most frequently the site of treatment failure with manifest distant
metastases. Some investigators have suggested that patients treated
loco-regionally for hepatic metastases die more often from systemic
spread of the disease. These facts might form arguments to add systemic
chemotherapy (5-FU; Mitomycin C) to loco-regional treatments in future
protocols.

The discussion led by Dr. Sugarbaker (NCI, USA) and Dr. Schein
(Washington, USA) were at the end of the workshop summarized by
Dr. Van de Velde (Leiden, The Netherlands) by listing the main topics

of the consensus for the major features of collaborative research
protocols in patients with hepatic metatastases (table 5).

Table 5

Major Features of the Matrix for Future Protocols

1. definition of the objectives of the study
2. uniform staging system
3. eligibility criteria
4. criteria for response
5. follow-up procedures
6. statistical analysis
7. no treatment control-group

These topics were considered by the Workshop group as essential for
the framework for future protocols, serving as a "matrix" into which
appropriate treatment modalities can be inserted.
This matrix has been chosen as one usable for all groups of investigators without introducing very specific requirements and/or equipments
that might lead to exclusion of institutes from participation.

Dr. Van de Velde stressed the need for no treatment controls in future
protocols. However, if a protocol shows improved survival in ongoing
studies used, it should serve as a control arm if a no treatment arm
cannot be taken into consideration for ethical reasons.
In coming meetings this protocol-matrix will be proposed in its more
definitive form; appropriate treatment modalities will than be discussed.

The interest of this group in research and treatment of hepatic metastasis, as manifested by the 55 accepted abstracts, the outstanding
lectures during the symposium and the active participation in the
workshop promises an encouraging approach to the improvement of results
of treatment of patients with liver metastasis.

REFERENCES

As a guideline for further reading.

Prognostic factors

1. Jaffe B.M., Donegan W.L., Watson F., Spratt J.S.
   Factors influencing survival in patients with untreated hepatic
   metastases. Surg. Gynec. Obstet., 1968, 127, 1.
2. Wood C.B., Gillis C.R., Blumgart L.H.
   A retrospective study of the natural history of patients with
   liver metastases from colorectal cancer.
   Clinical Oncology, 1976, 2, 285.
3. Lahr C.J., Soong S.J., Cloud G., Smith J.W., Urist M.M., Balch C.M.
   A multifactorial analysis of prognostic factors in patients with
   liver metastases from colorectal carcinoma.
   J. Clin.Oncology, 1983, 1, 720.
4. Bedikian A.Y., Chen T.T., Malahy M.A., Patt Y.Z., Bodey G.P.
   Prognostic factors influencing survival of patients with advanced
   colorectal cancer: Hepatic-artery infusion versus systemic intravenous chemotherapy for liver metastases.
   J. Clin.Oncology, 1984, 2,3, 174.

Diagnosis and staging

1. Sorokin J.J., Sugarbaker P.H. Zamcheck N. et al.
   Serial carcinoembryonic antigen assays, use in detection of cancer
   recurrence. JAMA, 1974, 228, 49.
2. Herrera M.A., Chu T.M., Holyoke E.D.
   Carcinoembryonic antigen (CEA) as a prognostic and monitoring test
   in clinically complete resection of colorectal carcinoma.
   Ann.Surg., 1976, 183, 5.
3. Snow J.H., Goldstein H.M. Wallace S.
   Comparison of scintigraphy, sonography and computed tomography in
   the evaluation of hepatic neoplasms. AJR, 1979, 132, 915.

4. Bronstein B.R., Steele G.D. Ensminger W.D., Kaplan W.D., Lowenstein M.S.,
   Wilson R.E., Forman J., Zamcheck N.
   The use and limitations of serial plasma carcinoembryonic antigen
   (CEA) levels as a monitor of changing metastatic liver tumor volume
   in patients receiving chemotherapy.
   Cancer, 1980, 46, 266.

5. Knopf D.R., Torres W.E., Fajman W.J., Sones Jr P.J.
   Liver lesions: Comparitive accuracy of scintigraphy and computed
   tomography. AJR, 1982, 138, 623.

6. Smith T.J., Kemeny M.M., Sugarbaker P.H. Jones A.E. Vermess M.,
   Shawker T.H., Edwards B.K.
   A prospective study of hepatic imaging in the detection of
   metastatic disease. Ann Surg, 1982, 195, 4, 486.

7. Wallace S., Chuang V.P.
   The radiologic diagnosis and management of hepatic metastases.
   Radiology 1982, 22, 56.

8. Alderson P.O., Adams D.F., McNeil B.J., Sanders R., Siegelman S.S.,
   Finberg H.J., Hessel S.J., Abrams H.L.
   Computed tomography, ultrasound and scintigraphy of the liver in
   patients with colon ore breast carcinoma: A prospective comparison.
   Radiology, 1983, 149, 225.

9. Lokich J.J., Ellenberg S., Gerson B.
   Criteria for monitoring carcinoembryonic antigen: Variability of
   sequential assays at elevated levels.
   J. Clin. Oncology, 1984, 2, 2, 181.

10. Liver Metastasis. Edited by L. Weiss and H.A. Gilbert, 1982.

Staging

1. Bengmark S., Jeppsson B.
   Staging of liver metastasis. In: Liver Metastasis, Edited by
   L. Weiss and H.A. Gilbert, 1982; Chapter 15, page 268.

2. Gennari L., Doci R., Bozzetti F., Veronesi U.
   Proposal for a clinical classification of liver metastases.
   Tumori, 1982, 68, 443.

3. Pettavel J., Leyvraz S., Douglas P.
   The necessity for staging liver metastases and standardizing treat-
   ment response criteria. The case of secondaries of colo-rectal origin.
   Proceedings of the International Symposium on Liver Metastasis, 1984,
   Chapter 15.

Treatment modalities

1. Cady B. Selection of treatment for liver metastases.
   In: Liver Metastasis, Edited by L. Weiss and H.A. Gilbert, 1982;
   Chapter 16, page 275.
2. Fortner J.G. et al
   Major hepatic resection using vascular isolation and hypothermic
   perfusion. Ann. Surg. 1974, 180, 644.
3. Wilson S.M., Adson M.A.
   Surgical treatment of hepatic metastases from colorectal cancers.
   Arch.Surg., 1976, 111, 330.
4. Fortner J.G., Kim D.K., Maclean B.J. et al
   Major hepatic resection for neoplasia : Personal experience in 108
   patients. Ann. Surg. 1978, 188, 363.
5. Foster J.H.
   Survival after liver resection for secondary tumors.
   Am.J.Surg., 1978, 135, 389.
6. Wanebo H.J. et al.
   Surgical management of patients with primary operable colorectal
   cancer and synchronous liver metastases.
   Am.J.Surg., 1978, 135, 81.
7. Cady B. et al.
   Elective hepatic resection. Am.J.Surg., 1979, 137, 514.
8. Adson M.A., Van Heerden J.A.
   Major hepatic resections for metastatic colorectal cancer.
   Ann.Surg., 1980, 191, 576.
9. Bengmark S. et al.
   Metastatic disease in the liver from colorectal cancer. An appraisal
   of liver surgery. Surg., 1982, 6, 61.

10. Logan S.E. et al
    Hepatic resection of metastatic colorectal carcinoma. A ten year
    experience. Arch.Surg., 1982, 117, 25.
11. Rajpal S. et al.
    Extensive resections of isolated metastasis from carcinoma of the
    colon and rectum. Surg.Gynec.Obstet., 1982, 155, 813.
12. Fortner J.G., Silva J.S., Golbey R.B., Cox E.B., Maclean B.J.
    multivariate analysis of a personal series of 247 consecutive pa-
    tients with liver metastases from colorectal cancer.
    I. Treatment by hepatic resection. Ann.Surg., 1984, 199, 3, 306.

Regional chemotherapy

1. Sullivan R.D., Zurek W.Z.
   Chemotherapy for liver cancer by protracted ambulatory infusion.
   JAMA, 1965, 194, 481.
2. Watkins E., Khazei A.M., Nahra K.S.
   Surgical basis for arterial infusion chemotherapy of disseminated
   carcinoma of the liver. Surg.Gynec.Obstet., 1970, 130, 581.
3. Cady B., Oberfield R.A.
   Regional infusion chemotherapy of hepatic metastases form carcinoma
   of the colon. Am.J.Surg., 1974, 127, 220.
4. Ansfield F.J., Ramirez G., Davis Jr.H.L., et al.
   Further clinical studies with intrahepatic arterial infusion with
   5-fluouracil. Cancer, 1975, 36, 2413.
5. Buroker T., Samson M., Correa J. et al.
   Hepatic artery infusion of 5-FUDR after prior systemic 5-fluorouracil.
   Cancer Treatment Rep., 1976, 60, 1277.
6. Sullivan R.D.
   Systemic and arterial infusion chemotherapy for metastatic liver
   cancer. Int.J. Radiation Oncology Biol.Phys., 1976, 1, 973.
7. Ariel I.A., Padula G.
   Treatment of symptomatic metastatic cancer to the liver from primary
   colon and rectal cancer by the intraarterial administration of
   chemotherapy and radioactive isotopes.
   J.Surg.Oncol., 1978, 10, 327.

8. Grage T.B., Vassilopoulos P.P., Shingleton W.W., Jubert A.V., Elias E.G. Aust J.B., Moss S.E.
   Results of a prospective randomized study of hepatic artery infusion with 5-fluorouracil versus intravenous 5-fluourarcil in patients with hepatic metastases from colorectal cancer: A central oncology group study. Surgery, 1979, 86, 4,550.

9. Oberfield R.A., McCaffrey J.A., Polio J., Clouse M.E., Hamilton T.
   Prolonged and continuous percutaneous intraarterial hepatic infusion chemotherapy in advanced metastatic liver adenocarcinoma from colorectal primary. Cancer, 1979, 44, 414.

10. Taylor I., Rowling J., West C.
    Adjuvant cytotoxic liver perfusion for colorectal cancer.
    Br.J.Surg., 1979, 66, 833.

11. Buchwald H., Grage T.B., Vassilopoulos P.P., Rohde T.D. Varco R.L., Blackshear P.J.
    Intra-arterial infusion chemotherapy for hepatic carcinoma using a totally implantable infusion pump. Cancer, 1980, 45, 866.

12. Patt Y.Z., Mavligiti G.M., Chuang V.P. et al.
    Percutaneous hepatic arterial infusion (HAI) of mitomycin C and floxuridine (FUDR): an effective treatment for metastastic colorectal carcinoma in the liver. Cancer, 1980, 46, 261.

13. Ensminger W.D., Niederhuber J., Dahhil S., Thrall J., Wheeler R.
    Totally implanted drug delivery system for hepatic arterial chemotherapy. Cancer Treatment Rep., 1981, 65, 393.

14. Patt Y.Z., Wallace S., Freireich E.J., Chuang V.P. Hersh E.M., Mavligit G.M.
    The palliative role of hepatic arterial infusion and arterial occlusion in colorectal carcinoma metastatic to the liver.
    Lancet, 1981, 349.

15. Reed M.L., Vaitkevicius V.K., Al-Sarraf M., Vaughn C.B., Singhakowinta A., Sexon-Porte M., Izbicki R., Baker L., Straatsma G.W.
    The practicallity of chronic hepatic artery infusion therapy of primary and metastatic hepatic malignancies: Ten year resutls of 124 patients in a prospective protocol. Cancer, 1981, 47, 402.

16. Barone R.M. Byfield J.E., Goldfarb P.B., Frankel S., Ginn C., Greer S.
    Intra-arterial chemotherapy using an implantable pump and liver irradation for the treatment of hepatic metastases.
    Cancer, 1982, 50, 850.

17. Ensminger W.D., Niederhuber J., Gyves J., Thrall J., Cozzl E., Doan K.
    Effective control of liver metastases from colon cancer with an implanted system for hepatic arterial chemotherapy.

18. Levin B., Karl R., DuBrow R. et al.
    Regional hepatic chemotherapy for metastatic cancer with an implantable drug infusion system.
    Clin.Res., 1982, 30, 783A.

19. Plasse T., Ohnuma T., Bruckner H., Chamberlaim K., Mass T., Holland J.F.
    Portable infusion pumps in ambulatory cancer chemotherapy.
    Cancer, 1982, 50, 27.

20. Balch C.H., Urist M.M., Soong S.J., McGregor M.
    A prospective phase II clinical trial of continuous FUDR regional chemotherapy for colorectal metastases to the liver using a totally implantable drug infusion pump.
    Annals of Surgery, 1983, 198, 5, 567.

21. Oberfield R.A.
    Intra-arterial hepatic infusion chemotherapy in metastatic liver cancer. Sem.in Oncology, 1983, 10, 2, 206.

22. Ensminger W.D., Gyves J.W.
    Regional cancer chemotherapy. Cancer Treatment Rep., 1984, 68, 1, 101.

23. Fortner J.G., Silva J.S., Cox E.B., Golbey R.B. Gallowitz H., Maclean B.J.
    Multivariate analysis of a personal series of 247 patients with liver metastases from colorectal cancer.
    Ann.Surg., 1984, 199, 3 317.

24. Fortner J.G. et al
    Treatment of primary and secondary liver cancer by hepatic artery ligation and infusion chemotherapy.
    Ann. Surg., 1973, 178, 162.

INDEX OF SUBJECTS

INDEX